Addiction Research Methods

Edited by

Peter G. Miller

John Strang

Peter M. Miller

WILEY-BLACKWELL

A John Wiley & Sons, Ltd., Publication

Addiction **Press**

This edition first published 2010
© 2010 Blackwell Publishing Ltd

Blackwell Publishing was acquired by John Wiley & Sons in February 2007. Blackwell's publishing programme has been merged with Wiley's global Scientific, Technical, and Medical business to form Wiley-Blackwell.

Registered office
John Wiley & Sons Ltd, The Atrium, Southern Gate, Chichester, West Sussex, PO19 8SQ, United Kingdom

Editorial offices
9600 Garsington Road, Oxford, OX4 2DQ, United Kingdom
2121 State Avenue, Ames, Iowa 50014-8300, USA

For details of our global editorial offices, for customer services and for information about how to apply for permission to reuse the copyright material in this book please see our website at www.wiley.com/wiley-blackwell.

Library of Congress Cataloging-in-Publication Data

Addiction research methods / edited by Peter G. Miller, John Strang, Peter M. Miller.
   p. ; cm.
   Includes bibliographical references and index.
   ISBN 978-1-4051-7663-7 (pbk. : alk. paper) 1. Substance abuse–Research–Methodology.
I. Miller, Peter (Peter Graeme)   II. Strang, John.   III. Miller, Peter M. (Peter Michael), 1942–
   [DNLM: 1. Substance-Related Disorders.   2. Research–methods.   WM 270 A22403 2010]
   HV5809.A33 2010
   616.86′027–dc22

                                                                            2009033610

A catalogue record for this book is available from the British Library.

Set in 10/12.5 pt Sabon by Aptara® Inc., New Delhi, India

1   2010

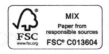

CONTENTS

Section V: Specialist Methods

CONTRIBUTORS

David Ball
Social Genetic and Developmental Psychiatry Centre, King's College London, and South London and Maudsley NHS Foundation Trust, London, UK

David Best
Department of Psychiatry, University of Birmingham, Birmingham, UK

Gerhard Bühringer
Institut für Therapieforschung, Parzivalstraße 25, München, Germany

Adrian Carter
School of Population Health, University of Queensland, Herston, QLD, Australia

Jonathan P. Caulkins
Heinz College and Qatar Campus, Carnegie Mellon University Pittsburgh, PA USA and Doha, Qatar

Kenneth R. Conner
Department of Psychiatry and Canandaigua Veterans Administration Center of Excellence, University of Rochester Medical Center, Rochester, NY, USA

Ross Coomber
University of Plymouth, Plymouth, Devon, UK

Shane Darke
National Drug and Alcohol Research Centre, University of New South Wales, Sydney, NSW, Australia

Ed Day
Department of Psychiatry, University of Birmingham, Birmingham, UK

Louisa Degenhardt
National Drug and Alcohol Research Centre, University of New South Wales, Sydney, Australia

Paul Dietze
Burnet Institute Centre for Epidemiology and Population Health Research and Monash Institute of Health Services Research, Melbourne, VIC, Australia

Krista Drescher-Burke
School of Social Welfare, University of California, Berkeley, CA, USA

John W. Finney
Center for Health Care Evaluation, VA Palo Alto Health Care System (152MPD), Menlo Park, CA, USA

Anton Goldmann
Department of Anesthesiology and Intensive Care Medicine, Charité – University Medicine of Berlin, Germany

Steven R. Goldberg
Preclinical Pharmacology Section, Behavioral Neuroscience Research Branch, Intramural Research Program, National Institute on Drug Abuse, NIH/DHHS, Baltimore, MD, USA

Paul Griffiths
European Monitoring Centre for Drugs and Drug Addiction, Lisbon, Portugal

Irene Guerrini
South London and Maudsley NHS Foundation Trust, London, UK

Wayne Hall
School of Population Health, University of Queensland, Herston, QLD, Australia

Lisa Kakinami
Department of Community and Preventive Medicine, University of Rochester Medical Center, Rochester, NY, USA

Benjamin Ladd
University of New Mexico, Albequerque, NM, USA

Jim Lemon
National Drug and Alcohol Research Centre, University of New South Wales, Sydney, Australia

Nick Lintzeris
Department of Addiction Medicine, Faculty of Medicine, University of Sydney, Australia

Barbara S. McCrady
University of New Mexico, Albequerque, NM, USA

Lorraine T. Midanik
School of Social Welfare, University of California, Berkeley, CA, USA

Peter G. Miller
School of Psychology, Deakin University, Victoria, Australia

Peter M. Miller
Center for Drug and Alcohol Programs, Medical University & South Carolina, Charleston, SC, USA

Katherine Mills
National Drug and Alcohol Research Centre, University of New South Wales, Sydney, Australia

David Moore
National Drug Research Institute, Curtin University of Technology, Perth, Australia

Jane Mounteney
Bergen Clinics Foundation, Bergen, Norway and European Monitoring Centre for Drugs and Drug Addiction, Lisbon, Portugal

Anne Moyer
Department of Psychology, Stony Brook University, Stony Brook, NY, USA

Tim Neumann
Department of Anesthesiology and Intensive Care Medicine, Charité – University Medicine of Berlin, Germany

Jeremy Northcote
School of Marketing, Tourism and Leisure, Edith Cowan University, Joondalup WA, Australia

David Nutt
Department of Neuropsychopharmacology and Molecular Imaging, Imperial College London, London, UK

Rosalie Liccardo Pacula
RAND Drug Policy Research Center, RAND Corporation, Santa Monica, CA, USA

Leigh V. Panlilio
Preclinical Pharmacology Section, Behavioral Neuroscience Research Branch, Intramural Research Program, National Institute on Drug Abuse, NIH/DHHS, Baltimore, MD, USA

Alastair Reid
Specialist Community Addiction Service – Bucks (SCAS-B), Oxfordshire and Buckinghamshire Mental Health NHS Foundation Trust, High Wycombe, UK

Tim Rhodes
Department of Public Health and Policy, London School of Hygiene and Tropical Medicine, London, UK

Monika Sassen
Institut fuer Therapieforschung, Munich, Germany

Charles W. Schindler
Preclinical Pharmacology Section, Behavioral Neuroscience Research Branch, Intramural Research Program, National Institute on Drug Abuse, NIH/DHHS, Baltimore, MD, USA

Julie Steele
University of New Mexico, Albequerque, NM, USA

Cathy A. Simpson
Department of Health Behavior, School of Public Health, University of Alabama, Birmingham, AL, USA

Tim Slade
National Drug and Alcohol Research Centre, University of New South Wales, Sydney, Australia

Claudia Spies
Department of Anesthesiology and Intensive Care Medicine, Charité – University Medicine of Berlin, Germany

Scott H. Stewart
Center for Drug and Alcohol Programs, Medical University of South Carolina, Charleston, SC, USA

Mark Stoové
Addiction Research Foundation, Toronto, Ontario, Canada

John Strang
National Addiction Centre (Institute of Psychiatry, Kings College London and South London and Maudsley NHS Foundation Trust), London, UK

Jalie A. Tucker
Department of Health Behavior, School of Public Health, University of Alabama, Birmingham, AL, USA

Leah Vermont
University of New Mexico, Albequerque, NM, USA

Robert West
Department of Epidemiology and Public Health, University College London, London, UK

Jason White
Department of Clinical and Experimental Pharmacology, University of Adelaide, Adelaide, SA, Australia

ACKNOWLEDGEMENTS

We are profoundly grateful to Kate Wisbey, Jenny Strang and Gay Miller, without whose support, tolerance and almost pathological patience, nothing would have been possible.

Chapter 1

INTRODUCTION

Peter G. Miller, John Strang and Peter M. Miller

1.1   Introduction

The addictions and alcohol and other drug (AOD) sector covers a vast array of disciplines and methodologies. Many of the techniques used in the understanding of drug use are essentially the same as those used in other fields, while others are special in both their design and their samples. In no other field of enquiry has there been such a multidisciplinary approach to the development of research methods and sampling techniques. For many in the field, this multidisciplinary reality is perplexing, making it challenging to truly understand the relationships and synergies between very different pieces of research on the same topic. And yet, each piece of research adds its own distinctive contribution. For example, attempts to reduce HIV in any given community require in-depth long-term ethnographic research to understand how social networks interact to increase or reduce blood-borne virus transmission and survey research to determine the prevalence and incidence of HIV in the community, just as it requires animal studies and pharmacological research to understand basic mechanisms and responses, and clinical trials to develop the appropriate medicines and schedules for treatment. Without one of these pieces of research, resources can be wasted, and lives can be lost, as a result if targeting the wrong people with the wrong intervention at the wrong time. But when research perspectives from all fields are considered, the best possible outcomes are achieved.

This book draws on the insights of an international assortment of leaders in the AOD field to document the major issues and techniques involved in each subdiscipline and to signpost the major works in the field. The book will also serve to help readers understand the fundamental principles of many of the disciplines in the AOD field and will lead to greater cooperation between disciplines and improved methodological flexibility and sophistication.

1.2   Where to start?

The research enterprise has many facets and it is often overwhelming when starting out to know which issue to address. The first question for any investigative team is often, 'what are we trying to find out?' This query often leads to a great many other issues around elements of the larger question, for example, how the research could and should be conducted, what theories or values are informing the question, what ethical issues should be considered.

In the initial stages, researchers should:

1. Take it slow – be over-inclusive to begin with – take your time in reaching a final set of questions – do not overlook alternative possibilities and strategies.
2. Subdivide questions – split questions into component parts – disentangle different questions from each other.

3. Order questions in terms of importance, size, practical considerations and interest.
4. Investigate theory/review literature/conduct observations.
5. Develop hypotheses.

This process of careful planning and brainstorming is often best accomplished in groups since contributions of individual members of the research team can advance the thinking of the group as a whole. Time spent at this stage is a good investment since it will help to avoid problems that could arise once the research is underway. It is important to remember that, with every research investigation, 'the devil is in the detail' and the devil must be given his due as early as possible to prevent later regrets. Without careful planning, an important variable may be overlooked, resulting in a serious methodological flaw that might later render the research results unconvincing.

1.3 Does theory matter?

For most types of research an important place to start is with theory. Sadly, this is often not the case, or more commonly, individuals will focus only on theories from their own discipline. There is much to learn from looking at other disciplines and methodological approaches when considering how best to answer a question. Theories can provide a framework for different types of research and the factors on which one should focus. Ideally, theory-driven research follows the process of deduction (Box 1.1) (see Figure 1.1).

1.3.1 How to ask the right question

Asking the right question is one of the most important elements of the research process. This book contains a raft of examples of different research methods and glimpses into the disciplines from which they come. For each of these methods, the process of asking the right question is the end of a different process. However, for many of the disciplines (definitely not all), using evidence and theory is the best way to develop a strong hypothesis (see Figure 1.1). This is most usually through the process of developing a hypothesis. 'A hypothesis is a predicated answer to a research question' (Bryman, 2004, p. 38).

Box 1.1   What are deduction and induction?

Deduction: In the process of deduction, you begin with statements, called 'premises', that are assumed to be true. You then determine what else would have to be true if the premises are true. The premises themselves, however, remain unproven and unprovable; they must be accepted at face value, or by faith, or for the purpose of exploration.

Induction: In the process of induction, you begin with data, and then determine what general conclusion(s) can logically be derived from those data. In other words, you determine what theory or theories could explain the data. Induction does not prove that the theory is correct. Ultimately, interactive logic demonstrates that the theory does indeed offer a logical explanation of the data.

Deduction and induction by themselves are inadequate for a scientific approach. While deduction gives support to the theory, it never makes contact with the real world; i.e. there is no place for observation or experimentation and no way to test the validity of the premises. Similarly, while induction is driven by observation, it never approaches actual proof of a theory. Ultimately, the development of the scientific method involves a gradual synthesis of these two logical approaches.

Theory

⇩

Hypothesis

⇩

Data collection

⇩

Findings

⇩

Hypothesis confirmed or rejected

⇩

Revision of theory

Figure 1.1 The process of deduction (Bryman, 2004).

However, there are many other considerations when contemplating a question, not least of which is 'can it be answered?' Unfortunately, most questions we have, particularly in the addictions field, are unanswerable through any one study, or possibly ever. Asking the right question can also be guided by knowing whether someone has asked the same or similar questions before, what tools are available and what methods have failed before. This is most commonly achieved through conducting a literature review.

1.4   The literature review

The literature review is a vital part of any good research project, and if not conducted properly, the project can end up needlessly replicating previous research or following directions already found unhelpful. There are numerous texts and websites which outline the best practice for conducting literature reviews (e.g. Ridley, 2008). However, there are a number of major elements worth addressing to ensure a good literature review.

1.4.1   Where to search?

A well-conducted literature review will cover the most likely and reputable sources of information. Simply conducting a quick web search on a single search engine is not acceptable. The highest level of evidence in any field comes from articles in peer-reviewed journals. Within the addictions field, there are over 80 specialist journals. No one database will allow you to search the content of all of these journals. Further, many important articles are published in more general medical, psychological, anthropological and other journals. However, for general topics within the addiction-related fields, the major search engines are PubMed (general health and medical content), CSA Illumina Databases (Sociological Abstracts), PsycInfo, PAIS, Worldwide Political Abstracts, etc. Search multiple databases at once, including full text as well as bibliographic databases, Web of Science (multidisciplinary content from highly cited/ranked journals), Scopus (the largest academic database in the world), Expanded Academic (multidisciplinary content) and JSTOR (full-text searches of digitised back issues of several hundred well-known journals, dating back to 1665 in the case of the *Philosophical*

Transactions). While these databases are easily found on the internet, if you have institutional links to a university, the most valuable resource when trying to determine where you should search may be your friendly librarian. Many libraries have specialist librarians for different subject areas, and a brief discussion with such an expert can save you a great deal of time and ensure you get to the sources you need.

There are a number of characteristics which make a good literature review. These include a clear organisation of concepts and topics, a clear idea of the chronology of ideas, a good summary of the major themes and trends in the phenomenon being studied and a consideration of the different methodologies used to investigate the topic. A good literature review makes interpretations of the available sources backed up with evidence, but does not go overboard, selecting only the most important points in each source to highlight in the review. The use of quotes should always be done sparingly, and it is better to use you own words to summarise and synthesise the literature, rather than supplying a series of quotes. Caution should always be taken to ensure that you report the author's information or opinions accurately and in your own words. A correctly conducted literature review will allow you to move to the next stage of your research – planning your methodology.

1.5   Which method suits my question – is a screwdriver better than a saw?

Different questions require different methods to answer them. Further, the way in which a question is asked can have implications for what needs to be done to answer it. It is important to remember that methods are not neutral since they are linked strongly to the way in which individuals view the world and how it should be examined (Bryman, 2004). It makes sense that we spend most of our time on what we think is most important. On the other hand, most scientists tend to strive for objectivity, and while preference is often obvious, it will seldom negate the worth of the piece of work. A sociologist looking into the causes of addiction would frame the question very differently to a geneticist. While the sociologist might look at issues such as class, employment status and gender, the geneticist may look into alleles and genomes. Increasingly, multi-methods are being used to investigate the same question from different angles. For example, the IMAGEN study combines cognitive, behavioural, clinical and neuroimaging data from adolescents and their families and teachers in a longitudinal design over 5 years (http://www.imagen-europe.com/en/imagen-europe.php). Research methods will include self-report questionnaires, behavioural assessment, interviews, neuroimaging of the brain as well as blood sampling for genetic analyses.

A good way to achieve the right fit between questions and methods is to ensure that the content of the research, or the research questions, comes before the methodological considerations. Put simply, asking 'what would we like to know?' is usually better than looking for a question that can be answered by a certain type of method. Unfortunately, this does not always happen and many researchers stand accused of 'methodolatry' – a combination of method and idolatry, which selects and defends specific methods, regardless of the question being asked (Punch, 2005).

This book is designed to give the reader a wide overview of the methods currently being used in addictions and other AOD-related research globally. By having these different perspectives available in a single volume, we hope that the readers can avoid sticking only to the methods they know and will be more confident about thinking beyond single disciplinary studies to develop complex methods to answer the complex questions posed by addiction. Depending on the method you require to answer your question, your reading of this book may vary.

1.6   Focus and structure of the book

The book is written to cater for a wide audience, including students, academics and clinical practitioners, but it is envisaged that the reader will already have some basic knowledge of research methods. The book is primarily divided into six major sections: (1) Research Fundamentals, (2) Basic Toolbox, (3) Real World Research Methods, (4) Biological Methods, (5) Specialist Methods and (6) Beyond Research. Research Fundamentals contains information on the basic concepts needed in most research, such as Gerhard Bühringer and Monika Sassen's discussion of the concepts of validity and reliability, and how they apply to addiction-related research. The section also covers sampling issues in Chapter 3 by Lisa Kakinami and Kenneth Connor – a vital question for any good research project as well as a chapter by Robert West looking at the issues associated with conducting experimental research in the addictions-related field. Tim Rhodes and Ross Coomber provide an insightful overview of qualitative research and its theoretical underpinnings, as well as giving guidance on how qualitative research has brought a different perspective to the many complex dynamics surrounding addictive behaviour and substance use. Finally, in a chapter by Peter G. Miller, Adrian Carter and Wayne Hall, the section looks at some of the ethical issues which commonly face addictions researchers and can be unique to our field.

The 'Basic Toolbox' section includes Chapter 7 on surveys and questionnaire design by Lorraine T. Midanik and Krista Drescher-Burke, which provides the reader with the basic issues associated with designing surveys and questionnaires. This is followed by the equally important instructions and suggestions on 'interviewing techniques' by Barbara S. McCrady, Benjamin Ladd, Julie Steele Seel and Leah Vermont. In Chapter 9, Shane Darke provides advice on the main tests and scales for addictions research and the contexts in which they might be appropriate. Chapter 10 on biomarkers of alcohol and other drug use by Scott H. Stewart, Anton Goldmann, Tim Neumann and Claudia Spies adds the dimension of biological testing to the research encounter. Finishing off the basic toolbox is Chapter 11 on quantitative analysis by Jim Lemon, Louisa Degenhardt, Tim Slade and Katherine Mills.

Building on this section, the following 'Real World Research Methods' section focuses on the issues faced in applied settings in Chapter 12, 'Applied Research Methods' by David Best and Ed Day, looking at how to conduct applied research in treatment system research, and in Chapter 13, 'Conducting Clinical Research' by Jalie A. Tucker and Cathy A. Simpson.

The 'Biological Methods' section focuses on the more specialised and predominantly lab-based techniques, which focus on the biological aspects of addiction and substance use. Jason White and Nick Lintzeris provide an overview of the most common type of research in the field, psychopharmacology. In Chapter 15, David Nutt and Alastair Reid give us an overview of one of the more recent methods to be used in the study of addiction using imaging technology to observe reactions and structures of the brain. Following this, David Ball and Irene Guerrini show us a small part of the vast work being commenced on relating addiction to genetics, and finally, Leigh V. Panlilio, Charles W. Schindler and Steven R. Goldberg give us an important insight into the use of animals and how they can and have been used to help us understand addiction and substance use in humans.

The 'Specialist Methods' section covers a number of disciplines, which play a very significant role in the study of addiction and require more detailed explanation for the readers to understand their unique contribution and challenges. In Chapter 18, 'Understanding contexts: Methods and analysis in ethnographic research on drugs', Jeremy Northcote and David Moore give the reader an insight into the complex and often all-consuming world of the ethnographer and highlight the unique benefits of this method and the challenges faced by the ethnographer. Mark Stoové and Paul

Dietze then provide us with an overview of one of the most used and policy-relevant disciplines in the study of addiction in Chapter 19, 'Epidemiology'. Chapter 20 on meta-analysis and/or Cochrane reviews by John W. Finney and Anne Moyer gives us an insight into this increasingly important way of synthesising evidence to reach stronger conclusions – a role vital in a discipline which often has contrary findings in different settings and substances. Chapters 21 and 22 describe the often related methods of drug trend monitoring and drug policy research. Paul Griffiths and Jane Mounteney give a comprehensive overview of the ways in which data on drug trends are collected around the world as well as the limitations of these data. Jonathan P. Caulkins and Rosalie Liccardo Pacula finish off the section with a description of the complex world of drug policy research and its modelling techniques. We finish the book with a brief note on publishing and other issues worth considering at the end of the research process.

All chapters contain descriptions of actual, definitive studies that have helped shape the field, as well as a set of recommended readings, and a set of exercises which will help readers develop their skills.

This book is specifically international in its focus. We have sought to include authors from a number of different countries to give us a perspective, which is as wide as possible. This means there are a number of terminological and definitional issues which might arise when reading the text.

1.7 Terminology

Words are, of course, the most powerful drug used by mankind.

Rudyard Kipling

When writing and editing an international book, the importance of words and terminology chosen becomes apparent. Different countries use different terms, and these terms can have a meaning which is far beyond those defined in dictionaries and lexicons, despite the best intentions of many. Certainly, there is a wide gap between the common usage of many words by the general public and their defined meaning used in academic text. However, words also represent theories and many of these theories are hotly debated. They also reflect social and cultural norms and viewpoints around acceptable behaviour, many of which can be traced back to pagan rituals and religious rites many centuries ago. During the process of editing this book a number of different meanings and interpretations became apparent and we, the editors, were required to make a decision about whether terminology should be standardised or whether to simply acknowledge difference. Ultimately, we have chosen the latter. However, a brief discussion of some of the different terms and common usages is warranted.

We recommend that readers refer to the World Health Organization (WHO) lexicon of alcohol and drug terms (World Health Organization, 1994). In 1994 the WHO developed a lexicon which aims to provide a set of definitions of terms concerning alcohol, tobacco and other drugs, which is useful to clinicians, administrators, researchers and other interested parties in this field. The definitions of two contested terms are instructive (abuse and addiction – see Boxes 1.2 and 1.3).

Ultimately, you will see the words 'substance use' and 'abuse' used interchangeably, despite different cultural interpretation of the appropriateness for a judgement of 'abuse'. Similarly, addiction and dependence are used according to the preference of the authors. Certainly, 'addiction' carries very different constructs and agendas in the UK, than it does in the United States, both of which differ to that in Australia. Another set of words with similar issues surrounds the appropriate terminology for people who access treatment services. Whether they are called patients, service users or clients differs in different countries, and while there is evidence to suggest that many actually prefer being

Box 1.2 Abuse

Abuse (drug, alcohol, chemical, substance or psychoactive substance): A group of terms are in wide use but of varying meaning. In DSM-IIIR,[a] 'psychoactive substance abuse' is defined as 'a maladaptive pattern of use indicated by . . . continued use despite knowledge of having a persistent or recurrent social, occupational, psychological or physical problem that is caused or exacerbated by the use [or by] recurrent use in situations in which it is physical1y hazardous'. It is a residual category, with dependence taking precedence when applicable. The term 'abuse' is sometimes used disapprovingly to refer to any use at all, particularly of illicit drugs. Because of its ambiguity, the term is not used in ICD-I0 (except in the case of non-dependence-producing substances – see below); harmful use and hazardous use are the equivalent terms in WHO usage, although they usually relate only to effects on health and not to social consequences. 'Abuse' is also discouraged by the Office of Substance Abuse Prevention (OSAP, now CSAP – Center for Substance Abuse Prevention) in the United States, although terms such as 'substance abuse' remain in wide use in North America to refer generally to problems of psychoactive substance use.

In other contexts, abuse has referred to non-medical or unsanctioned patterns of use, irrespective of consequences. Thus, the definition published in 1969 by the WHO Expert Committee on Drug Dependence was 'persistent or sporadic excessive drug use inconsistent with or unrelated to acceptable medical practice' (*see* misuse drug or alcohol)[b].

[a] *Diagnostic and Statistical Manual of Mental Disorders* (revised), 3rd edn. Washington, DC: American Psychiatric Association, 1987.
[b] WHO Expert Committee on Drug Dependence, Sixteenth report. Geneva: World Health Organization, 1969 (WHO Technical Report Series, No. 407).

Box 1.3 Addiction

Addiction, drug or alcohol: Repeated use of a psychoactive substance or substances, to the extent that the user (referred to as an addict) is periodically or chronically intoxicated, shows a compulsion to take the preferred substance (or substances), has great difficulty in voluntarily ceasing or modifying substance use and exhibits determination to obtain psychoactive substances by almost any means. Typically, tolerance is prominent and a withdrawal syndrome frequently occurs when substance use is interrupted. The life of the addict may be dominated by substance use to the virtual exclusion of all other activities and responsibilities. The term 'addiction' also conveys the sense that such substance use has a detrimental effect on society, as well as on the individual; when applied to the use of alcohol, it is equivalent to alcoholism. Addiction is a term of long-standing and variable usage. It is regarded by many as a discrete disease entity, a debilitating disorder rooted in the pharmacological effects of the drug, which is remorselessly progressive. From the 1920s to the 1960s, attempts were made to differentiate between addiction and 'habituation', a less severe form of psychological adaptation. In the 1960s, the WHO recommended that both terms be abandoned in favour of dependence, which can exist in various degrees of severity. Addiction is not a diagnostic term in ICD-10, but continues to be very widely employed by professionals and the general public alike (*see also* dependence, dependence syndrome).

called 'patients' in the UK (Keaney et al., 2004), this would appear different in Australia where most are called 'clients', despite not paying directly for their treatment. On the other hand, the book will not use the term 'marijuana' in place of its scientific name 'cannabis'. The racist undertones of the term have been discussed widely in the literature (Manderson, 1997), and although the term is often seen to mean simply the leaf form of cannabis, we choose to only use 'cannabis'.

1.8   The need for a wider perspective and more careful selection of study design

Basically, the choice of design is influenced by many factors, including the nature of the question, the type of answer sought and the different possible outcomes of interest. Different research questions in differing clinical, political and research contexts will point to the need for different types of study design – and that is how it should be (Mills, 1959). A substantial body of work in the area of addiction research is focussed on treatment outcomes. While this is an essential issue of many types of addictions research, we decided that a separate chapter on treatment outcomes would be redundant since many of the chapters in this book deal with elements of assessing treatment outcomes. Thus, treatment outcome studies fall under the banner of a number of chapters, including Conducting Clinical Research, Applied Research Methods, Scales for Research in the Addictions, and others. However, some of the other methods discussed have been to great benefit in understanding treatment outcome, such as qualitative and ethnographic methods (Koutroulis, 1998), and there are no doubt combinations of genetics and animal studies are on the horizon. We mention this topic here because we wanted to emphasise that studying the outcomes of treatment is a complex and important topic for research and it is vital that design choices need to be made in a careful and considered manner. Certainly, treatment outcome research should reflect measures which accurately assess the improvement (or otherwise) of an individual's well-being (Miller & Miller, 2009). This outlook on research is also the message we hope you take away from this book – that, in general, taking a wide perspective on the question you are facing will help you to find the method most appropriate for answering the question you are asking, and you should not fear to step beyond disciplinary specialities in the search for more innovative and appropriate methods.

References

Bryman, A. (2004) *Social Research Methods*. New York: Oxford University Press.

Keaney, F., Strang, J., Martinez-Raga, J., Spektor, D., Manning, V., Kelleher, M., Wilson Jones, C., Wana-garatne, S. & Sabater, A. (2004) Does anyone care about names? How attendees at substance misuse services like to be addressed by health professionals. *European Addiction Research*, 10(2), 75–79.

Koutroulis, G. (1998) Withdrawal from injecting heroin use: thematizing the body. *Critical Public Health*, 8(3), 207–225.

Manderson, D. (1997) Substances as symbols – race rhetoric and the tropes of Australian drug history. *Social and Legal Studies*, 6(3), 383–400.

Miller, P. G. & Miller, W. R. (2009) What should we be aiming for in the treatment of addiction? *Addiction*, 104(4), 685–686.

Mills, C. W. (1959) *The Sociological Imagination*. New York: Oxford University Press.

Punch, K. F. (2005) *Introduction to Social Research: Quantitative and Qualitative Approaches*, 2nd edn. London: Thousand Oaks, CA: Sage Publications.

Ridley, D. (2008) *The Literature Review: A Step-by-Step Guide for Students*. London: Sage.

World Health Organization (1994) *Progress towards Health for All: Statistics of Member States*. Geneva: World Health Organization.

Section I
Research Fundamentals

Chapter 2
RELIABILITY AND VALIDITY

Gerhard Bühringer and Monika Sassen

2.1 Introduction

In this chapter we cover two quality criteria for study findings, *reliability* as an indicator of measurement consistency or reproducibility (do we receive the same findings in repeated measurements?) and *validity* as an indicator of construct concordance (do the findings reflect what we intended to study?). Flaws in both properties may lead to completely false conclusions or at least may limit the generalisability of our findings to the real situation in the universe; for example, if a newly developed alcohol use questionnaire reveals past month average daily beer consumption of 0.25 L in a first measurement and 0.5 L for the same period in a second measurement, our questionnaire is not very reliable, and – as a consequence – long-term measurement differences of beer consumption in a cohort study cannot be interpreted as valid changes.

2.2 Background: Reliability and validity in addiction research

2.2.1 Threats to reliability and validity: Dr Newcomer's seminal alcohol consumption study

Drawing inferences (conclusions) from study findings to the 'truth' in the real world is a core purpose of research. But many decisions have to be made in the process of designing and implementing research studies, which affect scope and quality of conclusions from our study results to the real world. Core quality criteria are the reliability and validity of our findings. We demonstrate this dependence of conclusions on study characteristics in a virtual example.

Dr Newcomer from Bordeaux has got some money from the French brewery industry and wants to study the impact of high alcohol consumption on work performance of adults in France. He hypothesises (1) that average daily alcohol use in France is comparably low and (2) that high daily drinking amounts do not reduce work output, so the new French government's prevention programme is not needed. He designs a cross-sectional study with one group of young students (age 18–24) from his seminar on Basis Statistics (Figure 2.1). To increase the number of cases, he includes students from two other seminars with the same topic but different teachers. One of them is known to have extremely high failure rates in his seminars.

The predicting variable is the number of glasses of beer. He asked in a questionnaire, 'What was the average daily number of glasses of beer you drank from Monday to Friday in the last 3 months?' The outcome variable is the failure rate in the last seminar test. The questionnaire was filled out by the students during a seminar. The rate of missing information was very high, and therefore one junior researcher completed some missing questionnaires with his estimations of the students' beer consumption. Further on, he did not get enough cases and asked some people in a pub to fill out the questionnaire as well.

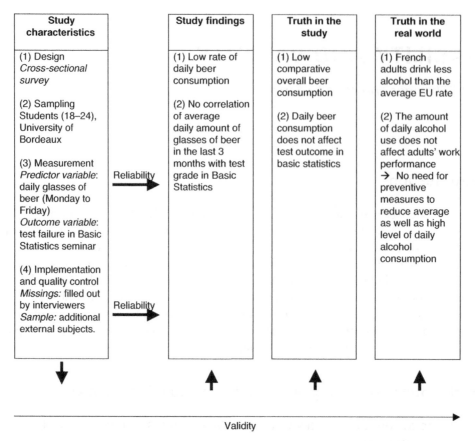

Study characteristics		Study findings	Truth in the study	Truth in the real world
(1) Design *Cross-sectional survey* (2) Sampling Students (18–24), University of Bordeaux (3) Measurement *Predictor variable*: daily glasses of beer (Monday to Friday) *Outcome variable*: test failure in Basic Statistics seminar (4) Implementation and quality control *Missings*: filled out by interviewers *Sample*: additional external subjects.	Reliability → Reliability →	(1) Low rate of daily beer consumption (2) No correlation of average daily amount of glasses of beer in the last 3 months with test grade in Basic Statistics	(1) Low comparative overall beer consumption (2) Daily beer consumption does not affect test outcome in basic statistics	(1) French adults drink less alcohol than the average EU rate (2) The amount of daily alcohol use does not affect adults' work performance → No need for preventive measures to reduce average as well as high level of daily alcohol consumption

Validity

Figure 2.1 Challenges in addiction research for the reliability and validity of conclusions from study findings to the truth in the real world: Dr Newcomer's seminal 'French Alcohol Use and Work Performance Study'.

Dr Newcomer's findings (1) that daily beer consumption among students is generally low and (2) that higher amounts of daily beer intake do not cause increased failure rates were published in the famous journal for weird research results. He concluded that indeed the amount of adult daily alcohol consumption does not have an impact on work performance in France and especially that high doses do not cause negative effects. He also concluded that preventive programmes to reduce alcohol consumption are not necessary. What is wrong with the study? (See Box 2.1)

2.2.2 Definition of core terms and concepts

Concepts and definitions of reliability and validity were developed in the context of test theory (de Gruijter & van der Kamp, 2007). As part of psychometric theory, a major topic of research interest in test construction is the measurement of psychological constructs and items in the social and psychological sciences, such as intelligence or personality traits. Classical test theory assumes that, because of imperfect measurements, an assessed (measured) score always consists of a *true score* and a *measurement error*. The larger the error, the lower the reliability. The goal is to detect the true value of a certain variable.

Measures ought to be as objective, reliable and valid as possible. The degree of *objectivity*[1] of a measurement indicates to what extent results are independent of the person applying the

---

Box 2.1 Frequent reliability and validity flaws in addiction research – exemplified with Dr Newcomer's study

Study design	Impact on
Cross-sectional design	
→ Impossible to draw conclusions concerning causality	Validity
Sampling	
Sample of 18- to 24-year-old students	Validity
→ Does not cover total French adult population	
→ No conclusion for total adult population can be drawn	
Sample of three seminars on basic statistics	
→ Seminars differ systematically in test failure rates due to different teacher styles: a moderating factor impacts on the relation of beer consumption and failure rate	
→ No causal or correlational conclusion can be drawn without controlling for systematic failure rate differences between seminars	Validity
Measurement	
'Average daily number of glasses of beer in the last 3 months'	Validity
→ No indicator for alcohol consumption in general, only for beer consumption	Validity
→ Disregarding the consumption of other alcoholic beverages (especially wine in a culture like France) leads to the underestimation of consumption	
→ Asking for average daily values over longer periods results in inconsistent alcohol consumption results[a]	Reliability
Reference period: Monday to Friday	
→ Alcohol consumption is likely to be higher on weekends	Validity
→ Disregarding weekends leads to underestimation of consumption	
Implementation and quality control	
Faking missing data	
→ No true results	Reliability
→ Limits analysis of causal or correlational relations	Validity
Adding subjects outside the sample	
→ Limits interpretation of results and conclusions	Validity

[a]A frequency–quantity index-based question would lead to more reliable data (see Gmel & Rehm, 2004).

---

measurement. *Reliability* describes the reproducibility of measured results on trustworthiness of the measuring method, and *validity* reports in what way the instrument measures what it pretends to do (Box 2.2).

Reliability

Reliability is related to the *precision* of data collection and measures the proportion of the true variance on the measured variance. Reliability is scored '1' when the measured variance and the true variance are the same, meaning that the variance of the measurement error is '0'. When the measured variance merely consists of measurement error, reliability is '0'. Reliability is calculated by correlating different measurements.

Three subtypes can be differentiated according to time and method of measuring (Table 2.1):

> **Box 2.2 Definition of objectivity, reliability and validity**
>
> *Objectivity*[1]
> Measurement results are independent of the person applying the measure (during conduction and during analysis).
>
> *Reliability*
> Core criterion: reproducibility of measuring outcome. Measurement reveals consistent results when circumstances remain the same.
>
> Reliability = true variance/measured variance (0.00 = zero reliable; 1.00 = totally reliable, no measurement error). Reliability of a measure is indicated by the correlation of equal measurements.
>
> *Validity*
> Measurement detects what it is intended to detect.

1. *Parallel-test reliability* is obtained by conducting two tests with similar measuring instruments at the same time and correlating the results of Instrument 1 with the results of Instrument 2. Two questionnaires on 'preparedness' to stop cigarette smoking should preferably lead to the same or very similar results when administrated at the same or similar time.

2. *Test–re-test reliability* registers stability of the measuring method over time. Therefore, the same measure is repeated in the same sample after a certain period. A questionnaire on self-efficacy to refuse alcohol offers after abstinence therapy should result in equal or similar results after repeated exposure, if the 'real' degree of self-efficacy did not change. This property is a prerequisite for all cohort and clinical trial studies with repeated measurements to detect possible (long-term) changes. Correlating the two measures indicates the test–re-test reliability. Different aspects have to be considered when taking into account the period between two tests. On the one hand, it should be long enough to exclude effects due to the day's condition and remembrance, which could influence the results. On the other hand, it should not be too long because real changes can occur between the two test intervals. A major problem for the test–re-test method is that real changes cannot be controlled. For example, scales can indicate a different weight because of low reliability of the measure or because of a real change in weight.

3. The most commonly used methods to estimate reliability involve dividing the test. Bisecting the test leads to 'parallel' tests, with each having a reduced number of items compared to the original test version. The so-called *split-half reliability* is calculated by correlating the two halves. However, this correlation underestimates reliability because the correlation coefficient grows with the number of items. This can be mathematically corrected by using the Spearman–Brown formula (de Gruijter & van der Kamp, 2007). Furthermore, each item can be considered to be a parallel measure and reliability can be calculated through mean correlation of items (Cronbach's α).

Table 2.1 Different approaches for reliability calculations

	Measuring time	
Measuring method	**Simultaneous**	**Repeated**
Same	—	Test–re-test reliability
Different	Internal consistency/split-half reliability	Parallel-test reliability

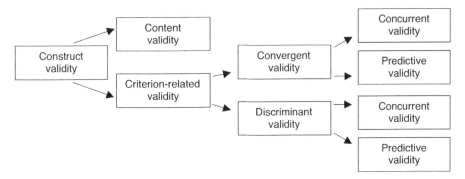

Figure 2.2 Different kinds of validity concepts.

It is worth noting that the different methods of testing reliability being described may lead to different results. Generally, reliability should at least be 0.80 (range 0.00–1.00) in order to be considered reasonable.

Validity

Validity describes the *accuracy* of research and can be subdivided into different concepts (Figure 2.2):

- *Construct validity* exists when a construct measures what is intended to be measured. It demands a theoretically justifiable relation of the construct with other variables and asks for hypotheses that can be confirmed empirically. The focus is on predicting as many criteria values as possible, which are measured independently and connected via a net of theoretical position instead of on a single external criterion.
- *Content validity* is a specific aspect of construct validity. It is achieved when the measured items embody a representative sample of the content, which the items intend to measure. For example, an intelligence test is content valid if its questions are representative for all aspects of intelligence. The ASI (Addiction Severity Index; McLellan et al., 2006) complies with the concept of content validity as all areas of possible negative substance use consequences are systematically covered by relevant items.
- *Criterion-related validity* is another element of construct validity, meaning the degree to which the measure correlates with a relevant external criterion. Measurements of one construct ought to be highly related to each other (*convergent validity*). For example, the outcome of a new alcohol disorder screening instrument for the general population should be highly correlated with clinical diagnoses by trained experts for the same subjects. Additionally, relations between measurements of different constructs should be smaller than relations between measurements of the same constructs (*discriminant validity*).
- A further differentiation exists between *concurrent validity*, that is measurement and criterion are collected at the same time, and *predictive validity*, meaning the criterion is collected after the measurement.

Interaction of reliability and validity

Quality criteria are ordered hierarchically with objectivity being a necessary but not sufficient requirement for reliability and therefore the weakest criterion of a measure. Scales are perfectly objective when different persons agree on the same weight being measured, but might be not reliable if they display different weights in repeated measurements, although no change in weight has occurred. Reliability, in turn, is necessary, but not sufficient regarding validity. Just because an instrument is objective and reliable, does not mean it is valid as well. For example, scales that measure weight changes reliably with an overestimation of several pounds are still not valid (indicating the right weight). Therefore, the main aim is to develop valid measures. With reliability – and indirectly objectivity – being necessary preconditions, the degree of validity is restricted according to their extent. More precisely, the validity coefficient of a measure concerning any criteria cannot exceed the square root of the reliability coefficient (validity coefficient $\leq \sqrt{\text{reliability coefficient}}$).

2.3   Reliability and validity in addiction research

Classical examples in the addiction research field are the measurement of quantity and frequency of alcohol intake or the use of psychotropic medicines. But validity issues are also very relevant for all steps in designing and implementing research studies (see Figure 2.1).

2.3.1   Study design

Defining research questions

There is no shortage of research questions, but the process from a general research interest to a specific research question and related study plan has many pitfalls, which might limit the reliability and validity of our study. The selection of a research question is more or less limited by time, money, staff, access to study subjects and other resources. Often one has to adapt the scope of a question to the feasibility of a related research concept. Study questions often have to be modified in an iterative process to compromise between research interest, ethical aspects, given research conditions and scientific state of the art.

Selecting study designs

Design limitations may restrict outcome validity. If a treatment study is to analyse the long-term course of self-efficacy and long-term effects of a new behaviour therapy programme on smoking behaviour, one has to (1) provide enough points of measurement to analyse changes (minimum three, more is better) and (2) include a long follow-up period according to scientific standards in the given field. In general, the design has to be selected according to the research question:

- *Observational studies*: This type of study observes behaviour of subjects in natural environment without any systematic intervention.
- *Cross-sectional studies*: They measure information at one point of measurement and allow only correlational analyses of data (e.g. the correlation of alcohol dependence and comorbidity).
- *Case-control studies*: They are a subgroup of cross-sectional studies and compare two groups that differ in one aspect (e.g. subjects with high and low daily alcohol intake in terms of liver diseases). Any causal interpretation of such correlational data would be invalid.
- *Cohort studies*: They include long-term observation with several points of measurement and allow causal interpretations with some restrictions; for example, if subjects with cigarette smoking develop more cases of lung cancer than non-smokers, a causal conclusion – cigarette smoking causes lung cancer – is possible, if no other factors exist which differentiate the two

groups. Examples are age, sex, general life style and general health behaviour. Cohort studies always have limitations for causal interpretations as one never knows all relevant intervening variables. But for ethical reasons, many research questions cannot be studied experimentally – as in the case described.

- *Randomised clinical trial:* Two or more groups are randomly allocated to control or intervention condition(s). By this procedure, ideally, outcome differences between groups are only caused by the intervention(s) as all other possible intervening variables are equally distributed in all groups and therefore do not have differential effects on group outcome. Blinding patients, therapists and researchers about hypotheses, intervention and placebo conditions will further eliminate any group-specific effects, but are often not feasible in addiction research interventions. Given possible restrictions by missing blinding procedures, randomised clinical trials allow the strongest causal interpretations.

2.3.2 Sampling

Sampling of study subjects

We cannot study the whole population of people or animals. Therefore, we need sampling rules to reduce the number of subjects to a feasible number. But this procedure bears many risks for the validity of our study (see Chapter 3). As a general rule, sample subjects should represent the total population of people as exactly as possible on whom we want to draw inference from for our study results. If Dr Newcomer wants to make a statement on adult alcohol consumption in France, he has to sample male and female subjects from the total adult population and not just students from age group of 18–24 years. Or, he has to limit his study question and related conclusions to French students in that age group. There are two major errors in subject sampling which affect validity:

1. *Conceptual errors:* The planned sample not covers the population of subjects on whom we want to draw conclusions, for example we are interested in the full range of cannabis use disorders for a treatment study, but looks only for subjects with cannabis dependence.
2. *Sampling errors:* Selecting study subjects from the population of subjects leads to a biased distribution; for example, we are interested in a random sample of factory workers and take every tenth worker from the morning shift and not from the late shift, which might limit the validity (generalisability) of our results to all workers (unless we control for differences in relevant variables between workers from the morning and late shifts).

Especially in treatment studies we differentiate between external and internal validity:

- *Internal validity:* Within a defined sample (e.g. all new admissions in the next 3 months with alcohol dependence), all patients are excluded (by exclusion criteria) who have further disorders or other specific characteristics (e.g. unemployment) in order to study a 'pure' sample of alcohol dependents. This procedure maximises internal validity (e.g. the significance of effects between treated patients and controls), but minimises the generalisability of the study results to the 'real' population of alcohol dependents.
- *External validity:* All patients (with the full range of other disorders) are included in the study. This strategy risks reducing or losing significant effects.

There is no perfect solution to this dilemma, and decisions must be made according to the state of scientific knowledge and to the study targets. In many cases, a long-term research strategy will be a good compromise: first, trial with highly selected subjects to test a new intervention, and then – if effective – further studies with more 'realistic' patients (more complex disorders) to test the feasibility of the health care service system (translational research; see Hulley et al., 2007, Chapter 2). In addition, there are always 'objective' exclusion criteria; for example, if we study a new outpatient treatment, we cannot include subjects who need inpatient care.

Other sampling procedures

Sometimes we have to sample other items for a study, for example time frames for observational studies. If we want to study gambling at slot machines, observing people only during workday mornings would not allow generalisation to all gamblers.

2.3.3 Measurement

Measurement issues are also a major concern when considering reliability and validity. Figure 2.3 depicts the different kinds of variables, which we strive to measure in addiction research, either to describe the type, intensity and pattern of a set of items or to analyse correlational or causal relationships between items. All the variables in Figure 2.3 are prone to be measured inadequately, leading to unreliable and invalid results. This is especially the case since a variety of different measurements can be used to study a single research question. For example, for measuring possible gambling-related problems, various sets of questions have been developed (among others, the South

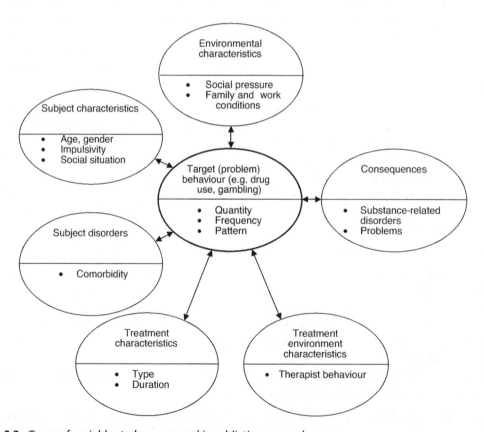

Figure 2.3 Types of variables to be measured in addiction research.

Oaks Gambling Screen – SOGS, Lesieur & Blume, 1987; the DSM-IV-MR-J, Fisher, 2000). Depending on the measure and its application, the results are trustworthy and useful or worthless and do not allow to answer the research question properly.

It is beyond the scope of this chapter to cover all areas in Figure 2.3. But we discuss a highly relevant and intensively researched set of variables: the measurement of (problem) alcohol-use behaviour. There is broad evidence that questions on the amount of use lead to clear under-reporting caused by factors such as hiding possible problems, neglecting, misunderstanding of instructions or fear of prosecution (e.g. drunk driving). Consequently, all feasible approaches to measure amount and pattern of use will never be totally reliable. Therefore, we always strive to gain data as reliable as possible in a given context (see Box 2.3).

To obtain valid and therefore useful information, it is helpful to follow certain rules:

- Apply questionnaires or items that have been examined and considered reliable and valid in previous research (gold standard).
- If you use newly developed items/questionnaires, try to implement some type of reliability control (e.g. include already tested items/questionnaires for comparisons).
- Cohort studies with repeated measurements need variables which are highly reliable to avoid a (non-interpretable) mix of measurement (random) errors and true changes.
- Do not try to answer a research question that cannot be answered with the data you have collected.

2.3.4 Implementation and quality control

Implementation and quality control are also needed to obtain reliable and valid results. No matter how well design and measurement are planned, no valid results can be obtained if the research study is not conducted properly. Various mistakes can occur at this stage of the research process:

- *Adding subjects outside the defined sample*
  Interviewers might be keen to finish their work within a certain time frame. Therefore, they might deviate from a specified sampling procedure (e.g. every third person entering the gambling venue or every second 20- to 30-year-old woman ought to be surveyed) and instead interview every person who is willing to participate. Doing so limits interpretability of results and conclusion because a different than the indented population is measured for which the research question was originally developed.
- *Faking data*
  Missing data can be faked by the interviewer. This can happen for different reasons: either some questions have not been asked because of imprecision in the observer technique or because the interviewer thinks asking a certain question is embarrassing. Or nobody is willing to participate, but the observer wants to finish research work in time. In the first case, the questionnaire is 'filled up' by the interviewer with some data in order to provide a complete dataset. Faking data is unethical and unprofessional and can ruin a career in science.

2.4 Strengthening the quality of your results and conclusions: A brief checklist to improve reliability and validity

2.4.1 Study design and sampling

Box 2.4 summarises relevant topics for improving study design and sampling issues.

Box 2.3 Recommendations for measuring alcohol-use behaviour (see Gmel & Rehm, 2004; Rehm et al., 2007)

Individual level	Country level
Measurement by customary drinking habits	*Measurement of national consumption*

Measurement by customary drinking habits

- Quantity–frequency index
    Two separate questions on:
    1. Usual frequency of drinking
    2. Usual quantity when drinking
- Extended quantity–frequency instrument
    Quantity–frequency questions on:
        Workdays and weekends separately
        Different drinking situations (bar, home)
- Semi-quantitative food frequency questionnaires
    One question for alcohol consumption:
        In general or per beverage
        Frequency of consuming a drink: 'once a week' – 'daily' (several options)
- Risky single-occasion drinking: +5, +8, +12
    'How often in the past 12 months did you have 5/8/12 or more drinks in the course of a day?'
- Graduated frequency and proportions of occasions
    Questions on:
        Beverage-specific frequency of drinking
        Proportion of different drinking quantities: +5, 3–4, 1–2 units; 'never' – 'nearly every time'

Measurement by listing amounts in recent drinking occasions
- Most recent drinking occasion approach
    List all drinking on the last occasion (last two, three, four occasions)
- Survey period approach
    List all drinking in a specific period
- Diaries
    Information on:
        All frequencies and quantities
        Beverage-specific frequencies and quantities

Measurement by objective measures
- Blood alcohol concentration
    Measured in serum, breath or urine
    Marker only for recent alcohol consumption
    Less measurement errors than verbal reports

Measurement of national consumption

- Adult per capita consumption of recorded alcohol
    Total consumption of pure alcohol per inhabitant aged 15 and above in litres in a given year
    Based on sales and production records
- Adult per capita consumption of unrecorded alcohol
- Prevalence of abstention by age and sex:
    Usually the past year
    Assessed by surveys
- Prevalence of different categories of average volume of alcohol consumption by age and sex
- Score for patterns of drinking
    Comprises four different aspects of heavy drinking:
    1. Quantity of alcohol per occasion
    2. Frequency of festive drinking
    3. Proportion of drinking occasions when drinkers get drunk
    4. Distribution of the same amount of drinking over several occasions
And two other questions:
    1. Drinking in co-occurrence with meals
    2. Drinking in public places

Box 2.4   Checklist for improving the validity of study design and sampling issues

1. *Study design*
Study questions
It is helpful to ask the following questions in the process of formulating study questions (in addition to ethical considerations, scientific novelty and relevance; see Hulley et al., 2007, Chapter 2):
   ○ What is the exact definition of my target population?
   ○ Can I draw representative samples of adequate size?
   ○ What are the risks of receiving biased samples?
   ○ Do I have adequate (reliable and valid) instruments to measure the needed variables?
   ○ Do the selected instruments cover the full topic of my research questions?
   ○ Do I have all further resources to plan, implement and analyse the study for my study question?

Study design
   ○ Does the study question require causal or correlational analyses?
   ○ Is the method appropriate?

2. *Sampling*
   ○ Will the sample be representative of the study population?
   ○ Does the sampling procedure minimise the risk of biased (non-representative) study subjects?
   ○ Given the state of scientific knowledge and feasibility aspects, what are needs, advantages and disadvantages of more internal or external validity (for defining exclusion and inclusion criteria)?
   ○ Is the size of the study group large enough to detect possible significant differences between groups (power analysis needed)?

2.4.2 Measurement

In order to improve reliability and validity of measurements, several different steps have to be considered (Hulley et al., 2007). Implementing the strategies of Box 2.5 reduces random (reliability) as well as systematic (validity) errors that may occur.

- *Standardisation of measurement methods* is based on written operational instructions on the process of interview preparation and conduction as well as on environment, instrument and subject. This standardised procedure is used as guidelines throughout the entire process of the study to help carrying out the research unvaryingly.
- Reliability of a measurement can be improved by *training the observer* to constantly apply the measurement in the same way.
- Lack of clarity and potential misunderstandings of questionnaires can be smoothed by *refining the instrument* and writing it down.
- *Automating the instrument* can reduce variations in the way the observer makes measurements.
- *Repeating the measurement* increases the reliability of the obtained results since the influence of random error diminishes.
- *Unapparent measurement* (for subjects) results in information that is unbiased regarding the behaviour of subjects. Since they are unaware of the measurement, they cannot consciously influence the results.
- Repeated *adjustment of the instrument* to a so-called gold standard assures that the intended aspect is measured, increasing the validity of the measurement.

Box 2.5   Strategies to reduce errors in order to increase reliability and validity of measurements (modified after Hulley et al., 2007)

Strategy to reduce errors	Source of errors	Possible *random* errors	Possible strategy to prevent the error	Possible *systematic* errors	Possible strategy to prevent the error
Standardisation of measurement methods	Observer	Variation in registered alcohol level due to variable observer techniques	Specify and pilot test instructions for behavioural observations	Consistently high registered alcohol level due to the observer estimating 'drunkenness'	Use operational definition and criteria for 'drunkenness'
	Subject	Consistently high registered alcohol level due to recent consumption	Specify that the subject does not drink for an hour before measurement	Consistently high registered alcohol level due to recent consumption	Specify that the subject does not drink for an hour before measurement
Training the observer	Observer	Variation in registered alcohol level due to variable observer techniques	Train the observer in standard techniques	Follow procedures specified in operations manual	The trainer checks accuracy of the observer's registration
Refining the instrument	Observer and instrument	Variation in registered alcohol level due to digit preference (e.g. the tendency to round number to a multiple of 5)	Design instrument that conceals registered alcohol level	Consistently high registered alcohol level due to only ask for consumption of beer and fail to ask for consumption of spirits	Ask for all kinds of alcoholic beverages
Automating the instrument	Observer	Variation in registered alcohol level due to variable observer techniques	Use electronic methods or self-administered question-naires	Tendency of the observer to estimate 'drunkenness'	Use automatic alcohol test

(Continued)

Box 2.5 *(Continued)*

Strategy to reduce errors	Source of errors	Possible *random* errors	Possible strategy to prevent the error	Possible *systematic* errors	Possible strategy to prevent the error
	Subject	Variation in registered alcohol level due to emotional reaction to the observer by the subject	Use automatic alcohol test	Tendency to behave sober due to proximity of the attractive technician	Use automatic alcohol test
Repeating the measurement	Observer, subject and instrument	All measure-ments and all sources of variations	Use mean of two or more self-administered question-naires concerning alcohol consumption	—	—
Unapparent measurement	Subject	—	—	Tendency to show expected behaviour (e.g. unclear language after alcohol consumption)	Measure alcohol in blood
Adjustment of instrument	Instrument	—	—	Consistently high registered alcohol level due to alcohol test being out of adjustment	Calibrate each month (particularly electrical devices and instruments that change over time)
Blinding	Observer	—	—	Tendency to treat study groups differently	Use double-blind strategy
	Subject	—	—	Overestimation of (side) effects if known to have consumed alcohol	Use double-blind strategy

- *Blinding* is a classical strategy to rule out that one group is biased more than the other. When using a double-blind strategy, neither the subjects nor the observers are informed on the study's conditions (e.g. if and in which experimental group, a placebo is applied instead of medicines). This means that any occurring imprecision is the same in the different groups.

2.4.3   Implementation and quality control

The improvement of reliability and validity of research results by using a certain study design, sampling and measurement is enhanced by ensuring implementation and quality control. One strategy to guarantee the most reliable and valid results as possible is to *train* observers according to necessary guidelines (see Section 2.3, 'Reliability and validity in addiction research') and *check* on their performance. For example, when conducting an interview, a more experienced interviewer can *monitor* the observer and the way the interview is carried out (e.g. video samples). As a kind of quality management, *feedback* on their work can be given.

2.5   Summary

Drawing inferences from study findings to the 'truth' in the real world is a core purpose of research. But many decisions have to be made in the process of designing and implementing research studies, which affect scope and quality of such conclusions. The core quality criteria are *reliability* and *validity*. Reliability is calculated by correlating different measurements, which should result in nearly similar figures. Reliability is relevant not only for selecting appropriate instruments during research planning process but also for implementing and carrying out a study properly. Validity describes the accuracy of research and is a key quality criterion for all study aspects such as determining study questions, design, sampling of subjects (e.g. is the sample representative of the population?), measurement and implementation/quality control. Flaws in either or both properties may lead to false conclusions or may limit the generalisability of our findings to the real situation.

Note

1. Objectivity is the third criterion for good measurement and a precondition of reliability and validity. For further information, see Kirk and Miller (1986).

References

Fisher, S. (2000) Developing the DSM-IV-MR-J criteria to identify adolescent problem gambling in non-clinical populations. *Journal of Gambling Studies*, 16, 253–273.

Gmel, G. & Rehm, J. (2004) Measuring alcohol consumption. *Contemporary Drug Problems*, 31, 467–540.

De Gruijter, D. N. M. & Van der Kamp, L. J. T. (2007) *Statistical Test Theory for the Behavioral Sciences*. Boca Raton, FL: Chapman & Hall.

Hulley, S. B., Cummings, S. R., Browner, W. S., Grady, D. & Newman, T. B. (2007) *Designing Clinical Research*, 3rd edn. Philadelphia, PA: Lippincott Williams & Wilkins.

Kirk, J. & Miller, M. L. (1986) *Reliability and Validity in Qualitative Research*. Thousand Oaks, CA: Sage University Paper.

Lesieur, H. R. & Blume, S. B. (1987) The South Oaks Gambling Screen (SOGS): a new instrument for the identification of pathological gamblers. *American Journal of Psychiatry*, 144, 1184–1188.

McLellan, T. A., Cacciola, J. C., Alterman, A. I., Rikoon, S. H. & Carise, D. (2006) The Addiction Severity Index at 25: origins, contributions and transitions. *American Journal on Addiction*, 15(2), 113–124.

Rehm, J., Klotsche, J. & Patra, J. (2007) Comparative quantification of alcohol exposure as risk factor for global burden of disease. *International Journal of Methods in Psychiatric Research*, 16(2), 66–76.

Recommended readings

Hulley, S. B., Cummings, S. R., Browner, W. S., Grady, D. & Newman, T. B. (2007) *Designing Clinical Research*, 3rd edn. Philadelphia, PA: Lippincott Williams & Wilkins.

An excellent monograph on all aspects of designing and implementing (not addiction related) clinical research, with many practical suggestions and examples.

Gmel, G. & Rehm, J. (2004) Measuring alcohol consumption. *Contemporary Drug Problems*, 31, 467–540.

A comprehensive journal publication on reliability and validity issues in the context of measuring individual and national alcohol consumption (e.g. frequency, quantity and pattern of use, measurement approaches, biological markers, comparison of instruments, survey errors and reasons for undercoverage).

Recommended websites

http://www.emcdda.europa.eu/themes/key-indicators

The European Monitoring Centre for Drugs and Drug Addiction (EMCDDA)

The EMCDDA is the European centre for collecting, analysing and disseminating all types of data on prevalence, prevention and treatment of (illicit) drug use. It provides a wide range of papers and tools for the measurement of so-called key indicators of drug use and related actions.

http://www.nida.nih.gov/researchers.html

The National Institute on Drug Abuse (NIDA)

http://www.niaaa.nih.gov/

The National Institute on Alcohol Abuse and Alcoholism

NIDA and NIAAA are central organisations in the United States for promoting research and research dissemination into practise. Both websites provide access to methodological projects and publications related to reliability and validity issues.

http://www.consort-statement.org/index.aspx?o=1011

Consolidated Standards of Reporting Trials (CONSORT Statement)

CONSORT is a set of guidelines and regulations for publishing relevant information on randomised clinical trials. They were developed to better assess reliability and validity of study outcomes and indirectly indicate research quality guidelines.

http://www.trend-statement.org/asp/statement.asp

Transparent Reportings of Evaluations with Non-randomized Designs (TREND Statement)

The purpose of TREND is similar to CONSORT, but for reporting results from non-randomised designs, for example public health interventions.

Chapter 3

SAMPLING STRATEGIES FOR ADDICTION RESEARCH

Lisa Kakinami and Kenneth R. Conner

3.1 Introduction

3.1.1 Purpose of the chapter

Throughout the chapter we describe specific sampling strategies, including their strengths and weaknesses, illustrate each strategy through a study published in the substance abuse field, discuss many of the considerations in choosing a sampling approach and briefly discuss sample size (power) calculation. The chapter is intended to assist students, researchers and clinicians in recognising and understanding major sampling issues that affect the design and interpretation of substance abuse studies. We focus on quantitative methods of sampling and also touch upon qualitative sampling.

3.1.2 Types of sampling

1. *Probability sampling.* This is a type of quantitative sampling that requires a list of all members (a *sampling frame*) to be available in order to randomly sample and accurately calculate the probabilities of selection. With the properties of random selection and known probability of selection, probability samples are theoretically unbiased estimates of the population. The main probability sampling strategies include (1) simple random, (2) systematic, (3) stratified and (4) cluster sampling. Each is discussed
2. *Non-probability sampling.* The probabilities of selection are unknown because this type of quantitative sampling does not use a sampling frame. It is used when probability sampling is impractical or impossible and/or as a lower cost or more convenient alternative. The most commonly used non-probability sampling approaches include (1) convenience, (2) snowball, (3) time-space, (4) respondent-driven and (5) targeted sampling.
3. *Qualitative sampling.* We briefly touch upon sampling in qualitative studies that may provide in-depth, rich information about population members.

3.1.3 Definitions of key concepts

We introduce and discuss several terms relevant to sampling throughout the chapter. Brief definitions for key terms are provided in Table 3.1. These concepts are discussed in greater depth in the text.

3.2 Probability sampling

3.2.1 Introduction

Planning prevention or intervention relevant to a population requires that the population is well understood. While a census would provide information on all members of the population, a census

Table 3.1 Definitions of key sampling concepts

Term	Definition
Bias	The difference between the sampling value and the true population value
Cluster	Mutually exclusive groups of units
Convergence	In respondent-driven sampling, when the sample population characteristics stabilise such that further waves of recruitment are expected to yield subjects with similar features, suggesting that further waves are not required
Equal allocation	In stratified sampling, selecting an equal number of respondents per stratum
Generalisability	The extent to which the results of a study population can be extrapolated to the general population or target population
Heterogeneous	Individuals in a population or sample that are dissimilar to one another in key characteristics
Hidden population	Individuals who are difficult or impossible to identify using routine sampling methods
Homogeneous	Individuals in a population or sample that are similar to one another in key characteristics
Masking	In snowball sampling, respondents do not provide referrals to the study staff to protect the confidentiality of their peers
Non-response	Missing responses either due to subjects' non-participation or non-responses to measurement items
Optimal allocation	In stratified sampling, selecting more respondents from strata with greater variance
Oversampling	Can refer to (a) sampling additional respondents from a subgroup to ensure adequate representation of that group in the sample or (b) sampling heavily from a single network of peers, resulting in a homogeneous sample that is not representative of the target population
Periodicity	Both the sampling frame and the sampling strategy are non-randomly arranged, producing a sample that is not representative
Post-stratification	Stratification after sampling
Primary sampling unit	The sampling unit chosen for the first stage of cluster sampling
Probability	The likelihood of an event occurring
Probability proportional to size	Probability of selection is based on the sampling unit size, with larger units having a larger probability of being selected than smaller units
Proportional allocation	In stratified sampling, selecting the number of respondents per stratum proportionally to the target population
Reliability	The consistency of a measurement tool or result
Response rate	The percentage of persons who agree to participate in a sample compared to the total number approached
Sample population	The population studied that is theoretically representative of the target population
Sampling frame	A listing of 'units' from which the sample is drawn such that every unit has an equal probability of being selected

Table 3.1 (*Continued*)

Term	Definition
Sampling interval	The ratio of the target population to the sample population, represented by k
Sampling unit	Unit in the sampling frame, most often an individual but could also be a zip code, school classroom, treatment programme, among other units
Sampling without replacement	Once a unit is selected for the sample, the unit cannot be selected again for the same sample
Sampling with replacement	Units can be selected multiple times into a single sample
Seed	The initial respondents in a study using snowball sampling or respondent-driven sampling who help recruit additional respondents
Selection bias	Probability of selection differs between respondents and leads to an unrepresentative sample of the target population
Standard error	Indicates how precise the results are, with larger SEs denoting less precision in the sampling estimates
Strata	Subgroups of population of interest (e.g. strata based on gender, ethnicity and geographical region)
Target population	The population the results of the study will generalise to
Validity	The degree to which the results obtained accurately represent the true population
Variance	The dispersion around an estimate, with larger variance denoting greater variability
Weighting	A data analysis step that adjusts for units having different probabilities of selection

is generally impractical. Surveying a sample of representative individuals can be used to extrapolate valuable information to the population. Quantitative methods are generally used, with probability sampling strategies theoretically preferable to non-probability sampling because they are more likely to be unbiased estimates of the population. In addition, probabilities of selection and corresponding confidence intervals around the estimates can be calculated. However, as these strategies require a sampling frame, they tend to be costlier and more time-consuming than non-probability strategies. This chapter is a non-statistical primer on sampling, and a researcher wishing to better understand the statistics underlying sampling is encouraged to refer to Levy and Lemeshow (1999).

3.2.2 Simple random sampling

Simple random sampling (SRS) is the most basic probability sampling strategy. SRS is analogous to pulling names out of a hat as each respondent is randomly selected and has a known, non-zero and equal probability of being selected. Random selection of respondents can be conducted using computer-generated random numbers with software such as SAS (http://www.sas.com/) or Systat (http://www.systat.com/) or the random number table provided in the appendix of many statistical

---

Box 3.1   SRS example

Drabble et al. (2005) analysed the relationship between alcohol use and sexual orientation. In order to create the sampling frame, the authors used a list-assisted number generator. For telephone surveys, a list-assisted method helps create the sampling frame by selecting clusters of 100 phone numbers defined by their area code and first five digits of their telephone numbers. Participants of at least 18 years old were then randomly selected from all 50 US states. With a response rate of 58% and 7612 respondents, data were weighted to adjust for factors such as number of independent phone numbers and number of adults living in the household. The authors showed that alcohol use did not differ among men based on sexual orientation, but that lesbian and bisexual women were less likely to abstain from alcohol and were more likely to experience alcohol-related social consequences than heterosexual women. The results underscored the necessity of taking into consideration sexual orientation when examining the prevalence of alcohol use and impairments among women.

---

textbooks, including Levy and Lemeshow (1999). As SRS assumes that each respondent in the population has an equal chance of being selected, SRS is inefficient for studying rare characteristics because proportionately few cases can be anticipated. Although the nature of randomly selecting respondents increases the likelihood of having an unbiased estimate of the population, SRS is not free of sampling error. By chance, a sample can be selected that has a proportion of a particular characteristic that is not representative of the population. All other things being equal, sampling error declines as sample size increases (Box 3.1).

3.2.3   Systematic sampling

Systematic sampling selects every kth respondent for the sample with the first respondent being selected randomly between 1 and k. The value of k is calculated as the largest integer in N/n, where N represents the total number of units and n represents the number of units to be sampled. Systematic sampling can be useful when a total list of respondents is not known a priori but is approximated. A simple example of this approach is selecting every third patient seen in a clinic. However, estimates from this sample will only be unbiased if the selection of the N/n is an integer (e.g. if the population is 20 and every third person is selected, the estimate will be biased because not every third person had an equal chance of being selected), but with increasing sample sizes, this becomes less of a concern. A greater concern with this sampling strategy is cyclic variation, also referred to as periodicity. Periodicity occurs when the sampling frame is non-randomly arranged in a pattern and the sampling strategy matches the same pattern. In these situations, every kth individual is different from the rest of the population and systematic sampling is not appropriate as the sample is not likely to be representative. Repeated systematic sampling can help decrease the likelihood of periodicity pervading the sample selection. Rather than conducting one systematic sample selecting every kth respondent, repeated systematic sampling uses multiple smaller systematic samples, each randomly starting at different points. When the sampling frame is randomly ordered, estimates using systematic sampling will be equivalent to those obtained using SRS (Box 3.2).

3.2.4   Stratified random sampling

In the situation in which multiple subgroups of interest exist (e.g. based on gender, ethnicity and age), stratified sampling helps ensure adequate numbers of each subgroup. The sampling frame is divided

---

Box 3.2 Systematic sampling example

Frone (2006) aimed to identify the prevalence of illicit drug use (marijuana, cocaine, sedatives and other psychoactive drugs) in the workforce, using a nationally representative sample of the US population. The author used a list-assisted method to generate a sampling frame and, more specifically, employed a method that eliminated numbers from clusters with low expected numbers of household residences. Frone's sampling frame of telephone numbers was among non-institutionalised adults 18–65 years of age residing in the United States. The numbers were then systematically sampled from the sampling frame, stratified by county. The study had a response rate of 57% and 2829 participants. Overall, 14.1% of employed adults reported illicit drug use in the past year, and 3.1% reported illicit drug use in the workplace. Prevalence of drug use varied based on occupation and age, among other factors, with individuals ages 18–30 years working in (1) food, construction, legal, maintenance or (2) arts/entertainment industries, showing the highest prevalence of illicit drug use in the past year (55.8 and 43.4%, respectively). Approximately 86% of the population surveyed reported no illicit drug use in the past year, and 97% reported no illicit drug use in the workplace. The low prevalence of illicit drug use in most occupations led to insufficient power for additional analyses, a concern with the use of probability sampling for the study of low base rate phenomena.

---

into homogenous but mutually exclusive strata, and the sampling for each stratum is conducted independently of the other strata (and, if selected randomly, is categorized as stratified random sampling). Selecting respondents for strata can be accomplished using equal, proportional or optimal allocation. Equal allocation selects an equal number of persons per stratum. Proportional allocation selects respondents so that the sampling strata maintain the proportions of the target population. Optimal allocation selects more respondents from strata with higher variability, making selection proportional to the variance of the strata. An advantage of stratified random sampling is that the standard errors (SEs) are rarely larger than that in SRS. It is preferable over SRS when the members are homogenous within a stratum and different between strata. However, the sampling frame requires more information than that needed for SRS. For instance, if ethnicity is the stratification variable, the ethnicity of all respondents would need to be known a priori, whereas SRS requires only the list of respondents available, with no demographic or further information being necessary for selection. It is also important to account for the stratification in the analysis, using weighted averages of the stratum-specific estimates. When it is impractical to stratify prior to collecting the sample, stratification after sampling (*post-stratification*) may be useful, as described by Cochran (1977). The post-stratification SEs may be only slightly larger than stratified random sampling when the stratification is done well with no misclassification of units (Box 3.3).

3.2.5 Cluster sampling

Clusters are groupings that occur naturally, such as based on geographic proximity (zip codes, counties, school districts) or time. Cluster sampling divides the population into clusters and a number of clusters are selected randomly. All respondents from selected clusters are then chosen for the sample. The selection of clusters can be conducted using a variety of the previously mentioned probability sampling strategies including SRS, systematic or stratified sampling. The method by which clusters are selected also affects the size of the SE, as random selection (simple cluster sampling) will have larger SEs than that of clusters sampled with a probability proportional to their size. Cluster sampling can be conducted as a single stage or more commonly in multiple stages with several levels

---

Box 3.3   Stratified random sampling example

Turner et al. (2004) investigated the utility of using estimated blood alcohol concentration (eBAC) as an index of negative alcohol-related effects among college students. The eBAC relies on self-report of number of drinks consumed and takes into account a person's gender, weight and time interval of consumption. Based on information from the registrar's office, e-mail addresses of the entire student body enrolled in the spring semester of 2003 at the University of Virginia were compiled and a random sample was identified. The random sample was drawn after stratifying, based on gender and class year. A stratified random sample of 4708 students yielded 2345 completed web-based surveys (51% response rate). Underclassmen, males and members of fraternities or sororities had significantly higher eBAC, and higher eBAC was associated with self-reported alcohol-related negative consequences. The study demonstrated the utility of the eBAC in identifying high-risk groups that can be targeted for intervention among the college populations. Although constructing a sampling frame can be difficult, captive audiences such as college students or patients at a hospital are well suited for random or stratified random samples because a sampling frame is likely to be available. Randomly selecting from a single institution, such as one university, limits the generalisability of the results. However, the extent to which authors can show that a university population is similar to that of other universities, for example, those in the same region and/or that serve students of similar characteristics, increases the likelihood (but does not guarantee) that the results are generalisable to subgroups of students and campuses that show similarities.

---

of clusters being selected (e.g. states → counties → cities → zip codes). As respondents in clusters tend to be homogeneous, the variability between different clusters is greater than the variability within respondents of the same cluster. Thus, multi-stage cluster sampling usually yields higher SEs than that of other methods using the same number of respondents. However, when cluster-level information is more easily accessible than the lists of all respondents in all geographic areas of interest, cluster sampling can be a valuable sampling tool. This may be particularly beneficial to surveys that cover large geographic areas as surveying clusters will be more cost-efficient and faster than surveying individuals spread out over large geographic regions. As a result, cluster sampling is widely used in large, national surveys (Box 3.4).

3.3   Non-probability sampling

3.3.1   Introduction

As non-probability strategies do not require a sampling frame of the population, the probability of selection is unknown and respondents are selected non-randomly. Because no sampling frame is used, non-probability strategies can be less costly and more efficient in recruiting participants than using probability sampling strategies. They can be particularly useful for obtaining participants from hard-to-reach populations (e.g. intravenous drug users), or when the population is so widely dispersed that cluster sampling would be inefficient (e.g. rural crack cocaine users). However, validity and reliability are more difficult to evaluate with this method, and non-probability sampling can be vulnerable to bias because recruiters may have no firm guidelines for selecting participants. In addition, without the information on probabilities of selection, sampling errors and the sampling distribution cannot be calculated. Within this approach, various purposive methods are used (snowball, time-space, respondent-driven, targeted), along with the use of convenience sampling.

Box 3.4 Cluster sampling example

Grant et al. (2004) implemented the National Epidemiologic Survey on Alcohol and Related Conditions (NESARC). NESARC is a longitudinal, nationally representative sample of civilian, non-institutionalised adults ages 18 and older. Primary sampling units (PSUs) consisted of all counties as well as areas that were not legally termed counties, but were statistically equivalent, and were based on the Census Bureau's Current Population Survey. The smaller PSUs were stratified according to factors such as population change, ethnic minority population and size of households living under the poverty line. Larger PSUs (defined as 250K+ residents) were automatically entered into the sample. Two PSUs per stratum were selected based on probability proportional to size. Households within the PSUs were then selected using a systematic sampling method. Individuals within the household were selected randomly. In addition, NESARC contained a separate sampling frame to include individuals with heavy substance use patterns. These subpopulations included people commonly under-represented in general population surveys such as those living in shelters, group homes and boarding houses. For the analysis, NESARC was weighted to adjust for non-response, probability of selection based on the sampling frame, as well as other factors to help create a nationally representative sample. The NESARC data have led to numerous publications. One example is a study by Hasin et al. (2007) investigating the prevalence and correlates of alcohol use disorders. From the 43 093 face-to-face interviews, the 1-year and lifetime prevalence of alcohol use disorders (alcohol abuse or alcohol dependence) was 8.5% (SE 0.24) and 30% (SE 0.77), with higher rates of lifetime alcohol use disorders among males and individuals ages 30–44. After adjusting for demographic factors, alcohol use disorders were associated with other drug use disorders, as well as mood, anxiety and personality disorders.

3.3.2 Convenience sampling

This type of non-probability sampling is the most vulnerable to bias. Using this approach, subjects may be chosen to promote feasibility, to minimise cost and/or to maximise efficiency. Since participants are selected without a structured mechanism, samples are often not representative of the target population. Thus, results and generalisability should be interpreted with caution. Although convenience sampling is not optimal, alternatives may not exist (e.g. in the study of rare events). Use of convenience samples in substance abuse research is common, and has been used in clinical, school, university and correctional venues. Investigators using convenience samples may implement steps to improve the quality of their sample. For example, researchers using convenience samples have demonstrated that study participants did not differ on a variety of measures from non-participants to suggest that recruitment within the venue was not biased (Wood et al., 2007) and have used unbiased procedures such as random selection to choose from among clinics (originally selected by convenience) to form the sample (Ross et al., 2005) (Box 3.5).

3.3.3 Snowball sampling

In snowball sampling (Goodman, 1961), a respondent in the sample is asked to identify other potential respondents. The study staff then attempts to recruit the participants that the respondent identified. Snowball sampling uses each respondent's contacts so that it is useful for studying hard-to-reach populations that are not accessible through conventional methods. However, there is a concern that larger social networks will be oversampled and respondents in smaller social networks will not be identified and accessed. Other concerns are that subjects may not want to disclose the identity or location of another individual (*masking*) or the investigator may be hesitant to put a subject in the position of doing so (e.g., for a study of illicit drug use). Theoretically, snowball

---

Box 3.5   Convenience sampling example

Wilsnack et al. (2008) used convenience sampling to investigate the relationship between drinking behaviour and lesbian sexual orientation among women. The authors explained how use of probability sampling would be impractical because of the low prevalence of lesbian sexual orientation, particularly given their desire to recruit subjects on whom meagre data are available including older women, women of colour and those of lower socioeconomic status. Using a variety of recruitment methods that included strategically placed flyers, newspaper advertisements and social networks, 447 sexual-minority women (mostly lesbian, exclusively lesbian, bisexual) were recruited. Heterosexual women ($n = 482$) from the National Study of All Health and Life Experiences of Women (a longitudinal study assessing drinking behaviour among women) were used as a comparison group. Exclusively heterosexual women had lower rates of heavy episodic drinking, intoxication, drinking-related problems, and alcohol-dependence symptoms than sexual-minority women. Exclusively heterosexual women were also less likely to be depressed or to have a history of sexual abuse. Bisexual women showed more hazardous drinking and depression than subjects who were mostly lesbian or exclusively lesbian, underscoring the heterogeneity on these measures among sexual minority groups.

---

sampling can start with a single initial respondent identified by the investigator, sometimes referred to as a 'seed', although in practice more than one seed is nearly always used. Because respondents are not drawn randomly, study results may be biased depending on the appropriateness of the initial sample (Box 3.6).

3.3.4   Time-space sampling

This form of sampling recognises that populations may gather together during certain times of the day; for example, intravenous drug users may congregate when a needle exchange programme opens. Time-space sampling uses qualitative methods such as ethnographic mapping and surveillance methods to identify the locations of interest (MacKellar et al., 1996). Sites are then randomly selected, and sampling is done with all or nearly all participants that are at the site at the specified time. The largest limitation of this strategy lies in the underlying assumption that respondents sampled in the time window are representative of the target population. This can lead to bias, as it is unlikely that all participants of interest congregate at the location consistently each time. This concern is mitigated by increasing the number of times the venue is sampled, although this may be constrained by project resources, time, staff work hours or safety concerns (e.g. it may be impractical to study subjects who congregate in a high-crime area late at night) (Box 3.7).

Box 3.6   Snowball sampling example

Boys et al. (2002) investigated reasons for substance use among youths between the ages of 16 and 22 years in southern England. Nine seeds were selected including students, a drug dealer and a waitress. These individuals were selected for their potential access to friends and acquaintances who had used illegal substances such as alcohol, cannabis, amphetamine and ecstasy. Using the snowball sampling technique, the authors were able to recruit 100 respondents in 4 months. For all substances, the perceived function of the drug (e.g. to relax, to boost confidence) was a better predictor of drug use than age, sex, gender or previously experienced negative effects. Moreover, perceived function of a drug was generally a superior predictor of its use than peer use of the drug, further supporting the importance of perceived reasons for drug use. The authors concluded that interventions should be tailored to address the different motivations for drug use.

Box 3.7 Time-space sampling example

Kelly et al. (2006) sought to characterise the prevalence and determinants of club drug use (e.g. ecstasy) based on gender, race and sexual orientation in New York City using time-space sampling. Preliminary fieldwork consisted of identifying the venues that attracted a minimum number of eligible individuals per hour for each day of the week. From this list of 71 appropriate venues, a number was assigned to each and a random number generator indicated which day and time a particular venue was to be surveyed. Once at the recruitment sites, systematic sampling was used, with every nth respondent being approached for the survey. Of the 5175 individuals approached, 2603 agreed to participate (50%), and of these persons 1914 were eligible (37%). Initially, recruiters had a difficult time recruiting one individual among a group of friends because the friends would tend to dissuade their peer from participating. To reduce the refusal rate, recruitment was modified and subsequently all club patrons were approached for the survey. Overall, 70% reported any previous experience with club drugs, and 22% reported club drug use in the past 3 months, with ecstasy and cocaine being the most common (45.2 and 41%, respectively), followed by lysergic acid diethylamide (25.5%) and ketamine (21%). Club drug use varied by race/ethnicity and sexual orientation. A pilot phase prior to implementation of the study may have been helpful in identifying the obstacle of peers dissuading a potential subject from participating.

3.3.5   Respondent-driven sampling

An offshoot of snowball sampling is respondent-driven sampling (RDS, Heckathorn, 1997). Whereas snowball sampling involves respondents providing names of referrals, RDS invites respondents to recruit subjects for the study from their personal network. Because potential subjects are informed about the study by their peers and only approach the researchers if they wish to participate, the identities of individuals who do not wish to be recruited are unknown to the researchers. Along with providing confidentiality, this approach may also reduce staff recruitment time and expense. Respondents are provided with an incentive for recruiting peers. To avoid the problem of individuals becoming 'professional recruiters', recruitment quotas are used in which each participant can only recruit a certain number of their friends for the study (e.g. up to three). Although the initial seeds are not selected randomly, data suggest samples typically reach *convergence* within 5–6 waves of recruitment. (Heckathorn, 1997). By identifying how successive respondents are linked to the recruiter, probabilities of selection can be calculated. For instance, if Bill knows ten people who are eligible for the study, the probabilities of an eligible friend being selected are 1/10 (Box 3.8).

Box 3.8 Respondent-driven sampling example

Wattana et al. (2007) used RDS to study injection drug use in Thailand. Sixteen active intravenous drug users residing in the Bangkok Metropolitan Administration area were the initial seeds. From the seeds, a total of 963 respondents were recruited for the sample. The authors gave each respondent 150 baht (approximately US$3.50) as their 'primary incentive', and 50 baht (approximately US$1.20) for each additional participant the respondent referred to the study. Twenty additional baht was provided for recruiting women and persons younger than 20 as these were perceived to be the most difficult intravenous drug users to identify and enrol. The sample converged after the fourth wave of recruitment, evidenced by the distribution of gender and IDUs who were in or outside the treatment remaining stable in subsequent waves. Never-treated intravenous drug users were more likely to be unemployed, female, younger than 35, or those who limited their injecting to heroin or methamphetamine.

Box 3.9 Targeted sampling example

Falck et al. (2007) reported the results of a natural history study of crack users residing in a county in Ohio. Before recruitment began, the relative density of crack users in the county was calculated. This was an important step for recruitment purposes so that recruitment quotas would reflect the numbers of users available. Sampling quotas were then created based on the proportion of crack users in that zip code as well as the formulation of global study quotas for gender and ethnicity. For instance, in areas with expected lower proportions of crack users (estimated based on data sources such as the number of arrests for crack use, divided by the number of total arrests), a lower percentage of respondents was expected in comparison to a zip code with a higher density of crack users. Among other analyses, trajectory of cocaine use over an 8-year period was investigated. Of the total sample of 401 respondents, 292 (73%) completed the 8-year follow-up. The mean years of crack use at study entry was 7.6 years, and the majority of users (63%) did not 'quit' (defined as abstaining for 6 consecutive months or more) at any time during the study period. Results illustrate the chronicity of crack use once a regular pattern of use is established.

3.3.6 Targeted sampling

Targeted sampling may employ probability and non-probability sampling techniques as well as qualitative strategies to obtain the sample (Watters & Biernacki, 1989). A list of specified populations is mapped out, and a plan is undertaken to recruit a particular number of cases or quota from each of the targeted populations. Targeted sampling aims to gather a minimum set of persons from each targeted area of interest, and so it may be more time-consuming to gather participants compared to other non-probability sampling strategies. Once the targeted populations are mapped out, the specific locations are then randomly selected, with quotas outlined beforehand for each subpopulation. Limitations of targeted sampling include the fact that it is contingent on valid mapping and quotas to identify the populations which can be uncertain. In addition, time and location used in recruiting participants may affect the results. Ideally, efforts should be made to approach respondents during various times and places throughout the day. This method is vulnerable to bias unless there is rigorous training and supervision of study staff in order to guard against a tendency to select subjects who are most available or approachable (Box 3.9).

3.4 Qualitative sampling

The main purpose of qualitative sampling is to identify information-rich cases (see also Chapter 5 on qualitative methods). Although many of the non-probability sampling strategies are used for recruitment of participants into qualitative research, the intent of the qualitative study can also affect the nature of recruitment. Several sampling strategies designed specifically for qualitative studies have been described by Patton (2002) and are mentioned briefly here:

1. *Extreme or deviant case sampling* uses severe examples so that lessons learnt can also be applied to the more typical programmes or persons.
2. *Intensity sampling* emphasises finding cases that are experiencing the phenomena in a lesser magnitude than those in the extreme sampling (but still intensely).
3. *Maximum variation sampling* uses heterogeneous samples in two ways. The similarities between cases can be studied as core experiences that transcend demographic differences, and the differences between cases serve as information-rich individual cases.

4. *Homozygous sampling* aims to describe one small subgroup in-depth. A commonly used homozygous sampling strategy is the use of focus groups, which use an open-ended interview with either a script or structured questions to a small group of people (usually five to ten people).
5. *Typical case sampling* seeks to describe what is 'typically' seen, for example for further research studies.
6. *Critical case sampling* identifies a critical case for which 'logical generalisations' can presumably be made of the larger group.
7. *Criterion sampling* reviews all cases that meet predetermined criteria. This sampling can be particularly effective for quality assurance purposes.
8. *Confirmatory and disconfirming case sampling* studies cases that are confirmatory in order to add depth and credibility to conclusions, whereas disconfirming cases may help to place boundaries between what was thought to be confirmed. Qualitative sampling is vulnerable to the same biases as convenience sampling.

3.5   Selecting your sampling approach

A detailed literature search is required before conducting a study. Your search may reveal that an appropriate database already exists to answer your research question. In this case, rather than devoting resources to obtaining a sample, you may determine that it would be more efficient to obtain and analyse the relevant database. Assuming that you decide to gather a sample, there are a number of considerations in choosing a sampling approach, and a given study may employ more than one strategy. Table 3.2 lists each approach with a brief description, and one (or two) major advantage(s) and disadvantage(s). It is typically beneficial to gather pilot data in order to demonstrate feasibility, estimate resources and costs that will be required, identify unforeseen problems and plan for necessary adjustments, and possibly inform sample size calculations. Sometimes the most optimal sampling design from a scientific standpoint will not be feasible due to practical (e.g. costs and time) or ethical/legal considerations. There are usually trade-offs in choosing one design over another, and there may not be a single best sampling design for a given study question. For example, Robinson *et al.* (2006) conducted a study comparing targeted sampling versus RDS strategies among injection drug users, and concluded that each approach yielded unique and valuable information. Thus, the best choice would depend on the specific goals of the project.

3.6   Technical considerations

3.6.1   Sample size

Assuming that sampling bias is minimised, increasing the number of respondents will increase the precision of the results (in other words, it will decrease the size of the SE). However, the increase in precision eventually becomes negligible with increased sample size and will not warrant the extra cost of additional recruitment. Determining the necessary sample size is based on several factors. It is important to conduct a **sample size calculation** because underpowered studies (where *n* is too small) result in imprecise estimates, whereas overpowered studies (where *n* is too large) waste time, money and personnel resources. The size of the sample depends on the purpose of the study, as well as the specific hypotheses. The nature of **power calculations** for studies with different purposes will be dissimilar (e.g. a randomised clinical trial detecting a treatment difference between groups is likely to require a different sample size compared to a study designed to show moderators of relationships

Table 3.2 Comparison of sampling strategies

Simple random sampling

Advantages	Most straightforward probability sampling strategy
Disadvantages	Requires a list of all potential respondents (sampling frame) to be available beforehand
	Can be costly and time-consuming for large studies

Systematic sampling

Advantages	Requires an approximated sampling frame a priori but not the full list
	When done correctly, will approximate the results of simple random sampling
Disadvantages	If periodicity exists, the sample will be biased
	If study participants deduce the sampling interval, this can bias the population as non-participants will be different from study participants

Stratified random sampling

Advantages	Ensures adequate representation of all subgroups
	When there is homogeneity within strata and heterogeneity between strata, the estimates can be as precise (or even more precise) as with the use of simple random sampling
Disadvantages	Requires knowledge of strata membership a priori
	Adds complexity to the analysis plan

Cluster sampling

Advantages	Is the most time-efficient and cost-efficient probability design for large geographic areas
Disadvantages	Requires group-level information to be known
	Commonly has higher SEs than the other sampling strategies

Convenience sampling

Advantages	Simplicity
	Helpful for pilot studies and for hypothesis generation
Disadvantages	Highly vulnerable to selection bias
	Generalisability unclear

Snowball sampling

Advantages	Ability to recruit hidden populations
Disadvantages	Oversampling a particular network of peers can lead to bias
	Respondents may be hesitant to provide names of peers and asking them to do so may raise ethical concerns

Respondent-driven sampling

Advantages	Safer and more cost-effective for staff than recruiting respondents directly
	Convergence of estimates occurs within five to six waves of recruitment
Disadvantages	Ineffective if the initial seeds do not know other members in the population of interest

Targeted sampling

Advantages	Ensures adequate representation of the subgroups of interest
Disadvantages	Can be vulnerable to recruitment bias

Time-space sampling

Advantages	Effective at capturing hidden populations that naturally congregate
Disadvantages	If only limited venues and times are used, it is vulnerable to bias as not everyone in the target population is likely to be available

Qualitative sampling

Advantages	Provides detailed, in-depth information
Disadvantages	Vulnerable to selection bias
	Maybe time-consuming

Table 3.3 Sample size calculation

Difference to detect between groups	Alpha	Power	Total sample size needed
0.5	0.015	0.80	390
0.4	0.015	0.80	328
0.5	0.05	0.80	286
0.5	0.015	0.90	500

or to one intended to describe the prevalence of disease in a population). Table 3.3 illustrates how sample size is affected by varying parameters in the calculation, illustrating that sample size is a trade-off between several factors. In this example, a randomised clinical trial aims to detect a difference of 0.4 or 0.5 in the means between a treatment group and a control group, assuming a SD of 1.5.

In determining sample size, researchers should ask themselves (1) what are the study's hypotheses, (2) how common are the phenomena under study (with rare phenomena requiring larger samples), (3) how homogeneous is the population (with larger samples needed for heterogeneous populations), (4) how small of a difference or magnitude of an association does the study wish to detect (smaller differences requiring larger samples) and (5) what is the desired alpha level (the probability of a false-positive error, with smaller alphas requiring larger sample sizes). Ultimately, a table or software is necessary to quantify the number of respondents needed for a study. Cohen (1988) and Kraemer and Thiemann (1987) provide statistical power tables. Online resources such as sample size calculators or freeware from the CDC (http://www.cdc.gov/epiinfo/) or Vanderbilt University are readily accessible (http://biostat.mc.vanderbilt.edu/twiki/bin/view/Main/PowerSampleSize). For qualitative studies, sample size may primarily be concerned with achieving redundancy in responses, rather than interviewing a predetermined number of respondents.

3.6.2 Technological assistance

Surveys may be conducted using computer-assisted self-interviewing (CASI) or audio-CASI (ACASI). Using respondents to input their responses directly into the computer, rather than in a face-to-face interview, can be advantageous as individuals tend to be more disclosing of sensitive information to a computer (also true of paper and pencil self-report). Softwares such as Questionnaire Development System (http://www.novaresearch.com/Products/qds/) or Computer-Assisted Survey Execution System (http://cases.berkeley.edu/) are particularly helpful as responses entered in directly are stored electronically in a database and do not require separate data entry.

For analysing quantitative data, SAS, STATA (http://www.stata.com/) or SPSS (http://www.spss.com/) are the most common software packages. All allow for line-by-line programming and the use of drop-down menus to select analysis options. For cluster sampling, in which weighted data must be taken into account in the analysis, SUDAAN (http://www.rti.org/SUDAAN/) is frequently used. RDSAT (http://www.respondentdrivensampling.org/) is commonly used for RDS. For qualitative studies, in which transcription of text and coding of themes are key, NVIVO (http://www.qsrinternational.com/products_nvivo.aspx) and Ethnograph (http://www.qualisresearch.com/) are often used.

3.6.3   Internet-based surveys and computer-assisted surveys

Depending on the research question, surveys conducted online may be a viable option. The main limitation is that surveys conducted in this fashion will not likely be representative of the target population. Duplicate entries are another concern. McCabe and Teter (2007) randomly sampled 5389 students from among undergraduates enrolled at a public university in 2005 and sent the sample population a postal letter, enclosed with US$2, and a unique password. By providing the incentive upfront, the likelihood of response may be increased, (James & Bolstein, 1990) and the unique password decreased the likelihood of duplicate entries, or entries by non-sampled respondents. Internet studies of substance abuse have also been conducted by mass emailing members of affiliated listservs (e.g. members of the Marijuana Policy Project) (Barnwell & Earleywine, 2006) but without requiring unique login or passwords. These studies have been unable to identify duplicate entries, a particular concern when an entrant can be eligible for prizes (e.g. through a drawing). With the growing use of the internet, the feasibility of internet-based surveys is growing and is a formidable source of substance abuse research in the future. Methods to maximise the quality of internet-based sampling may be expected to increase rapidly.

3.7   Conclusion

This chapter has provided an overview of sampling strategies along with technical and practical considerations that are important in designing a sampling plan. Understanding the differences in sampling strategies is vital for selecting a sampling plan that is feasible and appropriate, but is only one component of research. Readers are advised to not only delve further into sampling issues, but to also explore study designs and statistical methods in order to be better informed for developing a solid, comprehensive research plan.

Acknowledgements

The authors thank Susan Fisher, Ph.D., and Kay Spellane, MBA, for their helpful comments on an earlier draft.

Exercises

1. You wish to study the prevalence of drug use in your local community and decide to send questionnaires to all the licensed drug counsellors in the nearby hospitals. Are you concerned you might be introducing some biases into your study with your sample selection? Why or why not? Does your opinion differ depending on your response rate? (50% vs 95%)
2. Suppose you wish to conduct a statewide study assessing correlates of entering in drug rehabilitation programmes. You decide to do a cluster sample and have randomly selected three large hospitals in a single metropolitan area. Your colleague is concerned the hospitals may not be representative of the state, and suggests that you instead resample and select one hospital from an urban, rural and suburban area. Do you agree with your colleague's rationale? Why or why not?
3. You wish to better understand underage drinking on the local college campuses, but little information exists about the prevalence in this community. Although the college campus is of moderate size, you have limited resources and want to use them wisely. Should you use your resources conducting a large random sample that is representative, or qualitative studies to collect pilot data followed by a quantitative sampling method that is smaller in scale?

References

Barnwell, S. S. & Earleywine, M. (2006) Simultaneous alcohol and cannabis expectancies predict simultaneous use. *Substance Abuse, Treatment, Prevention, and Policy*, 1, 29.

Boys, A., Marsden, J. & Strang, J. (2002) The relative influence of friends and functions: modeling frequency of substance use in a non-treatment sample of 16–22 year olds. *Health Education*, 102(6), 280–288.

Cochran, W. G. (1977) *Sampling Techniques*, 3rd edn. New York: Wiley.

Cohen, J. (1988) *Statistical Power Analysis for the Behavioral Sciences*, 2nd edn. New Jersey: Lawrence Erlbaum.

Drabble, L., Midanik, L. T. & Trocki, K. (2005) Reports of alcohol consumption and alcohol-related problems among homosexual, bisexual and heterosexual respondents: results from the 2000 national alcohol survey. *Journal of Studies on Alcohol*, 66(1), 111–120.

Falck, R. S., Wang, J. & Carlson, R. G. (2007) Crack cocaine trajectories among users in a midwestern American city. *Addiction*, 102(9), 1421–1431.

Frone, M. R. (2006) Prevalence and distribution of illicit drug use in the workforce and in the workplace: findings and implications from a U.S. National survey. *The Journal of Applied Psychology*, 91(4), 856–869.

Goodman, L. (1961) Snowball sampling. *Annals of Mathematical Statistics*, 32, 245–268.

Grant, B. F., Dawson, D. A., Stinson, F. S., Chou, S. P., Dufour, M. C. & Pickering, R. P. (2004) The 12-month prevalence and trends in DSM-IV alcohol abuse and dependence: United States, 1991–1992 and 2001–2002. *Drug and Alcohol Dependence*, 74(3), 223–234.

Hasin, D. S., Stinson, F. S., Ogburn, E. & Grant, B. F. (2007) Prevalence, correlates, disability, and comorbidity of DSM-IV alcohol abuse and dependence in the United States: results from the National Epidemiologic Survey on Alcohol and Related Conditions. *Archives of General Psychiatry*, 64(7), 830–842.

Heckathorn, D. (1997) Respondent-driven sampling: a new approach to the study of hidden populations. *Social Problems*, 44(2), 174–199.

James, J. M. & Bolstein, R. (1990) The effect of monetary incentives and follow-up mailings on the response rate and response quality in mail surveys. *The Public Opinion Quarterly*, 54, 346–361.

Kelly, B. C., Parsons, J. T. & Wells, B. E. (2006) Prevalence and predictors of club drug use among club-going young adults in New York City. *Journal of Urban Health*, 83(5), 884–895.

Kraemer, H. C. & Thiemann, S. (1987) *How Many Subjects? Statistical Power Analysis in Research*. Newbury Park, CA: Sage Publications.

Levy, P. S. & Lemeshow, S. (1999) *Sampling of Populations: Methods and Applications*, 3rd edn. New York: Wiley.

MacKellar, D., Valleroy, L., Karon, J., Lemp, G. & Janssen, R. (1996) The Young Men's Survey: methods for estimating HIV seroprevalence and risk factors among young men who have sex with men. *Public Health Reports*, 111(Suppl 1), 138–144.

McCabe, S. E. & Teter, C. J. (2007) Drug use related problems among nonmedical users of prescription stimulants: a web-based survey of college students from a Midwestern university. *Drug and Alcohol Dependence*, 91(1), 69–76.

Patton, M. Q. (2002) *Qualitative Research and Evaluation Methods*, 3rd edn. Thousand Oaks, CA: Sage Publications.

Robinson, W. T., Risser, J. M., McGoy, S., Becker, A. B., Rehman H., Jefferson, M., Griffin, V., Wolverton, M. & Tortu, S. (2006) Recruiting injection drug users: a three-site comparison of results and experiences with respondent-driven and targeted sampling procedures. *Journal of Urban Health*, 83(7), i29–i38.

Ross, J., Teesson, M., Darke, S., Lynskey, M., Ali, R., Ritter, A. & Cooke, R. (2005) The characteristics of heroin users entering treatment: findings from the Australian Treatment Outcome Study (ATOS). *Drug and Alcohol Review*, 24(5), 411–418.

Turner, J. C., Bauerle, J. & Shu, J. (2004) Estimated blood alcohol concentration correlation with self-reported negative consequences among college students using alcohol. *Journal of Studies on Alcohol*, 65(6), 741–749.

Wattana, W., van Griensven, F., Rhucharoenpornpanich, O., Manopaiboon, C., Thienkrua, W., Bannatham, R., Fox, K., Mock, P., Tappero, J. & Levine, W. (2007) Respondent-driven sampling to assess characteristics and estimate the number of injection drug users in Bangkok, Thailand. *Drug and Alcohol Dependence*, 90(2–3), 228–233.

Watters, J. K. & Biernacki, P. (1989) Targeted sampling: options for the study of hidden populations. *Social Problems*, 36(4), 416–430.

Wilsnack, S. C., Hughes, T. L., Johnson, T. P., Bostwick, W. B., Szalacha, L. A., Benson, P., Aranda, F. & Kinnison, K.. (2008) Drinking and drinking-related problems among heterosexual and sexual minority women. *Journal of Studies on Alcohol and Drugs*, 69(1): 129–139.

Wood, P. K., Sher, K. J. & Rutledge, P. C. (2007) College student alcohol consumption, day of the week, and class schedule. *Alcoholism: Clinical and Experimental Research*, 31(7), 1195–1207.

Recommended readings

Faugier, J. & Sargeant, M. (1997) Sampling hard to reach populations. *Journal of Advanced Nursing*, 26(4), 790–797.

Levy, P. S. & Lemeshow, S. (1999) *Sampling of Populations: Methods and Applications*, 3rd edn. New York: Wiley.

Salganik, M. J. (2006) Variance estimation, design effects, and sample size calculations for respondent-driven sampling. *Journal of Urban Health: Bulletin of the New York Academy of Medicine*, 83(7), i98–i112.

Thompson, S. K. & Collins, L. M. (2002) Adaptive sampling in research on risk-related behaviors. *Drug and Alcohol Dependence*, 68, S57–S67.

Chapter 4

EXPERIMENTAL DESIGN ISSUES IN ADDICTION RESEARCH

Robert West

4.1 Introduction

Experiments usually provide the most secure information on causal relationships between variables of interest, but they usually also present the greatest challenges in terms of generalisability of findings and practical and ethical constraints. There are many different types of experimental design that can be used, each with its own useful features and limitations.

This chapter discusses the design options available and considers the circumstances in which they are most suitable. It also examines the other choices that need to be made when devising experiments, including choice of intervention and control conditions, selection of participants, sample size, choice of outcome measures and statistical analyses. In the space available, this chapter cannot aspire to be a comprehensive analysis of all the issues that arise, so the approach taken is to assume a basic knowledge of research methods in clinical and social sciences and to focus on what appear to be the key issues.

4.2 What constitutes an experiment?

The defining feature of an experiment is that the researcher does something deliberately and takes observations to see whether it made any difference to something of interest. It is distinguished from an observational study in which the researcher merely takes observations.[1]

Experiments are favoured as a way of ascribing causality because it can normally be assumed that the deliberate actions of the experimenter could not have been caused by the outcome of the experiment and that there can be no mechanism by which the actions of the experimenter and the outcomes of experiment arose from some common cause.

This is not always the case which is why certain kinds of experiment are more effective than others at establishing whether a causal relationship exists between two variables. The problem is particularly acute in the field of addiction where there are a multitude of factors that can influence outcomes of interest, and the role of one factor taken in isolation is very difficult to determine.

In these circumstances two key design features are of major importance: **use of comparisons**, and **randomisation**. Comparisons are needed because the outcome of interest will typically vary from one person to another or from one occasion to another without intervention, and so the mere observation of a difference or a change will not be able to be ascribed to something one has done. Randomisation means using a random process (such as toss of a coin) to decide whether to do the action whose effect one wants to observe or not, or to do one thing with one person and another thing with another. This is important because if one were to decide oneself, there would be a serious risk of bias.

Designing experiments involves a number of key choices, and making the wrong one can lead to a huge amount of wasted time, effort and money. Making the right choices relies on having an understanding of what is achievable in terms of the research question that can be answered. Once one has arrived at a research question, the key choices involve the following:

1. Is an experiment appropriate?
2. What kind of design should be used?
3. What interventions and comparison conditions should be compared?
4. What should be the target population and how should they be recruited and consented?
5. What should be the sample size?
6. What primary and secondary outcome measures should be used?
7. What statistical analyses should be undertaken?

The following sections address each of these in turn.

4.3　Is an experiment appropriate?

Experiments are appropriate when it is important to establish whether there is a causal relationship between two or more variables and possibly to estimate the extent of that association. They are not appropriate when simply describing phenomena or recording associations between events or characteristics. Neither are they appropriate when actively influencing outcomes in one way or another would be unethical or impracticable. They are also not appropriate when there is such a complex interplay of different causal elements that to produce useful results would require dozens of different comparisons, each involving hundreds of participants. They are inappropriate when it is not feasible to package up the interventions being compared into clearly identifiable and describable entities. Finally, experiments are not appropriate when the effect of an intervention being tested is likely to depend to a considerable degree on the context: thus, conclusions drawn from the experiment could not reasonably be generalised to populations or circumstances of interest.

If an experiment is not appropriate, it may still be possible to undertake an observational study. It will be necessary to temper any conclusions concerning causal relationships, but often one can use argumentation and statistical adjustment to compensate in part for the lack of experimental control.

4.4　What kind of experimental design?

Choice of experimental design is usually the starting point for any study. There are two main classes of experimental design used in addiction research:

1. **Between-group designs** apply different interventions to different groups of people and compare the effects on one or more outcome measures averaged over those groups.
2. **Within-group designs** apply different intervention to the same people at different times and compare the effects following those interventions.

These designs have many variants which are discussed in the following paragraphs, starting with the simplest and most commonly used in the field of addiction. For more information about these designs, see Craig et al. (2008).

4.4.1   Between-group designs

Individually randomised between-group design

This is the most straightforward design in many ways. Individuals are recruited into the study and then randomly allocated one at a time to two or more groups, each group being treated differently in some way (Box 4.1). The effects of this difference are then assessed on one or more outcome measure. The variable defining the difference in the way they are treated is called the '**independent variable**', while the outcome measure is called the '**dependent variable**'.

If a difference is observed in the dependent variable, this can be attributed either to '**chance**' or to the independent variable. Chance is ruled out for all practical purposes by doing statistical analysis to work out the probability that the size of difference in the dependent variable observed could have happened by drawing the groups randomly from exactly the same pool of observations. Typically, we say that if the probability of getting a difference of the size observed is less than 1 in 20 ($P < 0.05$), the presumption is that it must have been due to the difference in the way the groups were treated.

The **randomised controlled trial (RCT)** is an example of this type of design. This is used to evaluate the effectiveness of an intervention such as a treatment compared with either no intervention or another intervention believed to be less effective, often called a '**control**' or '**control condition**'. Alternatively, there may be several interventions all being compared against each other, in which case one may talk of two or more different '**intervention groups**' (e.g. in the field of smoking, see Nides et al., 2008).

Box 4.1   Possibly the most important study ever conducted of smoking cessation

Anthonisen and colleagues (2005) conducted a pragmatic randomised controlled trial of a combination of behavioural support and nicotine replacement therapy in smokers with mild-to-moderate chronic obstructive pulmonary disease. They showed a substantial benefit compared with usual care, not only on smoking cessation but on all-cause mortality at a 15-year follow-up.

Design: The Lung Health Study was a randomised clinical trial of smoking cessation. Special intervention participants received the smoking intervention programme and were compared with usual care participants. Vital status was followed up to 14.5 years.
Setting: Ten clinical centres in the United States and Canada.
Patients: 5887 middle-aged volunteers with asymptomatic airway obstruction.
Measurements: All-cause mortality and mortality due to cardiovascular disease, lung cancer and other respiratory disease.
Intervention: The intervention was a 10-week smoking cessation programme that included a strong physician message and 12 group sessions using behaviour modification and nicotine gum, plus either ipratropium or a placebo inhaler.
Results: At 5 years, 21.7% of special intervention participants had stopped smoking since study entry compared with 5.4% of usual care participants. After up to 14.5 years of follow-up, 731 patients died: 33% of lung cancer, 22% of cardiovascular disease, 7.8% of respiratory disease other than cancer and 2.3% of unknown causes. All-cause mortality was significantly lower in the special intervention group than in the usual care group (8.83 per 1000 person-years vs 10.38 per 1000 person-years; $P = 0.03$) (Anthonisen et al., 2005, taken from abstract).

Although this kind of design is optimal in an ideal world, there are many conditions in which it is not practicable. One of these is where there is risk of '**contamination**'. It may be impossible to prevent participants receiving one intervention from receiving elements of one or more other interventions. For example, if one wished to examine whether the effect of one form of smoking cessation advice on success at stopping was better than another, one might wish to train a number of advisers to deliver both forms of advice and then randomly decide which client would receive which one. The problem is that the advisers may inadvertently introduce elements of one form into the other. Or else, they may come to believe that elements in one form are effective and feel that it would be unethical to withhold those elements from both groups.

Contamination is a particular problem when it comes to evaluating interventions that are readily available. For example, suppose one wished to evaluate the effectiveness of an over-the-counter medication on craving for cigarettes over a 1-month period. It would be impossible to prevent participants allocated to a placebo condition from buying glucose tablets or sweets with a high glucose content. It is also easy to see how participants randomly allocated to receive take-home supplies of a medication to reduce alcohol cravings might swap medications with other participants if they know them and feel so inclined. There are other occasions in which it is not possible to target interventions to individuals: they can only be delivered to groups. Mass media campaigns are an obvious example.

Cluster-randomised between-group designs

Where it is impracticable to randomise participants individually to intervention and comparison conditions, it may be possible to randomise them in 'clusters'. For example, one may randomise by hospital or general practice where several or even hundreds of participants come from each cluster. This allows the intervention to be delivered in the same way to blocks of participants with reduced risk of contamination (e.g. Kaner et al., 2003).

There is a penalty to be paid for this kind of design. The statistical analysis cannot pretend that each participant is a completely independent source of data. There may be many reasons why outcomes from participants in the same cluster would be similarly quite apart from receiving the same intervention. For example, they may have sociocultural factors in common, or their physical and social environment may be similar. The statistical analysis needs to incorporate the clusters. The way this is done is usually to use what are known 'random-effects' models or 'multi-level' models. It is important to recognise that the fewer the clusters, the weaker the statistical power to detect an intervention effect, so it is important to put as much resource as one can into maximising the numbers of clusters.

Stepped wedge design

Quite often one wishes to examine the effectiveness of an intervention which is already in the planning stage. Many interventions in the field of addiction are implemented without having previously been subjected to experimental evaluation. Even where interventions have been developed on the basis of evidence from RCTs, there will often be the question of how effective these are in the 'real world'. The stepped wedge design offers the possibility of evaluating such interventions experimentally. This involves phasing the roll-out of the intervention so that different populations receive it after varying amounts of delay. The important thing is to be able to determine randomly the order in which different populations begin to receive the intervention (see Brown & Lilford, 2006).

Preference designs and randomised consent designs

A major problem with conventional RCTs is that they can only generalise to people who are willing to be allocated randomly to any of the intervention or comparison conditions being studied. If there are particular reasons why some people might prefer one intervention and others prefer another one, this can leave a very small and unrepresentative population from which to draw. There is no perfect way out of this difficulty, but two approaches are now commonly used to mitigate the problem.

One of these, the 'preference design', involves checking first of all whether potential participants would be willing to be randomised. Those that are willing are then allocated to intervention or comparison conditions as in the classical RCT. Those that are not willing are invited to participate in the study and receive the intervention that they prefer. The success of this method hinges on having significant numbers of participants agreeing to be randomised and choosing each of the experimental conditions. The statistical analysis involves assessing (1) the effect of the variable 'random allocation versus receiving preferred intervention', (2) the difference between the different intervention or control conditions and (3) the interaction between the two (see Janevic et al., 2003).

Another approach is not to give participants the choice but rather to randomise them before consent into one of the experimental conditions and then ask them whether they would like to take part in the study based on a clear understanding of what that will involve for them (Altman et al., 1995). This approach is increasingly used in situations where notifying participants of alternative interventions to which they might have been allocated could create disappointment once they see their own particular allocation. This could then lead to their dropping out of the study, which could easily lead to a bias in the results. There are clearly potential ethical issues with this approach, and ethics committees will weigh up any potential costs to participants against research objectives.

Fractional factorial designs

There are often occasions in experimental studies, particularly evaluations of interventions, in which one would like to test the effects of particular intervention elements, but it would be too costly to recruit enough participants to carry out a full-scale investigation in which every possible permutation of elements was represented. This is where fractional factorial designs can be useful (Collins et al., 2005; Nair et al., 2008; Strecher et al., 2008b). Suppose that one wishes to test the effects of five different treatment elements and the various combinations that may arise from these. In a full factorial design one would need 2 to the power of 5 experimental conditions, totalling 32 in all. Each condition may require 500 or more people in it if each element of the intervention is only presumed to have a small effect. This would make a full factorial design extremely expensive and unlikely to receive funding. A fractional factorial design involves choosing a particular subset of combinations of elements, which can answer most of the interesting questions that are of interest, including the average effect of each intervention element and whether there are some simple interactions between these elements.

4.4.2   Within-subject designs

There are occasions when one wishes to test the effects of interventions, and these effects are sufficiently short lived that one can use each participant as his or her own control (e.g. McKee et al., 2008). In the simplest possible case one might, for example, test the effect of a fast-acting medication on craving for a cigarette by having each participant take the medication on one day and a placebo on another. One would then measure craving on each day in question and compare the results.

This kind of design can be useful when there is a shortage of participants, but once a participant has agreed to take part in a study, he or she is willing to engage with all the interventions. It can also be useful when there are large individual differences but high-within individual consistency in the outcome measure. By using participants as their own controls, one can benefit from this within-individual consistency, substantially reducing the number of observations that one needs to make.

Very often in the field of addiction the limitations of within-subject designs preclude their use. They cannot be used when there is a risk of contamination from exposure to one intervention or observation to a later one. Thus, having experienced one intervention may well affect the way that participants respond to a later one. This can be addressed to a limited extent by counterbalancing the order in which interventions and comparison conditions are presented. However, in order to be able to test adequately for carry-over effects, one needs to look at the interaction between the order of presentation of interventions and the different interventions themselves. To have the statistical power to do this, one needs as many participants in the study as one would have if one had used a between-group design.

Another problem is that if participants drop out of the study before completion, one loses all their data. So this design is not appropriate where there is a significant risk of losing participants before they have completed all the experimental conditions. One way of helping to mitigate this problem is to reserve all or most of any financial or other compensation for the final session.

N-of-1 designs

Experiments in which one manipulates one variable with a group of people and looks at the average effect can fail to capture important cause–effect relationships that can only be observed in individuals. People bring to any situation a highly variable set of dispositions which can interact with the manipulation of interest to produce different effects. 'N-of-1' experimental designs offer the potential to address this problem. The principle is that one takes a series of measurements to establish a stable baseline, and then one introduces an intervention and takes a further series observations. One might then reverse the intervention (if that is possible) to see whether the observations return to their previous value and repeat the process a sufficient number of times for a statistical analysis on the set of observation to demonstrate a link between the intervention and changes in the observations. Alternatively, one might introduce an intervention randomly varying its timing across individuals in an analogous fashion to the stepped wedge design for groups.

This kind of design is well suited for situations in which one has the opportunity to collect a series of observation; it is reasonable to expect that in the absence of a specific intervention the observations will be relatively stable, and the effect of the intervention is reversible if it is withdrawn. This design has not been widely used in the field of addiction (but see Velicer, 1994) but has been used successfully elsewhere (e.g. Mahon et al., 1996).

4.5 What intervention and comparison conditions?

Having arrived at a suitable experimental design, there is the question of what intervention and comparison conditions to adopt. This depends on a number of factors.

A major issue that often arises is whether the question of interest is **pragmatic** or **theoretical**? For example, one may wish to know whether a particular multi-component intervention to attract heroin addicts into treatment is worth implementing. This intervention may have numerous elements, including providing incentives, use of word-of-mouth recommendation, offering home visits and leaflets. This is a pragmatic question and it would not be realistic to devise an experiment which individually tested the effect of each component and combination of components. If this intervention were not current practice, but rather was something that was being proposed, a typical comparison condition would involve current practice. However, this would leave open two important questions: first of all, would a somewhat cut-down version of the new intervention have been just as effective and, if so, which elements should be included; and secondly, if an effect is observed, to what extent is it simply a '**Hawthorne effect**', in which the novelty of doing anything different has an effect.

When answering theoretical questions, a great deal of ingenuity is often required to devise intervention and control conditions that genuinely test the hypotheses. The reason is that there are potentially so many factors that might contribute to the outcome that a negative result can rarely be considered to refute the hypothesis and a positive one always has another explanation. The history of psychology is littered with trails of experiments that have tried to test some important theory only for the series to peter out as people come to realise that there is not adequate resolution or they move on to another area of interest. The classic example is cognitive dissonance theory versus self-perception theory. The former argues that behaving in a way that runs counter to one's attitudes creates an unpleasant feeling and so people change their attitudes to bring them in line with their behaviour. The latter argued that people use their behaviour to infer their attitudes. It turns out to be remarkably difficult to disentangle these two explanations for experimental findings (for a discussion of some of the issues, see Crano & Prislin, 2006). It is important, therefore, to recognise the limitations of experiments in this field when it comes to theory testing. That is not to say that it cannot be done, but rather that a realistic appraisal of the link between observation and theory involves moving an imaginary pointer in one direction or another rather than making absolute statements about support and refutation.

Another issue in the choice of intervention and control conditions is ethicality (see DuVal, 2004). If there is strong reason to believe that a particular intervention is effective, it may be unethical to randomly allocate individuals to a control condition known to be ineffective. One might ask why one should want to conduct an experiment in such circumstances. However, this is quite a common scenario. The reason is that 'strong reason to believe' is not the same as 'direct evidence to support'. It is important to factor into this equation the value of the study for society. It can be ethical for an individual to volunteer for a study in which there is a risk of harm if there is a good prospect that there will be benefit for other people. In general, one would need strong ethical safeguards in such cases and err on the side of caution. It would also be particularly important for individuals who might be disadvantaged to be fully informed about the choice they were making in taking part in the study, to have their understanding checked and to gain their active consent.

Experimental evaluations of interventions to promote recovery from addictive disorders have mostly compared the proposed intervention with ones that are presumed to be minimally effective, such as a placebo. However, as the field matures, confidence is growing that certain interventions have a clinically significant effect and that raises the ethical question of whether it is acceptable to include a placebo or inactive control condition. Should one not always compare any new treatment with an active treatment comparator?

There are several reasons why this is not appropriate as a universal rule. First of all, the rationale for an active comparator is not always present. Thus, it is not necessary for a new intervention to be more effective on average than an existing one for it to have a significant public health benefit. A new intervention may have an important benefit just by helping the subset of individuals who are not helped by existing interventions. A new medication, for example, may be effective in individuals for whom existing medications are not. The new medication may not be better overall, but the public health gain of having both on the market would be considerable. One might argue that in this case, one should limit testing of the new medication to individuals who have not been helped with the existing one. However, this is not tenable because the link between outcomes and effectiveness of specific interventions is too tenuous in this field. Someone may, for example, not have been helped to stop smoking by a nicotine patch they were taking but stopped anyway, while another person may have been helped considerably but relapsed for some other reason. Therefore, we need to have a more sophisticated approach to gauging the benefit of a new intervention. This will typically involve demonstrating effectiveness compared with a placebo or inactive control in the first instance and then conducting further studies once it is in general use to establish what is the public health impact of introducing it.

A second reason for not always requiring 'active comparators' in trials of new interventions concerns the impracticability of setting up genuine comparisons. In the field of addiction, interventions can differ in many different ways and it is not feasible to equilibrate all these elements to determine inherent superiority or inferiority. For example, there is no study that could compare 'nicotine replacement therapy' (NRT) with, say, 'varenicline' to aid smoking cessation. NRT comes in many different forms, so which one does one choose? The dosing regimen typically starts on the quit date, while varenicline starts before the quit date. Should one then start the NRT before the quit date for comparability, but that would deviate from the current recommended regimen. Should one start varenicline on the quit date, but that would deviate from its regimen? NRT is usually continued for up to 8 weeks, while varenicline is continued for 12 weeks. To equilibrate these in a study might answer one question of theoretical interest, but it would not answer the crucial pragmatic question at issue. But to answer the pragmatic issue necessarily begs the question of whether it is the medication or the regimen that accounts for any difference. Moreover, NRT involves devices such as patches and gum while varenicline involves a tablet. It would be impracticable for a researcher or a company that was involved in manufacturing a tablet to set up a manufacturing plant for active and placebo devices, and it is unlikely that rival companies would assist them. These are just some of examples in the field of medication to treat addictive disorders. When it comes to behaviour interventions, the problems of what to choose as the active comparator are even greater.

A third reason for not always requiring an active comparator is that in the field of addiction even very small effect sizes are clinically significant. In the case of smoking, for example, a difference in 6-month continuous abstinence rates following a smoking cessation intervention of just 1 percentage point (e.g. raising the rate from 5 to 6%) is very important and could save a lot of lives (West, 2007). The cost of powering a study to detect a difference of this size would be prohibitive: the sample size required would run into the thousands, and the cost in the case of a medication trial would be beyond what any company would be willing or able to afford. Given that we have to be confident that an intervention has at least some efficacy, we generally have to power studies to detect effect sizes in the region of 5 percentage points compared with a placebo or minimal intervention control. This makes sense because we have to be assured that the intervention has at least some effect. However, when it comes to assessing effect size against an active comparator, it would be extremely optimistic to expect such a difference and to require such a comparison would be unreasonable.

4.6 What target population and recruitment strategy?

In the field of addiction research, there are a number of selection criteria that are typically applied to participants in experimental studies. The choices one makes concerning these criteria can fatally undermine the conclusions that can be drawn from the study, so it is extremely important to consider all the issues very carefully.

One issue concerns whether to choose individuals with a diagnosis relating to addiction. Logically, if one is interested in studying the effect of an intervention on people who are addicted, it makes sense to limit participation to that group. However, this is more problematic than might appear at first sight. First of all, addiction is clearly not a category but involves a continuum of severity, and the currently used diagnostic systems do not adequately capture that. Secondly, there may be question marks about what diagnostic system to use. In the case of smoking, for example, applying the DSM-IV criteria is almost certainly inappropriate because measures based on these criteria do not predict failure of attempts to stop smoking (West, 2006). The Fagerstrom Test for Nicotine Dependence (Heatherton et al., 1991) does quite a good job at predicting failure of attempts to stop smoking and is quantitative, but an arbitrary threshold would still need to be set. In practice, in trials of smoking cessation treatments it is common to limit participation to smokers of ten or more cigarettes per day.

There then arises the question of whether to exclude participants with other problems, for example use of other psychoactive drugs or psychological problems. The reason for doing this would be to attempt to study the effect of the intervention on the 'pure' case. However, such a case may not exist and in any case the attempt to narrow down participation to that ideal necessarily reduces generalisability to the population of interest (see Box 4.2). Of course, there may be occasions when one wants specifically to include participants with multiple problems, but then the question arises as how to define these and one comes up against similar problems to those encountered with diagnosing 'addicts' noted above.

In addition, there is the question of what 'state' the individuals should be in at the time they are being tested. When attempting to find out about cognitive or other functions of addicted individuals, should one test them while they are using an addictive drug in which case one may merely be observing the acute effects of the drug, or during withdrawal in which case one might be observing a temporary withdrawal state, or at some later time in which case one will only be able to test people

---

Box 4.2   The problem of eligibility criteria

Humphreys et al. (2005) investigated the eligibility criteria of 683 alcohol treatment outcome studies conducted between 1970 and 1998 were coded reliably into 14 general categories. Predictors of the use of eligibility criteria were then examined. Patients were most often ruled ineligible for research studies because of their level of alcohol problems (39.1% of studies), comorbid psychiatric problems (37.8%), past or concurrent utilisation of alcohol treatment (31.8%), co-occurring medical conditions (31.6%), and because they were deemed non-compliant and unmotivated (31.5%).

The number of eligibility criteria employed in studies increased from the 1970s through the 1990s, and was positively associated with funding from the US National Institute of Alcohol Abuse and Alcoholism and from the private sector, lack of an inpatient/residential treatment condition, presence of a pharmacotherapy and use of a randomised, multiple-condition design (Humphreys et al., 2005, taken from abstract).

The authors posit that the 'greater use of eligibility criteria in randomized trials and multiple condition studies may help explain a problem in technology transfer' and that 'it remains to be determined whether extensive use of eligibility criteria makes an important difference'. They note that 'most of the prevalent eligibility criteria in alcohol treatment studies are likely to exclude from research participation more poor prognosis than good prognosis patients' and believe this remains an important concern regarding much research in treatment outcome research (Humphreys et al., 2005, p. 1256).

who have succeeded in sustaining abstinence for an extended period? In practice, one has to accept that not every question one would like an answer to can be answered and one has to limit one's research question to one that is narrower and perhaps less interesting. A vain attempt to answer an unanswerable question can lead to a considerable waste of time and resources.

In the case of experiments testing interventions designed to get people to reduce or stop engaging in an addictive behaviour, a crucial distinction needs to be made between participants who have decided they wish to make the change and therefore the task is to help them achieve that goal, and participants who have not yet decided and where the task is to get them to initiate the change process (as well as perhaps supporting that process). For example, it is now clear that different motivations are important in making an attempt to stop smoking and succeeding in that attempt. Concern about harmful effects of smoking promotes quit attempts and enjoyment of smoking deters them, but neither of these predicts success of quit attempts (West, 2009). By contrast, degree of nicotine dependence has no bearing on whether people make quit attempts but plays a major role in their success. A study of an intervention that targeted smokers in general, regardless of whether they were currently making a quit attempt, would fail to address the key causal mechanisms involved and could produce very misleading results.

Striking a balance between pragmatics and sound experimental design principles is a common thread running through addiction research, and selection of participants exemplifies this well. It is common to see studies carried out on university students who drink alcohol when clearly the population of interest is excessive drinkers in the population. How far one should go in substituting convenience samples for samples of interest is a matter of judgement, but it is important to recognise that others reading the study protocol or manuscript arising from the study may well take a stricter view.

4.7   What sample size?

Far too many studies are planned without adequate power to detect an effect of a size that is realistic (see Box 4.3). It may often happen that recruitment is slower than expected and that planned sample sizes are not achieved. Studies where this happens should still be reported. However, it is a waste of resources to plan studies that have inadequate power. If cost or practical considerations make an adequately powered study impossible, the solution is to seek to address the cost or practical issue or address another research question: it is not to pretend that the problem does not exist.

A common fault with many studies, even ones that are published in high-quality journals, is to include more experimental conditions than are sustainable with a given sample size. It is tempting to try to include multiple conditions, but unless one does this in a factorial design, the loss of statistical power can easily invalidate the exercise such whatever pattern of similarities and differences one observes is impossible to interpret (see also Chapter 3).

Box 4.3   Sample size adequacy in smoking cessation trials (Ussher et al., 2008)

In a recent review of RCTs evaluating the effect of adding exercise classes or advice on exercise to smoking cessation counselling, only 4 of 13 studies had sample sizes greater than 200. It is extremely implausible that exercise counselling would increase the odds of smoking cessation by more than a factor of 2, and it would still be highly clinically significant if the odds ratio were as low as 1.5. Yet to have 80% power to detect an effect of this size would require sample sizes in excess of 500.

4.8 What outcome measures?

Almost no outcomes in the field of addiction can be measured with certainty and precision. For example, in a field study aimed at evaluating the effect of an intervention on alcohol consumption we are usually reliant on self-reported consumption, but we know that this may be subject to considerable bias and noise. In a randomised trial of an intervention to help smokers to stop, we typically rely on self-reported abstinence for a period supported by a biochemical test of abstinence at the time of follow-up (West et al., 2005). We have no way of being certain that the participants were completely abstinent throughout the follow-up period. The solution generally adopted is to follow what is generally regarded as best practice in that field. In the case of alcohol consumption, for example, self-report is regarded as acceptable despite its limitations because of the practical difficulty in using a more accurate measure. In the case of smoking, where it is practicable, biochemical tests of smoking are required accepting that these only provide a partial check. In the case of illicit drug use, self-report is sometimes used but urine screening for drugs would often be considered essential.

A second issue is that none of the interesting outcomes in the field can be uniquely identified as the only one of interest (see Chapter 9 for a discussion on many outcome measurement scales). For example, there are numerous measures of craving and withdrawal symptoms, numerous measures of problem drinking, etc. One would like to be able to say that there is little to choose between them but in practice they may actually measure quite different things, even though they have the same label. For example, the Questionnaire of Smoking Urges is a multi-item scale that includes questions about expectations of benefit from smoking (Tiffany & Drobes, 1991). One may also measure 'craving' or 'urges to smoke' using single ratings focusing just on those feelings (West et al., 2006). If one obtains different results with the two measures, this poses difficulties of interpretation. There is no resolution to this: no single measure is the right one because the constructs are socially defined. Where important differences emerge, it is necessary to go beyond the labels to a more detailed understanding of the phenomena in question. However, there are rarely the resources to do this. The solution usually adopted is the same as for the previous issue, to go with 'custom and practice'. But it is always important to be vigilant for ways in which this custom and practice can be improved.

In field trials evaluating interventions to promote recovery from addiction problems, a major issue concerns the **length of follow-up**. This is important because of the relatively high rates of relapse back to old behaviour patterns. There is probably no length of time beyond which one can say that there is not risk of relapse. One therefore has to choose a period of follow-up from which one can reasonably project into the future or which is in itself of sufficient interest because of the health or other gains that are evident during that period. In the case of smoking, the Cochrane Collaboration, sets a standard of 6 months because in general we can predict that the long-term success rate will be about 50% of this and we can undertake cost-effectiveness calculations on this basis. However, shorter follow-up periods are useful for proof of principle studies and longer ones may be required to acquire a marketing licence for smoking cessation medications. With smoking during pregnancy, it is reasonable to follow participants up to the birth of the baby because even if the mother relapses after that point there will still have been a major and quantifiable health gain. Similarly, with interventions designed to stop people smoking before surgical procedures, health gains arise immediately following surgery, so it is not essential to follow participants up for longer (though one might wish to do so in order to establish whether there will be further health benefits from the intervention).

It is common in experimental studies to employ multiple outcome measures. This presents potentially serious problems of 'false-positive' findings. The statistical significance level of $P < 0.05$ is based on a single test done in isolation. If multiple tests are done, for example, with different outcome measures, the chances of at least one of these yielding an individual P value of less than 0.05 can be very high. Yet there may be very good reasons for using more than one outcome measure. One may not know which outcome would be most sensitive to the intervention or several outcomes may be of clinical or public health interest. In RCTs, the solution adopted is usually to designate a single outcome measure as 'primary' and others as secondary. This has to be done when drawing up the study protocol. The primary outcome measure will be the one on which the main conclusions of the study will be based. Others will be considered supportive or of interest when it comes to interpreting this finding.

It is now recognised that there is a need to include variables that can explain why an intervention was or was not effective. These are often called **'process measures'** (Strecher et al., 2008a). Thus, there is usually a theory underpinning a presumed effect of an intervention on an outcome. If an intervention effect is detected, it is very important to know whether it achieved this by the mechanism proposed. Process measures can help with this. Thus, the medication, varenicline, is presumed to help smokers to stop by reducing craving and also by reducing the rewarding effect of nicotine if they lapse and smoke a cigarette. Collecting data on both of these variables allowed this hypothesis to be tested (West et al., 2008). It is equally important to measure process variables when interventions are not effective. Thus, the intervention may have failed because it did not influence one or more key variables in the causal chain. Of particular importance here are **'implementation checks'**. It could be that the intervention was not even delivered as planned. This can often happen for behavioural interventions that rely on clinicians or researchers to deliver them (Carroll & Rounsaville, 2007).

A further important issue in this field is **loss to follow-up**. This is very common and presents major challenges because we cannot assume that those lost to follow-up are similar to those who are followed-up. Thus, only using data from those from whom we have complete data may create a bias. For example, in smoking cessation research it is usually the case that participants who are traceable at follow-up but who do not re-engage with the study have resumed smoking. For this reason, researchers are usually required to count those lost to follow-up as treatment failures (Hughes et al., 2003). However, this will not always be the case. For example, even successes may not wish to take the time and trouble to attend the clinic to enable biochemical verification of their smoking status to be assessed. In that case, treating all those lost to follow-up as smokers would create a bias. There is no simple rule that will be applicable in all cases. The general principles are:

(1) to put as much resource as possible into maximising follow-up rates;
(2) to have documented rules that specify how exactly the same effort and resource will be put into following-up all participants regardless of experimental condition;
(3) where there is a reasonable presumption that loss to follow-up is confounded with treatment failure, to regard those lost to follow up as failures rather than dropping them from the analysis;
(4) where there is a reasonable presumption that loss to follow-up may be higher in one intervention than another (e.g. one treatment is more demanding than another), to analyse the findings using treatment completers as a sensitivity analysis to check whether this might explain the results;
(5) to ensure that the follow-up procedures are blind to allocation to intervention or comparison condition.

The final point in the last paragraph mentioned **'blinding'**. The scope for bias in addiction research is very high. This means that it is essential to take maximum precautions to minimise every source. Having researchers aware of allocation to experimental condition is a potentially important source of bias. When it comes to outcome assessment, it is important that any interviews or interactions with participants are undertaken, without the researcher being aware of the experimental condition of the participant concerned. This is often difficult or impossible to achieve, but the use of written questionnaires and computer-assisted interviews can help.

4.9   What statistical analyses?

Choice of statistical analysis for experimental studies must be made during the protocol design stage (see also Chapter 11 on quantitative analysis). There are many factors in the choice that are common to all quantitative studies, so this section focuses on those that are particularly relevant to experimental studies in the field of addiction.

One major issue is how to address pairwise comparisons when there are three or more experimental conditions. For example, one may have one inactive control condition and two active intervention conditions. One is interested to know (a) whether each intervention condition is better than the control and (b) whether the two intervention conditions differ from each other. In that event an overall analysis of variance (ANOVA) or comparable test of the overall difference between the conditions may emerge as non-significant because while both intervention conditions are different from the control, they are similar to each other thus reducing the overall variance between the three conditions. The appropriate analysis in this case is not an overall ANOVA but specific planned pairwise comparisons between each intervention and the control condition and between the two intervention conditions. It must be noted, however, that these are not independent comparisons, and so the P values attaching to them will not be statistically independent.

Note that this is not the same as undertaking an unplanned search through pairwise comparisons to see which, if any, are significant. In this case, it is essential to use one of the many available statistical methods for calculating P values for multiple post hoc pairwise comparisons.

It was noted earlier that experimental studies should normally cite a single primary outcome measure. However, there are occasions when one wishes to examine effects of an intervention on a basket of measures. It is often suggested in such cases that one should use a **Bonferoni correction**. This involves taking the P value arising from each individual analysis and multiplying it by the number of analyses one is undertaking. Thus, if there were four dependent variables and the analysis involving the first one yielded a P value of 0.01, a Bonferoni correction would adjust this to 0.04. This is a very conservative approach and likely to lead to false-negative results. It is also inappropriate in this instance because it assumes that the P values are independent – which they are not (Bland & Altman, 1995). There is no ideal solution to the problem, but it is usually acceptable to cite the original individual P values and note the fact that as a collection they are biased towards a positive finding and that replication will be important.

The final issue to be discussed concerns the use of '**interaction terms**'. When there is more than one independent variable, there exists the possibility that they will interact in some way in their effect on the outcome measure. For example, when examining the effects of behavioural support and medication for smoking cessation, it may be that medication is more effective when accompanied by behavioural support. It may also be the case that certain variables 'moderate' the effects of an intervention. For example, it may be that a treatment is effective in men but not in women. To claim such an interaction, it must be specifically tested. *It is not sufficient to find a significant effect in men and not in women*; one must show by a direct comparison that the effect in men is significantly greater than the effect in women. This is only rarely possible because the statistical power to detect interactions is much lower than to detect main effects (i.e. simple effects of independent variables). This means that it is rarely possible to make claims of an effect being larger in one case than another.

The best one can usually do is to say that an effect was detected in one case but not the other, but noting that this may be due to chance variation.

4.10   Conclusions

This chapter has identified a series of important issues that arise with regard to the design of experimental studies, although it is not exhaustive. Making the wrong choice of experimental procedure can be fatal for a study and lead to huge waste of time and resources. There are no perfect experiments, but choices can be made which make research finding more or less robust and generalisable. When in doubt, it is usually good practice to follow the same choices that have been made in major papers already published on the topic, whether this be in choice of overall design, intervention and comparison groups, study sample, outcome measures or analyses. Innovation is necessary for advancing science, but where possible the methods used to test ideas should be as close as possible to those in the most relevant body of literature. Where deviation is proposed, there should be a good justification for this.

Exercises

Under what circumstances is it appropriate to conduct an experiment?

What type of experimental design, what intervention and control conditions and what outcome variables would you use to examine the effect of a web-based self-help programme on cannabis dependence?

What are the ethical issues involved in the use of different types of experimental design when evaluating treatments for addictive disorders?

Note

1. 'Qualitative research' can be thought of as a particular kind of observational study in which the observations are typically responses to questions posed during interviews.

References

Altman, D. G., Whitehead, J., Parmar, M. K., Stenning, S. P., Fayers, P. M. & Machin, D. (1995) Randomised consent designs in cancer clinical trials. *European Journal of Cancer*, 31A(12), 1934–1944.

Anthonisen, N. R., Skeans, M. A., Wise, R. A., Manfreda, J., Kanner, R. E. & Connett, J. E. (2005) The effects of a smoking cessation intervention on 14.5-year mortality: a randomized clinical trial. *Annals of Internal Medicine*, 142(4), 233–239.

Bland, J. M. & Altman, D. G. (1995) Multiple significance tests: the Bonferroni method. *BMJ*, 310(6973), 170.

Brown, C. A. & Lilford, R. J. (2006) The stepped wedge trial design: a systematic review. *BMC Medical Research Methodology*, 6, 54.

Carroll, K. M. & Rounsaville, B. J. (2007) A vision of the next generation of behavioral therapies research in the addictions. *Addiction*, 102(6), 850–862; discussion 863–859.

Collins, L. M., Murphy, S. A., Nair, V. N. & Strecher, V. J. (2005) A strategy for optimizing and evaluating behavioral interventions. *Annals of Behavioral Medicine*, 30(1), 65–73.

Craig, P., Dieppe, P., Macintyre, S., Michie, S., Nazareth, I. & Petticrew, M. (2008) Developing and evaluating complex interventions: the new Medical Research Council guidance. *BMJ*, 337, a1655.

Crano, W. D. & Prislin, R. (2006) Attitudes and persuasion. *Annual Review of Psychology*, 57, 345–374.

DuVal, G. (2004) Ethics in psychiatric research: study design issues. *Canadian Journal of Psychiatry*, 49(1), 55–59.

Heatherton, T. F., Kozlowski, L. T., Frecker, R. C. & Fagerstrom, K. O. (1991) The Fagerstrom Test for Nicotine Dependence: a revision of the Fagerstrom Tolerance Questionnaire. *British Journal of Addiction*, 86(9), 1119–1127.

Hughes, J. R., Keely, J. P., Niaura, R. S., Ossip-Klein, D. J., Richmond, R. L. & Swan, G. E. (2003) Measures of abstinence in clinical trials: issues and recommendations. *Nicotine and Tobacco Research*, 5(1), 13–25.

Humphreys, K., Weingardt, K. R., Horst, D., Joshi, A. A. & Finney, J. W. (2005) Prevalence and predictors of research participant eligibility criteria in alcohol treatment outcome studies, 1970–98. *Addiction*, 100(9), 1249–1257.

Janevic, M. R., Janz, N. K., Dodge, J. A., Lin, X., Pan, W., Sinco, B. R. & Clark, N. M. (2003) The role of choice in health education intervention trials: a review and case study. *Social Science and Medicine*, 56(7), 1581–1594.

Kaner, E., Lock, C., Heather, N., McNamee, P. & Bond, S. (2003) Promoting brief alcohol intervention by nurses in primary care: a cluster randomised controlled trial. *Patient Education and Counseling*, 51(3), 277–284.

Mahon, J., Laupacis, A., Donner, A. & Wood, T. (1996) Randomised study of n of 1 trials versus standard practice. *BMJ*, 312(7038), 1069–1074.

McKee, S. A., O'Malley, S. S., Shi, J., Mase, T. & Krishnan-Sarin, S. (2008) Effect of transdermal nicotine replacement on alcohol responses and alcohol self-administration. *Psychopharmacology (Berl)*, 196(2), 189–200.

Nair, V., Strecher, V., Fagerlin, A., Ubel, P., Resnicow, K., Murphy, S., Little, R., Chakraborty, B. & Zhang, A. (2008) Screening experiments and the use of fractional factorial designs in behavioral intervention research. *American Journal of Public Health*, 98(8), 1354–1359.

Nides, M., Glover, E. D., Reus, V. I., Christen, A. G., Make, B. J., Billing, C. B., Jr & Williams, K. E. (2008) Varenicline versus bupropion SR or placebo for smoking cessation: a pooled analysis. *American Journal of Health Behavior*, 32(6), 664–675.

Strecher, V. J., McClure, J., Alexander, G., Chakraborty, B., Nair, V., Konkel, J., Greene, S., Couper, M., Carlier, C., Wiese, C., Little, R., Pomerleau, C. & Pomerleau, O. (2008a) The role of engagement in a tailored web-based smoking cessation program: randomized controlled trial. *Journal of Medical Internet Research*, 10(5), e36.

Strecher, V. J., McClure, J. B., Alexander, G. L., Chakraborty, B., Nair, V. N., Konkel, J., Greene, S., Couper, M., Carlier, C., Wiese, C., Little, R., Pomerleau, C. & Pomerleau, O. (2008b) Web-based smoking-cessation programs: results of a randomized trial. *American Journal of Preventive Medicine*, 34(5), 373–381.

Tiffany, S. T. & Drobes, D. J. (1991) The development and initial validation of a questionnaire on smoking urges. *British Journal of Addiction*, 86(11), 1467–1476.

Ussher, M. H., Taylor, A. & Faulkner, G. (2008) Exercise interventions for smoking cessation. *Cochrane Database Systematic Reviews*, 4, CD002295.

Velicer, W. (1994) Time series models of individual substance abusers. In: L. M. Collins & L. Seitz (eds) *Advances in Data Analysis for Prevention Intervention Research: NIDA Research Monograph 142*. Rockville, MD: USDHHS, pp. 264–302.

West, R. (2006) Defining and assessing nicotine dependence in humans. In: G. Bock & J. Goode (eds) *Understanding Nicotine and Tobacco Addiction*. London: Wiley, pp. 36–51.

West, R. (2007) The clinical significance of 'small' effects of smoking cessation treatments. *Addiction*, 102(4), 506–509.

West, R. (2009) The multiple facets of cigarette addiction and what they mean for encouraging and helping smokers to stop. *COPD* (in press).

West, R., Baker, C. L., Cappelleri, J. C. & Bushmakin, A. G. (2008) Effect of varenicline and bupropion SR on craving, nicotine withdrawal symptoms, and rewarding effects of smoking during a quit attempt. *Psychopharmacology (Berl)*, 197(3), 371–377.

West, R., Hajek, P., Stead, L. & Stapleton, J. (2005) Outcome criteria in smoking cessation trials: proposal for a common standard. *Addiction*, 100(3), 299–303.

West, R., Ussher, M., Evans, M. & Rashid, M. (2006) Assessing DSM-IV nicotine withdrawal symptoms: a comparison and evaluation of five different scales. *Psychopharmacology (Berl)*, 184(3–4), 619–627.

Recommended readings

Craig, P., Dieppe, P., Macintyre, S., Michie, S., Nazareth, I. & Petticrew, M. (2008) Developing and evaluating complex interventions: the new Medical Research Council guidance. *BMJ*, 337, a1655.

DuVal, G. (2004) Ethics in psychiatric research: study design issues. *Canadian Journal of Psychiatry*, 49(1), 55–59.

Chapter 5

QUALITATIVE METHODS AND THEORY IN ADDICTIONS RESEARCH

Tim Rhodes and Ross Coomber

5.1 Introduction

Addictions research places predominant emphasis on understanding drug use in relation to individual-level factors (Rhodes, 2009) and increasingly as a brain disease (Weinberg, 2002). Despite a rich heritage, the social science of drug use can remain a peripheral voice. The addictions research field is overwhelmingly quantitative in flavour, with qualitative methods often poorly understood.

Drug use and addictions are '*social constructions*' (Reinarman, 2005). This means that the effects of drugs, whether pleasurable or problematic, have a social basis, as does our knowledge about drug use. We know this, in part, because understandings of drug use and their effects vary by social and cultural context, as well as over time. Patterns of drug use and dependency, as well as the related effects of drug policies and interventions, do not obey universal laws, but are shaped by the social situations and conditions of their occurrence. We need qualitative research to understand how drug use and addiction have a social basis. We need qualitative research to capture how drug use and addiction are lived, and how such lived experience can differ according to social context.

We begin our chapter with some introductory theory. This is necessary, even if what we say relates more to qualitative research per se than to drug use research specifically. We then translate what is theoretically distinctive about qualitative research into some applied principles. We next offer some notes on methods of data generation and analysis. Our emphasis is not an overview of methods, for space does not permit, and these are available elsewhere (e.g. Silverman, 2001; Green & Thorogood, 2004).[1] Overall, we seek to emphasise the importance of using qualitative methods for particular *analytical purpose* in a *theoretically informed* approach to addictions research.

5.2 Theory

All researchers have a theoretical perspective, whether formalised or not, which shapes how they do research. Key considerations when thinking about qualitative research include whether theory guides research (deductive) or whether theory is an outcome of research (inductive), whether natural science models of research are suitable for the study of the social world (epistemology) and whether the social world is something external to researchers or something that researchers are in the process of creating (ontology). These seem like complex questions. But they are necessary ones. Social research 'does not exist in a bubble' and 'methods are not simply neutral tools' (Bryman, 2001). For researchers, 'there is no escape from philosophical assumptions' (Hammersley, 1992). While there is much (too much) published qualitative research which is undertheorised, this does not excuse side-stepping the need to reflect on how our theoretical proclivities inform how we do research and for what analytical purpose (Bryman, 2001).

5.2.1 Positivism and interpretivism

A key (epistemological) distinction is between research paradigms that are 'positivist' and 'interpretivist'. Although there are exceptions, qualitative research is usually aligned to interpretivism. Whereas positivism assumes that the study of humans and their world is analogous to that of the natural world, interpretivism says otherwise, since the objects of social science – people – think as well as attribute meanings to their behaviour and environments, whereas the objects of natural science – atoms, gases – do not. Humans reflect on their world. They do not act in law-like ways. This requires a research paradigm oriented to discovering the *subjective meanings* of social action and how these *social meanings* are made. Interpretivist research therefore discovers – and interprets – the 'taken-for-granted' schemes of interpretation used by participants.

Interpretivism has its roots in symbolic interactionism (Blumer, 1969). This emphasises that individuals continually interpret the symbolic meanings of their environment and the actions of others, and *act on the basis of these imputed meanings*. Actions related to drug use, and the meanings these have for participants, are derived from social interactions with others. This means that qualitative researchers aim to 'catch the process of interpretation through which [people] construct their actions' (Blumer, 1969, p. 188). The emphasis is on the 'person-in-context' (Agar, 1997, 2003) and the lived experience of 'being in the world' (Schutz, 1967). Most qualitative addictions research is 'social interactionist' in flavour, and the seminal studies by Lindesmith (1938, 1947), Becker (1953, 1967) and Denzin (1993) provide examples.

5.2.2 Deduction and induction

A second commonly drawn distinction is between 'deduction' and 'induction' (Box 5.1). Positivism emphasises that scientific knowledge is arrived at through the accumulation of facts, made possible by hypothesis testing. Science is a compendium of empirically established facts, and scientists get progressively closer to discovering the 'right' explanations. Here, the purpose of science is to generate hypotheses that can be tested, thereby allowing explanations to be assessed. This is *deduction*. The aim is to test theoretical propositions (usually of postulated causal connections) to deduce whether they are correct. If falsified, the hypothetical law must be modified, but if not falsified, it can be accepted until new evidence is found to refute it (Popper, 1959).

Where deduction offers *theory before observation* (putting theory to the empirical test), induction is *theory from observation*. No a priori assumptions are made as to the nature of laws or connections to be tested, but rather hypotheses are generated from, and *grounded* in, the data gener-

---

Box 5.1 Deduction and induction in research

Key stages in deduction
- Draw on existing theory
- Conjecture hypothesis
- Collect data
- Examine findings
- Confirm or reject hypothesis
- Revise theory

Key stages in induction
- Select general research question
- Select sites and participants
- Generate data
- Interpret data
- Develop concepts
- Repeat the above cycle
- Generate hypothesis

Box 5.2　Induction in the study of opiate addiction

Lindesmith's pioneering study of opiate addiction is a classic example of induction (1938, 1947). He based his inductive analysis on an attempt to discover negative evidence for his emerging generalisations (Silverman, 1985). He found that heavy morphine use among hospital patients was a negative case in his original understanding of addiction as borne out of physiological withdrawal distress. Such morphine use did not generally lead to opiate addiction, despite withdrawal symptoms. Whereas morphine users did not interpret their symptoms as withdrawal and therefore did not infer the need to use opiates to relieve them, street heroin users were expectant of withdrawal effects and used opiates consciously to alleviate them. This led to re-defining addiction as not simply a physiological process but also as a *social process*, involving context-based learning and meaning (Weinberg, 2002). Lindesmith found no negative cases to his reformulated hypothesis that 'if the individual fails to conceive of his distress as withdrawal distress brought about by the absence of opiates, he cannot become addicted' (Lindesmith, 1947, p. 165).

---

ated. Qualitative researchers usually begin with a general explanatory question or with preliminary concepts (rather than a specific hypothesis). They then collect data, observe patterns emerging in the data and organise these into a conceptual framework. This is done by systematically comparing empirical cases to see whether emerging hypotheses fit. If not, the hypothesis is reformulated (or the phenomenon re-defined to exclude the case). The discovery of negative cases disproves the explanation and requires a reformulation. This is *induction*. This cycle may be repeated several times until a conceptual framework is well developed, and until new data yield only minimal or no new information (Box 5.2).

But, of course, it is important to acknowledge that there are elements of deduction in qualitative research, as there is induction in quantitative research. The iterative process of moving between cases and hypothesis generation in qualitative research involves incremental deductive leaps as hypotheses are refined or rejected (some call this 'retroduction'; Bulmer, 1979). Very little quantitative addictions research is in fact hypothesis-testing, but tends towards description, arguably leading to generalisations or hypotheses for future testing or refinement.

5.2.3　Realism and critical realism

A third distinction is between 'realism' and 'critical realism'. This distinction is at the centre of the (ontological) question of whether the social world is external to researchers or something that researchers are in the process of creating. Strict positivists see reality as 'out there', as something external and waiting to be discovered. Here, the role of science is discovering unknown but *actual facts* about drug use and addiction, using methods which can describe reality as *objectively* as possible. Objectivity is secured by researchers being uninvolved in what they observe, the use of standardised measures and through techniques which check for validity and bias (see Chapter 2). Many qualitative researchers likewise do not question the existence of an objective material world. Many ethnographers, for example, claim to discover truth by 'digging deep'. This is research which claims *realism*.

But more critical traditions of qualitative research (as well as 'post-positivist' quantitative science) argue that the constructs which people use to understand the world are, in fact, social products. Their definition and meaning are derived through social interaction and subject to change over time and situation. Here, the role of social science is discovering the processes by which drug use and addiction come to have meaning, and *research is part of this process*. It is a fallacy of positivism to claim objectivity, since reality is constructed, and research an interpretation of it. This introduces the idea of *critical realism* (Hammersley, 1992). This, in our view, is where most critical social scientists working in addictions research are most comfortable. This position rejects naïve realism (claims to have unmediated access to objective truth) in favour of acknowledging that our access to reality is inevitably shaped by our understandings and depictions of it. Objectivity is unavoidably a social construction in which research is a key player.

This calls upon addiction researchers to describe the processes by which drug use and addiction realities are 'socially situated' for participants. It also calls upon them to be *reflexive* about how their own involvement in the research process shapes the interpretations they make. Conceptions of 'drug use', 'addiction', 'dependence', 'recovery' and 'drug-related harm' are each discursively constructed in part by the paradigms, methods and findings of research (Davies, 1992; Moore, 1992; Weinberg, 2002; Reinarman, 2005).

5.3   A recurring debate

Relevance for policy is increasingly the harbinger upon which qualitative research is justified. This is happening in a wider context of 'evidence-based' policy approaches, in which qualitative evidence is often sidelined. What does our call for theoretically informed qualitative research imply for multidisciplinary addictions research? There are usually three positions adopted here (see Murphy et al., 1998). The first envisages qualitative research as an *adjunct* to quantitative research. This assumes a weak role, in which qualitative research assists in the design or piloting of quantitative research and the interpretation of its findings. Second, there are advocates of a 'horses for courses' approach, wherein methods are envisaged as a kind of *toolbox*, with methods selected according to their feasibility and pragmatic purpose. Third, as we have suggested, methods may also be viewed as *epistemologically distinct*, as offering different ways of knowing drug use and addiction. For some, this might imply that qualitative and quantitative methods are not easily mixed. For others, it implies that truly *inter*-disciplinary research acknowledges, and learns from, differences in interpretation (Rhodes, 2000; Bourgois, 2002; Curtis, 2002; Agar, 2003).

Earlier discussions on multidisciplinary addictions research attempted to 'reconcile' differences between quantitative and qualitative methods. For example, McKeganey (1995) argued that quantitative–qualitative 'divides' are 'unhelpful' and that 'methodological identity' should not be preserved at 'the cost of greater understanding'. Differences can be unhelpful, but they are helpful too (Bourgois, 2002; Curtis, 2002). Moreover, epistemological differences cannot be resolved by *side-stepping* these in favour of a 'giving-up' of critical realism for realism. This dilutes considerably the contribution of qualitative research. Qualitative researchers inevitably have difficulties translating their methods and findings into terms understandable to quantitative realists who seek objective truths about addiction (Bourgois, 2002; Curtis, 2002). But it is important that multidisciplinary approaches do not require qualitative researchers to suspend their constructionist critiques on addiction science.

One consequence of the 'dumbing down' of addiction research methods *theory*, and the blurring of quantitative–qualitative differences, is the belief that qualitative addictions research can be readily conducted among those not trained in qualitative methods or the social sciences (Moore, 2002). Promisingly, there is growing momentum towards 'post-positivist' approaches in public health (Krieger, 2008), and towards 'ethno-epidemiology' and 'qualitative epidemiology' in the drug field (Agar, 1997, 2003; Bourgois et al., 2006; Rhodes, 2009).

Box 5.3   Applied principles for qualitative research

- Understanding *social action* as purposive and meaningful
- Understanding *processes* of social interaction
- Studying action in its *natural* setting
- Studying phenomena *in context*
- Assumes *multiple* perspectives on a phenomenon
- Emphasises learning through *progressive focusing*

5.4   Principles for practice

An orientation to interpretivism frames how qualitative research is done. Here, we identify six pragmatic principles, with examples from addictions research (see also Murphy et al., 1998; Bryman, 2001; Box 5.3).

First, qualitative research seeks to understand *social action*. As we have noted, qualitative researchers start from the premise that people differ from natural objects in their ability to *interpret* their own action and those of others, and act on the basis of these understandings. Drug use is seen as *purposive* and *meaningful*. The core questions for qualitative researchers are therefore 'how are things done?' and 'what are the *meanings* implicated in action?' Let us take the example of tobacco smoking. Smoking is a powerful 'identity tool', conveying information about who you are and who you are not (Nichter et al., 2006). It can function, for example, as a mechanism by which young women communicate their social status during transitions to adulthood (Haines et al., 2009). As such, becoming a smoker creates 'social capital', and can be an active and purposeful decision, borne out of social interactions in specific social contexts (Haines et al., 2009).

Second, qualitative research emphasises *process*. Because meanings and interpretations are generated through social interaction, they develop and change. Actors' identities are subject to the process of *becoming*, rather than being fixed. This means that no meaning or identity is assumed, as there are *various* definitions of 'what is going on' in almost every social situation. We therefore need to capture the processes of interaction through which meaning is made. Becker's study on becoming a marijuana user is a seminal example (Becker, 1953). He shows how social interaction provides the basis for learning how to use and respond to the drug and its effects. He shows that drug effects are not simply a product of pharmacology or psychopharmacology but also of 'social pharmacology' – that what we know about a drug and its effects powerfully impacts on how those effects are identified and made manifest, and that this knowledge is borne out of social interactions (Becker, 1953, 1967).

Third, there is emphasis on investigating *natural settings*. What people say and do depends on the social context in which they find themselves. An ideal, especially in ethnography, is to study everyday life as it 'naturally occurs'. People behave differently when being researched (the 'Hawthorne effect'), and so emphasis is given to capturing everyday 'natural' environments and describing 'real life'. Of course, this remains an ideal, as all research involves interpretation, and has some kind of reactive effect, and so attention is also given, especially in 'critical realist' approaches, to reflecting on how the research setting itself impacts on behaviour. Contemporary qualitative studies are much more 'critical realist' than they used to be, though many drug ethnographers hold tightly to the idea that they 'develop an organic relationship to a social setting where their presence only minimally distorts indigenous social interactions' (Bourgois, 1999, p. 2158).

Fourth, emphasis is placed on studying things *in context*. Drug use is understood within the general context of a setting, culture, subculture or organisation. Actions are shaped in relation to surrounding events, ideas and discourses, so they need to be understood in relation to these. We noted above that Lindesmith (1947) demonstrated through qualitative research that the meanings opiates have are context dependent, and so is opiate addiction. Zinberg (1984), like Becker (1953, 1967), identified the social settings giving meaning to drug use and their effects to be critical determinants in 'addiction' and 'recovery', showing for example, that in some social contexts regular heroin use need not lead to addiction. Following in this tradition, Reinarman et al. (1994) use qualitative data to explore the social basis of cocaine careers, showing that 'pharmacology is not destiny'. Public discourses about drug use – for instance, a 'war on drugs' discourse constructing drugs as danger – are likewise shaped by particular political and economic milieu (Reinarman & Levine, 2004).

Fifth, and fundamentally, qualitative research assumes there are *multiple perspectives* on action and its meanings, and thus seeks to describe *actors'* perspectives. This is what is meant by an 'emic' (insider) perspective. The aim is to gain access to 'the way the world looks' to the people being studied. This can help outsiders – such as researchers and policy makers – understand practices that, on the face of it, seem to be 'irrational' or otherwise difficult to understand. The sharing of used syringes, for example, may come about not as a consequence of cognitive dysfunction, failures in risk awareness or risk fatalism, but because of the context-dependent 'cultural logics' and meanings of such practices, which give rise to alternative perceptions of risk and benefit given the situation (Murphy, 1987; Rhodes, 1997; Bourgois, 1998).

Lastly, given an emphasis on *discovery* and *learning*, qualitative research works through a process of *progressive focusing*. Here, it is important to avoid coming up with specific hypotheses before a large amount of exploratory investigation has occurred. The development, refinement and perhaps redirection of research ideas occur in response to what is discovered as fieldwork progresses. This process of progressive focusing, which is in keeping with induction, means that qualitative designs are *flexible*.

5.5   Data generation

There are many ways to generate qualitative data, including interviews, group interviews, observations, visual data, documents and diaries, but first, some caveats. We refer to methods of 'data generation' rather than 'data collection'. This emphasises that data are not merely 'out there' waiting to be collected, but are in the process of being created *inter-subjectively* as part of a research process. We likewise emphasise the importance of being *reflexive* to the status of data and how it is *co-produced* by researchers with their participants. The key point we are making is that data produced in research do not provide an unproblematic window into an external reality or lived experience. Moreover, merely choosing a data generation method that has a 'qualitative' soubriquet does not ensure 'good' qualitative data. What is important is being theoretically informed about what data generation methods to use for what *analytical purpose*.

5.5.1   Interviews

We live in an interview age (Silverman, 2001). The interview is probably the most widely employed method of data generation in addictions qualitative research. There are different types of interview (Green & Thorogood, 2004). First, there are *structured* interviews, which tend to employ closed questions of fact or opinion, and which are usually used as part of surveys or interviewer-administered

---

Box 5.4   Pointers to doing in-depth interviews

- Concentrate on few topics in detail
- Keep questions 'open'
- Keep conversation 'non-directive', and do not 'lead'
- Do not make assumptions and turn any assumptions into questions
- Be responsive and allow the participant to facilitate direction
- Prompt for detail, by asking 'how?' and 'why?' questions
- Seek elaboration, by asking for a specific example and detail
- Seek clarification, by asking questions which compare and contrast
- Make a mental note of responses as you go

---

questionnaires (see Chapter 8). In structured interviewing, there is affinity with positivist approaches (see above) and an emphasis on the use of standardised questions, that seek to minimise bias. Second, there are *semi-structured* interviews, which are set by an agenda and include preset questions but which also enable more detailed and open-ended conversation. Third, there are *in-depth* interviews, which are topic-guided but emphasise open-ended conversation in which the interview account is also participant driven.

In-depth interviews focus on the exploration, through guided conversation, of few topics in detail (Box 5.4). They go for depth rather than breadth. Box 5.5 gives an example of a topic guide used in an in-depth study of cannabis use. Most fundamentally, in-depth interviews are '*open*' and '*non-directive*'. This means that interviewers are *responsive* to the language and concepts introduced by participants, and learning is accomplished without the researcher leading too much the nature of interview talk. Non-directive interviewing is most effective when there is *trust* and *rapport*. This explains the close attention given by qualitative researchers to reflecting on the dynamics of their relationships with research participants (Liamputtong, 2007). The empathetic researcher has to balance getting 'close' enough to accomplish trust and rapport while maintaining a 'critical distance', described by Patton (1990) as 'empathic neutrality'.

Non-directive and open interviewing can be difficult at the outset. For example, in a project investigating 'drinking behaviour', students might ordinarily start out by suggesting closed question formats, such as 'How many drinks would you have in an evening?', 'What kind of alcohol do you drink?' or 'Where do you go out drinking?' All these may be relevant questions, but a non-directive approach might seek to generate the participant telling his or her story, in his or her own language, by more open questions, such as 'Can you describe for me the last occasion when you went out for a drink?', with the idea of following-up with prompts to generate further elaboration, such as

---

Box 5.5   An in-depth topic guide

Topic guide: cannabis use (Lofland, 1971)
- First trying marijuana
- Circumstances surrounding first contact
- State of being following first contact
- Conditions for continual use
- Conditions for curtailment or stoppage
- Present situation
- Current attitudes towards usage

'Why was this?' or 'Can you say more about what happened?' Core to in-depth interviewing uses simple prompts, such as 'Why?', 'How?', 'Can you give me an example?' and 'Can you say a little more about that?' (Box 5.4). In addition, questions of *contrast* or *comparison*, such as 'Can you give me an example where things were different?', help to describe how cases differ according to context and situation.

But let us reflect upon what is going on in interviews. There is often the assumption that a non-directive and neutral approach provides an unproblematic window into participants' social worlds. But we think as we speak, and we think as we hear, so meaning and interpretation is co-produced during interviews (Green & Thorogood, 2004). It is not the case that an interviewer 'simply turns on his tape recorder and invites people to talk' and that researchers 'merely have to ask the right questions and the other's "reality" will be theirs' (Holstein & Gubrium, 1997, p. 115). Participants are not 'passive vessels of answers' but co-producers of data (Holstein & Gubrium, 1997, p. 115). Interviews then are not an unproblematic resource to the discovery of meaning and lived experience, but are *accounts* (Scott and Lyman, 1968; Dingwall, 1997). We know this intuitively because we accept that everyday interview accounts – for instance, those by politicians – contain 'a mix of the real and the representation' (Dingwall, 1997, p. 60). Participants' stories about what they *do* are only as valid as what they *say* in accounts. And in interviews, as with any social interaction, participants take into account who the researcher is, what they could be presumed to know and 'where' they are in relation to themselves in the world they describe (Baker, 1984, p. 109).

There is a growing interest in understanding interviews as *accounts* of drug use and users (Weinstein, 1980; Weinberg, 2000; Monaghan, 2002; Coxhead & Rhodes, 2006; Coomber, 1997). Consider the first two extracts in Box 5.6. These account for needle and syringe hygiene (Rhodes et al., 2007). Participants make distinctions between themselves as 'drug users' and riskier others

---

Box 5.6　Accounting for risk and drug use

Extract 1 (Rhodes et al., 2007)

I know we are addicts, yeah, but Smackheads are different. They don't even put the tops on their needles, and throw them anywhere. Kids could walk and pick them up. We bring our needles back in here [syringe exchange] when we are finished with them.

Extract 2 (Rhodes et al., 2007)

You walk down the street and there are needles on the floor. I've seen kids playing over the other side of the road. I pick it up with a piece of paper and drop them down the drain because I don't think it's right. I don't do it, and I don't see why anyone else should. Respect, isn't it?

Extract 3 (Martin & Stenner, 2004)

Me sister, like, me sister an' her boyfriend, they, um, they'd been doin' little bits, an' then, er, he got some money from, er, some royalties, like, from a single they had on this album, like, years ago, right, er, it was in the seventies, but he got these royalties through, so he decided to buy a big lump an' start dealin' a bit. And so an' they were stayin' at me Mum's, me Mum an' me Stepdad's house at the time, so it was there every day, like, an' every day they kept goin', y'know, 'Go on', y'know, 'It's not, just try a bit, it won't hurt. Just try a bit, it's alright'. I said, 'No', for ages, an', well, for months, like, y'know, I said, "No", an' then just one day I come back from the, I'd been out somewhere, had a few drinks an' that, an' came back, they were goin', 'Go on, Go on', so I thought I didn't want, 'I'll just do a bit to shut them up', really. An' that was it.

as 'smackheads', creating a distance between their presentations of self and others in relation to risk responsibility, also acknowledging a sense of shared perception of normative responsibility and expectation ('respect, isn't it?'). Accounts of risk – such as of actions under moral evaluation – are themselves risk managed (Rhodes & Cusick, 2002). Consider the third extract in Box 5.6. This is an account of initiation into heroin (Martin & Stenner, 2004). It emphasises that inducements to use were resisted before use occurred, thus mitigating against acceptance of bad behaviour, and emphasising agency and responsibility. It makes a commonsense appeal to self-control breaking down after 'a few drinks'. It offers a plausible explanation, giving a realistic effect of 'what actually happened'. In so doing, it neutralises possible accusations of 'excuse making', presenting the self in the best possible light.

This critique of 'realist' interviewing (see Silverman, 2001) shifts qualitative researchers towards a position of reflecting critically upon how interview data are co-produced, and in turn, towards envisaging interviews as a *topic of study*, not merely as a resource to meaning. Interviews can provide 'naturally occurring' data on how conversations are done (Silverman, 2001). This makes it possible to uncover underlying cultural categories and shared meanings, which people use to interpret, classify and describe their world of drug use and addiction. The focus 'is as much on the assembly as on the assembled', but 'without losing sight of the meanings produced or the circumstances that condition the meaning-making process' (Holstein & Gubrium, 1997, p. 127).

5.5.2   Group interviews

Group interviews provide access to *interaction* between participants, and this is their main analytical advantage over individual interviews. Coreil draws a distinction between focus groups and group interviews (Coreil, 1995). Whereas *focus groups* are usually purposively sampled groups (usually of six to eight individuals), which are formally facilitated and audio-recorded, and seek a broad range of perspectives on an open-ended topic, *natural groups* exist independently of the research, may be formal or informal, but are also usually open-ended. Focus groups are typically used to explore service user views as well as reactions to health promotion materials and/or emerging research findings. They may also be used to guide the development of ongoing qualitative research. Group interviews, especially those conducted informally, are oriented to the collection of 'ethnographic' data (see also Chapter 18).

The benefits of group interviews are that they allow data to be collected that might not otherwise be available: less confident individuals may feel more secure in their group, contributing more freely than in individual interviews; they help clarify the extent to which behaviours, meanings or events are socially accepted; they enable exposure to group language which may not emerge in individual interviews and which may help capture social norms; the research process itself can be less skewed regarding researcher/interviewee power relations than individual interviews; and most importantly, 'group dynamics' themselves can be observed, thus revealing how identities, hierarchies and meanings are negotiated.

5.5.3   Observation

Despite the strong North American track record in 'drugs ethnography' (e.g. Agar, 1973; Weppner, 1977), observation is underused. An emphasis upon interview data fosters reliance upon retrospective storytelling at the expense of 'naturally occurring' data captured through engagement in the field (Bourgois, 1999; Lambert & McKevitt, 2002). Qualitative studies in addictions research often make

---

Box 5.7 A field note: chasing the dragon

With a small pocket knife she takes a knife tip of heroin from the paper package and puts it on the oblong strip of aluminium foil that lies in front of her on the table. She takes the foil in her left hand, and with her right hand she puts a tube with a length of 7 cm and a diameter of 0.5 cm in her mouth. With the same hand she takes the disposable lighter from the table and lights it. Before holding the flame under the foil, she checks the height of the flame. Then she bends a little over and brings the foil at approximately 10 cm from her mouth, a little tilted and parallel to her body. The end of the tube is now 1 cm away from the little pile of light brown powder on the foil (Grund, 1993).

---

claims to be 'ethnographic', yet they rarely are (Bourgois, 1999; Moore, 2002). Observation is a defining feature of ethnography (see Chapter 18). Ethnography is distinct from other forms of qualitative research by its strong emphasis on learning through immersion in the social relations under study. Ethnographers argue that to understand the social worlds of drug users, they either need to 'encounter it firsthand' (Agar, 1986) or put 'themselves "in the shoes" of the people they study in order to "see local realities" through local eyes' (Bourgois, 1999, p. 2158). Observation captures very well the processes of social action. This has an immediate pragmatic value, for it helps to make sense of actions otherwise misunderstood or hidden from view. Consider, for example, the closeness to action provided by the field note extract in Box 5.7 (Grund, 1993). Probably the best-known contemporary example of drug ethnography is *In Search of Respect*, an ethnographic portrayal of everyday life and expectation in the context of crack use and dealing in East Harlem (Bourgois, 1995). For a detailed discussion, see Chapter 18.

5.5.4 Visual data

There is unrealised potential for the use of visual data in addictions research (Rhodes & Fitzgerald, 2006). Visual documentation offers a means to capture the detail and nuance of social interaction in context, sometimes more intensely than audio or written description. Images may present a case for policy change at least as forcefully as words. Visual data would seem a perfect fit for qualitative researchers interested in capturing 'life as it is lived, accurately recorded as it happens, and constantly available for playback and analysis' (Plummer, 2001). Developments in digital technology make visual data affordable as well as amenable to analysis.

We have outlined elsewhere how photographic, video and other visual data can be used (Rhodes & Fitzgerald, 2006; Parkin & Coomber, 2009a). These uses include: detailed visual documentation of drug use practices and related risk behaviours and how these unfold; analysis of symbolic meaning, including how meaning is attached to visual codes such as bodily appearance and gesture; and analysis of context, especially the unfolding process of naturally occurring interactions. Just as ethnography is a distinct form of qualitative research, there can be distinctions in how visual data generation is approached. In 'visual ethnography', the emphasis is on the visualisation of *participation* in social relations, where the camera is like an extension of the participant observer or even a co-participant in the action (McDougall, 1975). In other forms of qualitative visual documentation, the emphasis may be on the 'passive recording' of 'whole scene' events (Erickson, 1992). Other common techniques, which again make different epistemological assumptions about the status of qualitative data, include 'auto-photography', where participants are invited to make

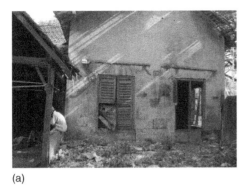
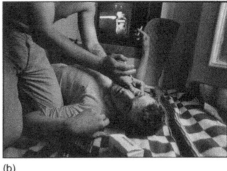

(a)   (b)

Figure 5.1 Visual data in qualitative research. (a) Photograph by Tim Rhodes, Chennai; (b) Photograph by John Ranard, Moscow, Copyright Ranard Family Estate.

a visual record of how they see their world (useful when trying to depict a hidden environment); visual diaries, which likewise are participant led and seek to capture social worlds from the 'ground-up'; 'photo-elicitation', where visual data are used as a means of encouraging interview talk and reflection; 'visualisation', such as concept maps, geographic maps, drawings and matrices; and analysis of existing visual data, such as that generated by documentary photography and film.

Figure 5.1(a) shows a semi-public environment frequented by heroin injectors and smokers in Chennai, India. There is no running water at this site, where homeless injectors also camp. Some injectors hide their injecting equipment at injecting sites for re-use rather than store their equipment at home or on their person. The image both documents and brings to life the social environment, which shapes day-to-day drug use. These kinds of data could be important when exploring how the environment, such as a public injecting environment, acts as a social context, shaping health and safety. Figure 5.1(b) shows an example of 'found data'. This was produced by the documentary photographer John Ranard. The image was taken in the suburbs of Moscow. Eye drops made from crushed anti-indigestion pills are used to counteract constriction of the eye pupils, a sign of heroin use, and enough to be stopped by the police. The image encourages an interpretive act regarding the making sense of how the local environment shapes perceptions of risk and fear among drug users in relation to the police.

5.5.5   Documents

Just like evidence from interviews and observations, documentary data capture a *perspective* – it provides an insight into how something is perceived and presented. By accessing various documents on a particular issue, a researcher can 'observe' how that issue was (or is being) represented to its audience. Analyses of texts, for example, may elucidate how scientific and media constructions of 'addiction' are situated in time and sociopolitical context as well as how these representations compete with one another (Davies, 1992; Berridge, 1999; Reinarman & Levine, 2004).

Documents are forms of 'text' in its widest sense. As well as books, papers, policy reports, health promotion materials, and written and visual media (including advertising), they may include minutes of meetings, drug treatment case notes, memos/emails or drug-related graffiti. All evidence something (whether explicitly or implicitly) about the time and moment of their production and the meanings surrounding drug use. Sometimes informal documentation (such as memos or emails) can tell us more about why or how something is happening than formal presentations or reports, as can the absence of documents and/or the censure of data within them (Prior, 2008). For examples of how drug researchers have engaged with different forms of documentary analysis, see Fraser on hepatitis C health promotion discourses (2004), Fraser on media reporting (2006) and Lalander (2002) or Boyd (2002, 2008) on film.

5.5.6   Diaries

It is common (and good) practice for qualitative researchers to keep a research diary (Charmaz, 2006). The research diary can operate as a reflective record of how the researcher's thoughts have developed through the experience of doing the research; it can record moments of inspiration or doubt; it can provide a record of key ideas, codes or concepts as they emerge out of the process; it can allow the reflexive researcher to mull over relationships with participants in the field as well as issues of validity, reliability and interpretation. The research diary is an important aide memoir, providing an invaluable audit trial of analytical thinking on how things were done as they were, and why. This is important given the flexible and inductive nature of qualitative designs.

As a means of participant data generation, there are a variety of diary formats (audio, written, oral) and uses (Alaszewski, 2006), including retrospective recording, as with life history, life grids and personal diaries of past events; prospective recording, as with lifestyle, drug use and drug treatment diaries; and within-interview diaries acting to encourage recall and reflection, for example, by using biographic points in time to situate accounts, or as a means of triangulation (Carney et al., 1998). For examples of drug research using diaries, see Hanson et al. (1985), Acocella (2005) and Albertin and Iniguez (2008).

5.6   Analysis

Both the selection of methods of data generation and how data are analysed bear close relationship to epistemological position (Mason, 1996). A discourse analysis of health promotion documents, for instance, makes assumptions about the role of discourse and language in shaping subjectivity and action. A focus group study makes assumptions regarding the role of group dynamics and norms in shaping attitudes. An ethnographic study of client–provider interactions in a methadone clinic makes assumptions regarding how these contextualise the drug treatment experience (Stimson & Oppenheimer, 1982). Analysis is not merely something to be accomplished once data are generated; it begins the moment a research question is posed and a study designed. The idea of *analytical thinking from the outset* is formalised through induction.

5.6.1   What can qualitative analyses do?

With its emphasis on induction and discovery, qualitative analyses help develop or refine *concepts*. As we noted above, qualitative research has led to some fundamental re-thinking regarding the concepts of addiction, dependency and drug-using careers (Lindesmith, 1938, 1947; Becker, 1953, 1967; Zinberg, 1984; Denzin, 1993). Second, qualitative analyses generate descriptive or analytical *typologies*. For example, Monaghan's (2002) study of steroid users generated a descriptive typology of forms of justification used among bodybuilders in defence of their steroid use. Third, qualitative analyses explore *associations*, as with research exploring links between drug use and gender (Maher,

---

Box 5.8   Pointers to doing qualitative analysis

- Compare coded categories to each other
- Compare coded data incidents to codes and to each other
- Make notes on how codes, themes and concepts were generated
- Make notes on the exceptions ('negative cases') to emerging codes
- Be prepared to refine and change codes
- Keep coding accessible to others
- Be as systematic as well as comprehensive as possible
- When coding, stick as closely to the data as possible
- When coding, look for in vivo codes and insider perspectives

Adapted from Charmaz (2006).

1997; Bourgois et al., 2004; Lindsay, 2006; Haines et al., 2009). Lastly, qualitative analyses help generate *explanations* (e.g. see Bourgois, 2002) (Box 5.8).

5.6.2   Descriptive thematic analysis

Most thematic analysis in addictions research is probably akin to 'framework analysis' (Ritchie & Spencer, 1994). This is not geared towards the generation of theory but to thematic description, useful in policy research. Five stages are distinguished: (1) familiarisation of the data (through writing field notes, listening to audio-recordings, re-reading and annotating transcripts, and generating analytical memos); (2) identification of a thematic framework; (3) coding (while refining the coding frame); (4) charting (listing the transcript details of codes by theme or case); and (5) interpretation (generating typologies or associations). In framework analysis, the key emerging themes across accounts and cases form the basis of codes, and these themes often have a close resemblance to the topic guide. These will combine with inductive and 'in vivo' (participant generated) codes. Box 5.9 gives an example of an in vivo code.

Thematic analyses usually distinguish two coding steps. First-level codes may be descriptive and broad as a means of generating a general coding frame. For example, in a study of injecting drug use, first-level codes might be as broad as 'share' (needle and syringe sharing) or 'sharing reasons' (accounts given for sharing). Second-level codes may be thematic or analytic, and seek to break down first-level codes into smaller units, which are useful for making comparisons across cases. In our fictitious study of injecting drug use, 'environment' might be a second-level code within the

---

Box 5.9   In vivo codes

'**Commonsense**' (Davis et al., 2004)

It sounds like you're pretty kind of careful. So where did this knowledge come from? What made you...?

... I just thought it was commonsense, just to clean it [the syringe] out, y'know, it's just common-sense really. I didn't really learn it from anywhere. I didn't read an instruction manual to know what to do. I just thought that sounds more sensible.

first-level code of 'share', and 'accidents' a second-level code within 'sharing reasons'. Interpretation begins the moment data give rise to thinking in relation to patterns, associations, concepts, new ideas or explanations. In a study of drug injecting, we might see links between 'sharing reasons' and 'risk responsibility', 'trust', 'environment' or 'agency', or we might see patterns on account of case or context, such as among women or the homeless.

5.6.3 Grounded theory analysis

Many published qualitative studies are described as 'grounded theory' (Glaser & Strauss, 1967), but like claims to 'ethnography', this is an oft-misused term (Green, 1998). Grounded theory (GT) is specifically oriented to the generation of theoretical propositions through induction and iteration. Theory here means *substantive theory*, such as that emerging from the immediate phenomenon of interest, such as a theory of 'shame' linked to drug use identity, or *formal theory*, extrapolated from substantive theory, such as a theory of stigma linked to social marginalisation.

GT is distinguished by its emphasis on *theoretical sampling* and *constant comparison*. Theoretical sampling means that researchers sample for theoretical relevance. This is an iterative process whereby cases are sampled successively to refine emerging grounded hypotheses. The two basic questions in theoretical sampling are "What groups or groupings does one turn to next in data collection?" and "For what theoretical purpose?" (Glaser & Strauss, 1967). Theoretical sampling involves:

> Choosing cases to study, people to interview, settings to observe, with a view to finding things that might challenge the limitations of the existing theory, forcing the researcher to change it in order to incorporate new phenomena. (Seale, 1999, p. 92)

Theoretical sampling proceeds alongside coding until *saturation* is reached. This is when the researcher 'sees similar instances over and over again', having purposively sought out potential negative cases, and there are no new data requiring the category of interest or the emerging hypothesis to be refined (Glaser & Strauss, 1967). In practice, it is often difficult to demonstrate that saturation has been achieved, and claims to saturation become a little artificial in studies of a fixed duration or when a target sample size is established a priori.

Constant comparison is critical in GT and strongly advised in any qualitative analysis (Green, 1998; Charmaz, 2006). This involves coding incidents in the data into categories so that the different incidents grouped together can be compared. This helps to generate ideas about the specific properties or attributes of a category. As data are gathered, and new data incidents coded, categories may be refined, some merging with others, some collapsing altogether. By comparing the properties of different categories, it also becomes possible to see how they interact. Throughout fieldwork, data are being compared with data, and categories with categories (Charmaz, 2006).

In GT, coding can be quite formalised (Strauss & Corbin, 1990; Charmaz, 2006). *Open coding* is done first. This is a summarising activity, noting what is in the data, especially 'in vivo' codes. As already noted, Box 5.9 gives an example of an 'in vivo' code, called 'commonsense', emerging in a study exploring hepatitis C risk perception (Davis et al., 2004). Key properties of this category included being of younger age and shorter duration of injecting career, and of having grown-up 'post-AIDS', in a context in which safer injecting practices were taken for granted (Davis et al., 2004). The key questions to ask when open coding are 'What is happening in the data?' and 'What category is this data an indicator of?' (Green & Thorogood, 2004). The key pointers to open coding include be open, stick closely to the data, let the data do the talking and code for actions and not only topics (Charmaz, 2006). The idea is to stimulate ideas, as codes can always be provisional.

Axial coding identifies central categories around which the open codes might be grouped. It synthesises open codes into larger categories. This involves 'wading through the notes and placing them into what [feel like] major categories' (Orona, 1990, p. 1249). The open code of 'commonsense' (Box 5.9) was grouped into a central category called 'hepatitis C prevention', alongside 11 other open codes. Axial coding thus also looks for relationships between codes.

Selective coding, which occurs towards the end of the coding process, and may not always be necessary, involves identifying the core category or concept, which provides a framework into which axial categories relate. Taken together, the coding process in GT shifts from open to more focused and theoretically sensitive coding. Arguably, the most important stage is open coding. It is often recommended to apply open codes *line by line*, at least initially, to get as close to the data and action in a story as possible (Charmaz, 2006). Some argue that axial and selective codings are not so much distinct coding stages as simply 'further elaborations of open codes through a method of constant comparison' (Seale, 1999, p. 100).

5.6.4   Narrative and discourse analysis

Given that interviews function as accounts (see above), analyses can give specific attention to how accounting is done and how meaning is *locally produced* through the language of the interview. Two themes characterise discourse and narrative analysis: *structure* (how accounts are put together) and *function* (for what purpose). Rather than coding to segment data thematically, narrative analysis involves treating narratives as complete, starting out by identifying the core narratives and dominant narrative structure of each interview, before identifying the narrative forms used by participants and the functions these serve. For examples of discourse analyses in addictions research, see Martin and Stenner (2004), Fraser (2006) and Davies (1997). For examples of narrative analysis, see Steffen (1997), Singer et al. (2001) and Skårberg et al. (2008).

5.7   Conclusions

Qualitative methods provide an essential means of exploring the social basis of drug use and addictions. Drug use and addictions are *context-based* phenomena. They are *socially situated*, varying according to time and place. To side-step this observation in favour of an addictions science which promises the discovery of objective universal truths, is to fail to acknowledge how drug use and addiction are *lived*, and how such lived experience impacts on the nature of drug use and addiction itself. Qualitative research promises an understanding – at least an interpretation – on the lived experiences of drug use and addiction, of how these come to have meaning for participants in the context of their everyday lives. This kind of knowledge is increasingly recognised as being important for practice and policy (Rhodes, 2000).

5.7.1   Method

Most qualitative research on drug use and addiction relies upon the interview, but it does so without critically reflecting upon the status of interview data, which is commonly presented as a 'given'. We have emphasised that empirical data are 'co-produced' between researchers and participants. There is a need for greater recognition of this in the addictions field. Interview data provide a resource for understanding participants' perspectives on drug use and addiction, as well as a means to exploring *how* these perspectives are generated. We also call for greater emphasis on using observational and visual data, as well as documents and diaries. Taken together, we emphasise the importance of using particular methods of data generation for specific *analytical purpose*. We draw distinctions between descriptive and theoretical approaches to grounded data analysis, oriented respectively to the advancement of policy and theory.

5.7.2 Theory

What we *know* about drug use and addiction is context based. Knowledge about drug use and addiction is always in the process of being 'made' through *social interaction*, of which research is a part. It is a naïve and fallacious claim of positivism to hold on to the idea that research on human behaviour can be objective and value free, and that certain methodological approaches give unmediated access to capturing the 'truth' of drug use or addiction. All researchers have a theoretical perspective, and this informs the kind of addiction research knowledge produced. We have called upon addiction researchers to stand back from their engagement in the research process to reflect upon how their interpretations shape the knowledge they produce. We have cautioned against a previous tendency in addictions research to 'side-step' the important (epistemological) differences between quantitative and qualitative methods, for these differences are not only fundamental and irresolvable, but *useful*. We envisage and encourage an interdisciplinary addictions research, which accepts competing theoretical perspectives. Qualitative research offers a *critique* on how addiction sciences produce evidence, and this is important to protect in multi-method approaches. We believe it is damaging to attempt to avoid theory regarding how research is done, and find it of concern that so much addictions research – including qualitative – proceeds as if 'theory free'. Qualitative methods are essential in a multidisciplinary model of theoretically informed addictions research.

Excercises

Exploring the added value of qualitative research

Exercise 1
Read Bourgois et al. (2004).

1. What does this study contribute to an understanding of how 'disease' is transmitted, which might not be captured by an epidemiological survey?
2. What are the specific cultural and other environmental influences which render women in this context vulnerable to hepatitis C transmission?
3. Consider – in the context of your own work and research – how qualitative methods might be employed to enhance understanding.

Exercise 2[a]
Take an example of quantitative research exploring human behaviour (e.g. an epidemiological study of injecting risk behaviour) that you consider important. Re-read the study and then consider the following:

1. What are the primary assumptions being made about the topic being researched? Could the topic question have been approached from another perspective, which would have suggested a different set of questions?
2. What questions does a re-reading of the research raise for you? Specifically, what areas would benefit from greater insight into the motivations and experiences of those being studied?

3. Think about how a qualitative study might approach the same topic. Essential to this would be the aim to increase *depth* of understanding.
4. Reflect upon the extent to which the original study would have benefited from using a qualitative approach either alone or in tandem with the original approach.

[a]Adapted from Silverman (2000).

Note

1. Given space restrictions, we do not cover here issues of ethics, fieldwork access, critical appraisal or writing up.

Acknowledgements

We would like to thank John Ranard and the Ranard family for permission to use the photographic image taken by the late social documentary photographer John Ranard in Figure 5.1.

References

Agar, M. (1986) *Speaking of Ethnography (Vol. 2)*. Beverley Hills, CA: Sage.

Alaszewski A. (2006) *Using Diaries for Social Research*. London: Sage.

Albertin, P. & Iniguez, L. (2008) Using drugs: the meaning of opiate substances and their consumption from the consumer perspective. *Addiction Research and Theory*, 16, 434–452.

Acocella, C. M. (2005) Using diaries to assess non-prescription drug use among university students. *Journal of Drug Education*, 35, 267–274.

Agar, M. (1973) *Ripping and Running: A Formal Ethnography of Urban Heroin Users*. New York: Academic Press.

Agar, M. (1997) Ethnography: an overview. *Substance Use and Misuse*, 32, 1155–1173.

Agar, M. (2003) Qualitative epidemiology. *Qualitative Health Research*, 13, 974–986.

Baker, C. (1984) The search for adultness: membership work in adolescent-adult talk. *Human Studies*, 7, 301–323.

Becker, H. (1953) Becoming a marijuana user. *American Journal of Sociology*, 59, 235–242.

Becker, H. (1967) History, culture and subjective experience: an explanation of social bases of drug-induced experiences. *Journal of Health and Social Behavior*, 8, 163–176.

Berridge, V. (1999) *Opium and the People*. London: Free Association Books.

Blumer, H. (1969) *Symbolic Interactionism*. Englewood Cliffs, NJ: Prentice Hall.

Bourgois, P. (1995) *In Search of Respect: Selling Crack in El Barrio*. New York: Cambridge University Press.

Bourgois, P. (1998) The moral economies of homeless heroin addicts: confronting ethnography, HIV risk, and everyday violence in San Francisco shooting encampments. *Substance Use and Misuse*, 33, 2323–2351.

Bourgois, P. (1999) Theory, method and power in drug and HIV prevention research: a participant'-observer's critique. *Substance Use and Misuse*, 33, 2323–2351.

Bourgois, P. (2002) Anthropology and epidemiology on drugs: the challenges of cross-methodological and theoretical dialogue. *International Journal of Drug Policy*, 13, 259–269.

Bourgois, P., Martinez, A., Kral, A., Edlin, B. R., Schonberg, J. & Ciccarone, D. (2006) Reinterpreting ethnic patterns among white and African American men who inject heroin: a social science of medicine approach. *PloS Med*, 10(e452), 1805–1815.

Bourgois, P. Prince, B. & Moss, A. (2004) The everyday violence of hepatitis C among young women who inject drugs in San Francisco. *Human Organization*, 63, 253–264.

Boyd, S. (2002) Media constructions of illegal drugs, users and sellers: a closer look at traffic. *International Journal of Drug Policy*, 13, 397–407.

Boyd, S. (2008) *Hooked: Drug War Films in Britain, Canada and the United States*. New York: Routledge.

Bryman, A. (2001) *Quantity and Quality in Social Research*. London: Unwin Hyman.

Bulmer, M. (1979) Concepts in the analysis of qualitative data. In: M. Bulmer (ed.) *Sociological Research Methods*. London: Macmillan.

Carney, M. A., Tennen, H., Affleck, G., Del Boca, F. K. & Kranzler, H. R. (1998) Levels and patterns of alcohol consumption using timeline follow-back, daily diaries and real-time 'electronic interviews'. *Journal of Studies on Alcohol*, 59, 447–454.

Charmaz, K. (2006) *Constructing Grounded Theory: A Practical Guide through Qualitative Analysis*. London: Sage.

Coomber, R. (1997) 'The Adulteration of Drugs: What Dealers Do, What Dealers Think', Addiction Research, Vol 5, No. 4. pp. 297–306.

Coreil, J. (1995) Group interview methods in community health research. *Medical Anthropology*, 16, 193–210.

Coxhead, L. & Rhodes, T. (2006) Accounting for risk and responsibility associated with smoking among mothers of children with respiratory illness. *Sociology of Health and Illness*, 28, 98–121.

Curtis, R. (2002) Coexisting in the real world: the problems, surprises and delights of being an ethnographer on a multidisciplinary research project. *International Journal of Drug Policy*, 13, 297–310.

Davies, J. B. (1992) *The Myth of Addiction*. London: Routledge.

Davis, M., Rhodes, T. & Martin, A. (2004) Preventing hepatitis C: 'common sense', 'the bug' and other perspectives from the risk narratives of people who inject drugs. *Social Science and Medicine*, 59, 1807–1818.

Denzin, N. K. (1993) *The Alcoholic Society*. New Brunswick, NJ: Transaction.

Dingwall, R. (1997) Accounts, interviews and observations. In: G. Miller & R. Dingwall (eds) *Context and Method in Qualitative Research*. London: Sage, pp. 51–65.

Erickson, F. (1992) Ethnographic microanalysis of interaction. In: M. LeCompte, W. Milroy & J. Presissle (eds) *The Handbook of Qualitative Research in Education*. San Diego: Academic Press.

Fitzgerald, J. (1993) Lived fictions: moving from pharmacology to ethnography. *Drug and Alcohol Review*, 12, 423–428.

Fraser, S. (2004) 'It's your life!': injecting drug users, individual responsibility and hepatitis C prevention. *Health*, 8, 199–221.

Fraser, S. (2006) Speaking addictions: substitution, metaphor and authenticity in newspaper representations of methadone treatment. *Contemporary Drug Problems*, 33, 669–698.

Fraser, S. & Valentine, K. (2008) *Substance and Substitution*. Basingstoke: Palgrave.

Glaser, B. G. & Strauss, A. (1967) *The Discovery of Grounded Theory*. Chicago: Aldine.

Green, J. (1998) Grounded theory and the constant comparative method. *British Medical Journal*, 316, 1064–1065.

Green, J. & Thorogood, N. (2004) *Qualitative Methods for Health Research*. London: Sage.

Grund, J-P. (1993) *Drug Use as a Social Ritual: Functionality, Symbolism and Determinants of Self-Regulation*. Rotterdam: Instituut voor Verslavingsonderzoek.

Haines, R. J., Poland, B. P. & Johnson, J. L. (2009) Becoming a 'real' smoker: cultural capital in young women's accounts of smoking and other substance use. *Sociology of Health and Illness*, 31, 66–80.

Hammersley, M. (1992) *What's Wrong with Ethnography?* London: Routledge.

Hanson, W., Beschner, G., Walters, J. & Bovelle, E. (eds) (1985) *Life with Heroin: Voices from the Inner City*. Lexington, MA: Lexington Books.

Harding, G. (1998) Pathologising the soul: the construction of a 19th century analysis of opiate addiction. In: R. Coomber (ed.) *The Control of Drugs: Reason or Reaction*. Amsterdam: Harwood Academic Publishers.

Holstein, J. & Gubrium, J. (1997) Active interviewing. In: D. Silverman (ed.) *Qualitative Research*. London: Sage.

Koester, S. (1996) The process of drug injection: applying ethnography to the study of HIV risk among IDUs. In: T. Rhodes & R. Hartnoll (eds) *AIDS, Drugs and Prevention: Perspectives on Individual and Community Action*. London: Routledge.

Krieger, N. (2008) Proximal, distal and the politics of causation: what's level got to do with it? *American Journal of Public Health*, 98, 221–230.

Lalander, P. (2002) Who directs whom? Films and reality for young heroin users in a Swedish town. *Contemporary Drug Problems*, 29, 65–90.

Lambert, H. & McKeviit, C. (2002) Anthropology in health research: from qualitative methods to multidisciplinarity. *British Medical Journal*, 325, 210–213.

Liamputtong, P. (2007) *Researching the Vulnerable: A Guide to Sensitive Research Methods*. London: Sage.

Lindesmith, A. (1938) A sociological theory of drug addiction. *American Journal of Sociology*, 43, 593–609.

Lindesmith, A. (1947) *Opiate Addiction*. Bloomington, IN: Principia Press.

Lindesmith, A. (1968) *Addiction and Opiates*. Chicago: Aldine.

Lindsay, J. (2006) A big night out in Melbourne: drinking as enhancement of class and gender. *Contemporary Drug Problems*, 33, 29–61.

Lofland, J. (1971) *Analyzing Social Settings*. Belmont, CA: Wadsworth.

Maher, L. (1997) *Sexed Work: Gender, Race, and Resistance in a Brooklyn Drug Market*. Oxford: Clarendon Press.

Martin, A. & Stenner, P. (2004) Talking about drug use: what are we (and our participants) doing in qualitative research? *International Journal of Drug Policy*, 15, 395–405.

Mason, J. (1996) *Qualitative Researching*. London: Sage.

McDougall, D. (1975) Beyond observational cinema. In: P. Hockings (ed.) *Principles of Visual Anthropology*. Chicago: Aldine.

McKeganey, N. (1995) Quantitative and qualitative research in the addictions: an unhelpful divide. *Addiction*, 90, 749–751.

Monaghan, L. (2002) Vocabularies of motive for steroid use among bodybuilders. *Social, Science and Medicine*, 55, 695–708.

Moore, D. (1992) Deconstructing 'dependence': an ethnographic critique of an influential concept. *Contemporary Drug Problems*, 19, 459–490.

Moore, D. (2002) Ethnography and the Australian drug field: emaciation, appropriation and multidisciplinary myopia. *International Journal of Drug Policy*, 13, 271–284.

Murphy, S. (1987) Intravenous drug use and AIDS: the social economy of needle sharing. *Contemporary Drug Problems*, 14, 373–396.

Murphy, E., Dingwall, R., Greatbatch, D., Parker, S. & Watson, P. (1998) Qualitative research in health technology assessment. *Health Technology Assessment*, 2(16).

Nichter, M., Nichter, M., Lloyd-Richardson, E., Flaherty, B., Cakoglu, A. & Taylor, N. (2006) Gendered dimensions of smoking in college students. *Journal of Adolescent Health*, 21, 215–243.

Orona, C. J. (1990) Temporality and identity loss due to Alzheimer's disease. *Social Science and Medicine*, 30(11), 1247–1256.

Parkin, S. and Coomber, R. (2009) 'Value in the Visual: On Public Injecting, Visual Methods and their Potential for Informing Policy (and Change)', Methodological Innovations Online, 4(2): 21–36. http://www.pbs.plym.ac.uk/mi/pdf/12-8-09/3. Parkin & Coomber MIO Final.pdf

Patton, M. Q. (1990) *Qualitative Evaluation and Research Methods*. London: Sage.

Plummer, K. (2001) *Documents of Life*. London: Sage.

Popper, K. (1959) *The Logic of Scientific Discovery*. London: Hutchinson.

Prior, M. (2008) Post-broadcast democracy: how media choice increases inequality in political involvement and polarizes elections. *International Journal of Public Opinion Research*, 20, 398–400.

Reinarman, C. (2005) Addiction as accomplishment: the discursive construction of disease. *Addiction Research and Theory*, 13, 307–320.

Reinarman, C. & Levine, H. G. (2004) Crack in the rearview mirros: deconstructing drug war mythology. *Social Justice*, 31, 182–199.

Reinarman, C., Murphy, S. & Waldorf, D. (1994) Pharmacology is not destiny: the contingent character of cocaine abuse and addiction. *Addiction Research*, 2, 21–36.

Rhodes, T. (1997) Risk theory in epidemic times. *Sociology of Health and Illness*, 19, 208–227.

Rhodes, T. (2000) The multiple roles of qualitative research in understanding and responding to illicit drug use. In: J. Fountain (ed.) *Understanding and Responding to Drug Use: The Role of Qualitative Research*. Lisbon: European Monitoring Centre for Drugs and Drugs Addiction.

Rhodes, T. (2009) Risk environments and drug harms: a social science for harm reduction approach. *International Journal of Drug Policy*, 20, 193–201.

Rhodes, T. & Cusick, L. (2002) Accounting for unprotected sex: stories of agency and acceptability. *Social Science and Medicine*, 55, 211–226.

Rhodes, T. & Fitzgerald, J. (2006) Visual data in addictions research: seeing comes before words? *Addiction Research and Theory*, 14(4), 349–363.

Rhodes, T. & Moore, D. (2001) On the qualitative in drugs research. *Addiction Research and Theory*, 9, 279–299.

Rhodes, T., Watts, L., Martin, A., Smith, J., Clarke, D., Craine, N. & Lyons, M. (2007) Risk, shame and the public injector: a qualitative study of drug injecting in South Wales. *Social Science and Medicine*, 65, 572–585.

Ritchie, J. & Spencer, L. (1994) Qualitative data analysis for applied policy research. In: A. Bryman & R. G. Burgess (eds) *Analysing Qualitative Data*. London: Routledge.

Seale, C. (1999) *Quality in Qualitative Research*. London: Sage.

Schutz, A. (1967) *The Phenomenology of the Social World*. Evanston, IL: Northwestern University Press.

Scott, M. B. & Lyman, S. M. (1968) Accounts. *Sociological Review*, 33, 46–62.

Silverman, D. (1985) *Qualitative Methodology and Sociology*. Aldershot, UK: Gower.

Silverman, D. (2000) *Doing Qualitative Research*. London: Sage.

Silverman, D. (2001) *Interpreting Qualitative Data*. London: Sage.

Singer, M., Scott, G., Wilson, S., Easton, D. & Weeks, M. (2001) 'War stories': AIDS prevention and the street narratives of drug users. *Qualitative Health Research*, 11, 589–611.

Skårberg, K., Nyberg, F. & Engström, I. (2008) The development of multiple drug use among anabolic-androgenic steroid users: six subjective case reports. *Substance Abuse Treatment, Prevention, and Policy*, 3, 24.

Steffen, V. (1997) Life stories and shared experiences. *Social Science and Medicine*, 45, 99–111.

Stimson, G.V. and Oppenheimer, E. (1982) Heroin Addiction: Treatment and Control in Britain, London: Tavistock.

Strauss, A. & Corbin, J. (1990) *Basics of Qualitative Research: Grounded Theory Procedures and Techniques*. Newbury Park, CA: Sage.

Weinberg, D. (2000) 'Out there': the ecology of addiction in drug abuse treatment discourse. *Social Problems*, 47, 606–621.

Weinberg, D. (2002) On the embodiment of addiction. *Body and Society*, 8, 1–19.

Weinstein, R. (1980) Vocabularies of motive for illicit drug use: an application of the accounts framework. *Sociological Quarterly*, 21, 577–593.

Weppner, R. S. (ed.) (1977) *Street Ethnography*. Beverly Hills, CA: Sage.

Zinberg, N. (1984) *Drug, Set and Setting*. New Haven, CT: Yale University Press.

Recommended readings

Agar, M. (1973) *Ripping and Running: A Formal Ethnography of Urban Heroin Users*. New York: Academic Press.

Becker, H. (1953) Becoming a marijuana user. *American Journal of Sociology*, 59, 235–242.

Bourgois, P. (1995) *In Search of Respect: Selling Crack in El Barrio*. New York: Cambridge University Press.

Green, J. & Thorogood, N. (2004) *Qualitative Methods for Health Research*. London: Sage.

Rhodes, T. (2000) The multiple roles of qualitative research in understanding and responding to illicit drug use. In: J. Fountain (ed.) *Understanding and Responding to Drug Use: The Role of Qualitative Research*. Lisbon: European Monitoring Centre for Drugs and Drugs Addiction.

## Chapter 6

ETHICAL ISSUES IN ALCOHOL, OTHER DRUGS AND ADDICTION-RELATED RESEARCH

Peter G. Miller, Adrian Carter and Wayne Hall

6.1 Introduction

Ethical review of human research has become increasingly important since the Nuremberg war crimes trial after World War II, which convicted German medical scientists for conducting research on unwilling participants who were harmed as a result. Over the subsequent 60 or so years, a consensus has gradually developed about the key ethical principles that should be respected in any research endeavour to protect human subjects from being used as 'guinea pigs'. However, ethical restrictions on research can conflict with the pressure for research to provide new insights into human illness, suffering and behaviour. Today's ethical regulation of research tries to encourage research without compromising the rights of individuals and communities. In some contentious areas (e.g. human embryonic stem cell research), there are no obvious 'right' answers. The best one can do is to ensure that all research receives independent ethical review to protect research participants and that researchers debate ethical issues with the aim of clarifying the issues and identifying solutions that are broadly acceptable. In planning research, it is vital that ethical considerations are considered at an early stage when ideas are less concrete and less resources have been expended.

Ethical review is especially important when research deals with vulnerable groups who are marginalised within the community, such as illicit drug users. The illegal nature of their drug use and the possibility of added stigmatisation and increased social harm arising from such research participation must be of paramount concern. The intersection between personal choice and freedom and public health creates a number of very difficult ethical quandaries for people doing research into drug use and addiction-related problems.

6.2 Key concepts

There are a number of key concepts used in contemporary social and medical research approaches to protecting the rights of research participants (e.g. National Health and Medical Research Council, 1999; Economic and Social Research Council, 2005). All these concepts are underpinned by a basic 'respect for persons'. This respect is manifested in a number of basic concepts. Firstly, the principle of **voluntary participation** requires that people should not be coerced into participating in research. This can be especially relevant where researchers deal with 'captive audiences' for their subjects, that is populations who are socially restricted or marginalised in some way (e.g. prison populations). Closely related to the notion of voluntary participation is the requirement of **informed consent**: prospective research participants must be fully informed about the procedures and risks involved in research participation before giving their free and uncoerced consent to participate. Researchers should also not expose participants to **risk of harm** – physical or psychological – as a result of their participation.

There are two standards that aim to protect the privacy of research participants. **Confidentiality** assures that any identifying information about participants will not be made available to anyone who is not directly involved in the research (e.g. law enforcement, employers). The protection of **anonymity** ensures that participants will remain anonymous throughout the study, often even to the researchers themselves. This protection is often used in studies of illicit drug use to ensure that participants do not experience any social harm from taking part in the research. Anonymity is sometimes difficult to ensure if participants are to be followed-up over time, for example in longitudinal studies.

No set of ethical standards can anticipate every ethical circumstance and people ultimately interpret ethical issues differently. In order to ensure that researchers consider all relevant ethical issues in formulating research, most institutions require independent review of research proposals by **Ethics Committees (ECs)** or **Institutional Review Boards (IRBs)**. These consist of panels of persons from different social and professional backgrounds who review research proposals with respect to ethical (and often legal) implications and decide whether additional actions need to be taken to protect the safety and rights of research participants.

6.3   Major ethical frameworks

There are a number of frameworks, which may prove useful for assessing whether a proposed piece of research can be conducted ethically. The range of frameworks reflects the reality that there is no consensus on a universal theory of ethics. The competing ethical frameworks available can make the job of resolving ethical dilemmas more difficult, particularly for clinicians looking for guidelines and frameworks that can help them make decisions that sometimes must be made in the heat of the moment. Two of the most commonly used frameworks in health-related research and clinical settings are **principlism** and **communitarianism**.

6.3.1   Principlism

Principlism emerged in the United States in the 1970s as a way of seeking common moral principles that could guide ethical decisions (Beauchamp & Childress, 2001). Its language still forms the backbone of many codes of ethics (see National Health and Medical Research Council, 1999). The four major ethical principles are *autonomy* (respecting the actions of rational persons and valuing informed voluntary consent, confidentiality and privacy), *non-maleficence* (minimising research risks and harms), *beneficence* (ensuring research/treatment benefits outweigh risks) and *distributive justice* (equitable distribution of risks and benefits of research participation) (National Health and Medical Research Council, 1999; Beauchamp & Childress, 2001) (Box 6.1).

A number of critics have pointed out that autonomy is the ascendant value within this framework, reflecting its libertarian origins (Callahan, 2003). It also features prominently in ethical discussions of addiction, which is seen as involving the loss of autonomy (see Section 6.4.3) (Cohen, 2002).

A major difficulty with principlism is resolving conflicts between the different principles. In the treatment of addiction, for example, respecting the autonomy of the addicted person to engage in drug use may conflict with the principles of beneficence and non-maleficence, which require us to minimise harm and do good. Some see this as warranting the mandatory treatment of addiction for

---

Box 6.1   White and Popovits' list of 'universal' values

White and Popovits (2001, p. 10) proposed the list of 'universal' values. This list expands on the more traditional list of four seen in other principlist models, but it is worthy of reviewing and ascertaining the degree to which it is repetitive, or whether you think something is missing:

Autonomy (freedom over one's own destiny)
Obedience (obey legal and ethically permissible directives)
Conscientious refusal (disobey illegal or unethical directives)
Beneficence (do good; help others)
Gratitude (pass good along to others)
Competence (be knowledgeable and skilled)
Justice (be fair; distribute by merit)
Stewardship (use resources wisely)
Honesty and candour (tell the truth)
Fidelity (keep your promises)
Loyalty (do not abandon)
Diligence (work hard)
Discretion (respect confidence and privacy)
Self-improvement (be the best that you can be)
Non-maleficence (do not hurt anyone)
Restitution (make amends to persons injured)
Self-interest (protect yourself)
Other culture-specific values

---

the 'addict's own good'. Principlism has also been criticised for blocking creative solutions to ethical dilemmas:

> Instead of inviting us to think as richly and imaginatively about ethics as possible, in fact it is a kind of ethical reductionism, in effect allowing us to escape from the complexity of life, and to cut through the ambiguities and uncertainties that mark most serious ethical problems. (Callahan, 2003, p. 289)

In its defence, principlism has two key virtues (1) it reflects the Western liberal, individualistic culture from which it emerged and (2) its simplicity in conceptualisation and application makes it attractive in guiding clinical decision-making. Few other ethical frameworks have shown the same utility and popularity as principlism in the clinical setting (Box 6.2).

6.3.2   Communitarian ethics

Communitarian ethics has been proposed as providing a way of solving some of the problems associated with principlism. Communitarianism 'is meant to characterise a way of thinking about ethical problems, not to provide any formulas or rigid criteria for dealing with them' (Callahan, 2003, p. 288). Communitarian ethics focuses more on the common good and public interests than on individual autonomy. The major problem with communitarian ethics in the drug field is reaching consensus on values about drug use (Keane, 2005; Loff, 2006). What is the 'common good' and which is the 'community' when referring to different forms of drug use? Communitarian ethics has also been criticised for reifying 'the community', assuming that societal agreement is likely, or even

> **Box 6.2   Should naltrexone implant treatment be mandated?**
>
> In a debate appearing on the pages of the journal, *Addiction*, Arthur Caplan and Wayne Hall and colleagues debated whether it was acceptable to mandate people to receive an invasive medical treatment, specifically naltrexone implants. Much of the argument ultimately focused on whether this specific treatment could be called 'safe'. Both agreed that 'it would not be ethical to force treatment upon anyone if there were significant risks involved with the treatment' (Caplan, 2008, p. 1918), although Hall et al. pointed out that there should be a range of treatments available for the patient to choose from. 'People who are truly addicted to alcohol or drugs really do not have the full capacity to be self-determining or autonomous. Standard definitions of addiction cite loss of control, powerlessness and unmanageability … An addiction literally coerces behavior. An addict cannot be a fully free, autonomous agent precisely because they are' (Caplan, 2008, p. 1918). He further argues that it is justified to override temporarily an addict's autonomy. However, Hall et al. argue that naltrexone is far from safe. Where Caplan perceived the treatment as 'safe and effective', Hall et al. pointed to 'its efficacy in unselected patients is no better than placebo' and 'doubts about the safety of oral naltrexone in treating unselected opioid-dependent patients' (Hall et al., 2008). These differing viewpoints highlight that even such basic considerations are open to interpretation in such debates.

possible, and that the views of all members of the community are equally represented in what is taken to be 'the community view'. Experience suggests this is unlikely to be the case (Keane, 2005). The behaviour of the uninformed and often uninterested majority towards a disenfranchised minority may not always be 'ethical'. However, if it is the process of seeking consensus that is truly important, then communitarian ethics adds a valuable element to the process of the ethical deliberation.

The communitarian ethics model also has a number of positives in dealing with addiction-related research. Firstly, it can add other ethical principles to autonomy, beneficence, non-maleficence and distributive justice, such as honesty and fidelity in deliberations about ethical dilemmas. Secondly, communitarian ethics accepts that there is often conflict between principles and attempts to resolve them by appealing to the ideal of 'community benefit' or shared values as a way forward. Some addiction-related research issues may however still require tailored responses that might not fit notions of community benefit. For example, reducing hepatitis C in injecting drug-using populations might possibly also mean an increase in discarded needles in public spaces and harm to the local resident community. In such situations it may be more helpful to engage in an ethical decision-making process of the type that we next discuss.

6.3.3   Ethical decision-making models

Two decision-making models have been suggested for use in the addiction sector (White & Popovits, 2001; Solai et al., 2006). Both include elements of principlism and communitarian ethics. They have, to date, been often used in assessing ethical issues in treatment settings, but may be readily adapted to the analysis of ethical issues in research contexts.

Solai et al. (2006) provide an ethical framework with the goal of reaching consensus on resolving ethical challenges within a treatment setting. It includes eight steps: (i) to identify the practical ethical problem; (ii) to identify the client's individual context as known to the staff member; (iii) to identify the responsibilities of each staff member in the care process; (iv) to identify the diverse values considered by each staff member as essential to reaching a favourable outcome to the problem;

(v) to identify the conflicts of values occurring in this situation; (vi) to identify alternative solutions to the ethical conflict identified; (vii) to choose the option which best allows the realisation of the objectives of the institution in a consensual way; and (viii) to give a justification for this choice (Solai et al., 2006, p. 19). An example of the use of this process is provided by the ethical issue of whether novice injectors should be able to access a drugs consumption room.

White and Popovits (2001, pp. 7–9) propose a systematic model of ethical decision-making that involves answering a series of three related questions to provide a structure for the analysis of ethical dilemmas:

1. Whose interests are involved and who can be harmed?
2. What universal or culturally specific values apply to this situation and what course of action would be suggested by these values? Which of these values are in conflict in this situation?
3. What standards of law, professional propriety, organisational policy or historical practice apply to this situation?

They also provide a basic checklist for ensuring ethical issues are addressed adequately. This framework is by no means perfect, particularly in its assumption of 'universal' values and its lack of consideration of power relationships. It does nonetheless supply a useful starting point for ethical decision-making with a list of 'universal' ethical values (White & Popovits, 2001, p. 28) that ensures a wide range of issues are considered. Importantly, this model explicitly includes organisational policy and historical practice that can often play a major role in clinical practice and in the assessment of research protocols.

6.4　Addiction-specific ethical issues

6.4.1　Informed consent

In all major research ethics statements, the respect for persons requires that individuals provide meaningful, fully informed and voluntary consent (i.e. of their own free will) to participate in research (Faden et al., 1986). Informed consent is the process whereby individuals agree to participate in research in full knowledge of its possible risks and benefits, and in the absence of any duress, coercion or undue inducement. This means that researchers ensure that participants have the capacity to:

- understand the risks and benefits of participating in research and what their participation will involve;
- appreciate the consequences of participating and care whether they occur or not; are not under some form of external or internal pressure, real or perceived; and
- are fully informed of the risks and benefits of participating in the research study, including choosing not to participate.

There are a variety of features of addiction that can affect the ability of addicted individuals to provide free and informed consent to participate in a research study. Acute intoxication with most drugs of addiction, such as opioids, alcohol, benzodiazepines, ecstasy and amphetamines, can produce behavioural and cognitive changes that undermine both an understanding and appreciation of the consequence of participating in research (Curran et al., 2001). The 'high' produced by these drugs can also affect individuals' interest in the consequences of research participation, thereby impairing their volitional capacity (i.e. their motivation to participate and consider the consequences).

Repeated use of most drugs of addiction can also lead to a withdrawal syndrome on cessation of drug use. The symptoms of withdrawal to some drugs, such as alcohol, nicotine and opioids (e.g. diarrhoea, nausea, dysphoria, severe headaches and seizures), can produce severe cognitive impairments (Carter & Hall, 2008). Relief of withdrawal symptoms can also be a potent motive for participating in research that involves drug consumption or subject payments that may be used to buy drugs. Therefore, it is widely accepted that individuals who are intoxicated or suffering acute withdrawal symptoms are unable to provide free and informed consent at that point in time (Smith et al., 2006). The symptoms need to have abated before they are able to provide free and informed consent to research participation. There are standardised scales for assessing symptoms of drug intoxication and withdrawal that should be used to assess the capacity of addicted individuals to give consent, such as the Mini-Mental State Examination (Smith et al., 2006), the Clinical Opiate Withdrawal Scale (Wesson & Ling, 2003) and the Clinical Institute Withdrawal Assessment for Alcohol (Ebbets, 1994).

Subjects with an addiction also experience a number of other social, economic and psychological conditions that can impair their ability to provide free and uncoerced consent. Individuals may have been convicted of a criminal offence and may even be incarcerated.[1] Individuals involved with the justice system, correctional services or child protection agencies may believe that they may be punished by refusing to participate in a study. It is therefore important that subjects be made aware that they are free to refuse to participate in a research study at any time without penalty.

The chronic use of addictive drugs can also cause significant cognitive deficits (e.g. Wernicke-Korsakoff syndrome) or psychiatric symptoms (e.g. psychosis, anxiety and depression) that may impair the capacity to provide informed consent. Consequently, it may be important for researchers involved in studies that put subjects at some risk (e.g. those that administer drugs) to use clinical diagnostic tests (e.g. Mini-Mental State Examination) to ensure that subjects have the capacity to consent to research participation (Smith et al., 2006).

6.4.2 Subject Payment

As individuals with an addiction often have low incomes, they could be argued to be particularly vulnerable to financial inducements to participate in research such as payment for research participation. On the other hand, it can be argued that addicted participants should be compensated for their time and inconvenience in the same way as any other research subject. A balance needs to be struck between adequately compensating subjects for their time and providing financial inducements that are large enough to make subjects unable to properly assess the consequences of participating in research (e.g. Hando & Darke, 1998).

There are a large number of studies that have used monetary rewards as compensation for heroin users' time. Some have argued that providing subject payments to addicted participants will lead to increased drug use and more social harm (i.e. the payment will be used to obtain drugs). Some have proposed that the use of vouchers provides a solution to this. Experience in the UK with vouchers suggests that this method of remuneration can have undesired effects for both the subject and the wider community. For example, some subjects may approach members of the public to exchange the vouchers for cash, usually at a reduced rate. This means that subjects receive less money and create a public nuisance. This practice also arguable violates the ethical principles of respect for autonomy and beneficence.

Another alternative would be to reimburse subjects on the basis of bus tickets, taxi receipts, etc. This approach is also problematic for this group of participants who may be less likely to be organised enough to return receipts or cash cheques. Many have temporary or unstable accommodation and some will be functionally homeless. For virtually all these subjects, $5–10 is a significant amount of their weekly income that they can ill afford to lose via an inconvenient reimbursement process. The consequence may be that subjects are either disadvantaged financially by taking part in the research, or will choose not to take part because of this disincentive. Both choices will mean that they will be discriminated against by not having an equitable opportunity to participate in research.

6.4.3   Autonomy and rational choice in addiction

Respect for autonomy is the respect for rational and cognitively competent individuals to make their own choices, free from outside influence. Addiction is a condition in which, by definition, autonomy is impaired: addicted persons continue to use drugs in the face of enormous negative consequences, and often despite an expressed wish to stop. Addiction is commonly understood as a 'loss of control' over or 'compulsive' drug use that generally consumes a great deal of an individual's time and resources to the detriment of other activities, such as working or caring for children. Neuroscience has shown that the chronic use of addictive drugs causes changes in the brain that focus attention on drug use (Yucel & Lubman, 2007) and evoke intense cravings to use drugs that overwhelm rational decisions not to use them (Volkow & Li, 2004). Consequently, the autonomous ability of people with drug dependence to refuse to use drugs is seen to be impaired. The question is when, under what circumstances and by how much?

The categorical notion of autonomy in which one is either autonomous or not is of limited use in discussions of the ethical recruitment of addicted subjects. While autonomous decision-making in addiction, particularly regarding choices to use drugs, is impaired, the loss is not complete (Levy, 2006). People with an addiction can, and often do, make choices not to use drugs. Consequently, some degree of autonomy remains. This view is consistent with legal judgements which hold people responsible for decisions made while under the influence of drugs or in order to obtain drugs. Given that individuals with a drug dependency possess a degree of autonomy, even though significantly impaired, how do researchers ethically obtain consent from addicted individuals in situations that involve decisions about whether to use drugs (e.g. research that administers addictive drugs)? An alternative conception of autonomy is required.

The concept of **relational autonomy** has arisen in reaction to the failings of the more traditional categorical understanding of autonomy. Relational autonomy proposes that individual autonomy is *socially dependent* and therefore stresses the importance of providing social conditions that foster autonomous action (Sherwin, 1998). In other words:

> the capacity and opportunity for autonomous action is dependent on our particular social relationships and the power structures in which we are embedded. Autonomy requires more than freedom from interference: it requires that one's relationships with particular individuals and institutions be constituted in such a way as to give one *genuine* opportunities for choice. (MacDonald, 2002, p. 283)

Relational autonomy enables researchers to develop and apply protocols that aim to maximise autonomy. We explore this approach in the case of addicted individuals consenting to participate in research that administers their drug of addiction.

6.4.4 Administering addictive drugs in research

The administration of addictive drugs, particularly to research participants, can provide valuable scientific information about the effects that these drugs have on behaviour and cognition. Such research also raises ethical challenges. Administering addictive drugs to drug-naïve participants could theoretically introduce individuals to addictive drug use. However, it is widely recognised that providing drug-naïve participants with an appropriate dose of an addictive drug in a laboratory setting by a qualified health professional does not increase the risk of developing an addiction or its associated harmful behaviours (Adler, 1995; Wood & Sher, 2000). Radioactively labelled psychotropic drugs are often administered to drug-naïve subjects in neuroimaging studies, but at doses so low as to not have any significant cognitive impact. Despite the negligible risk of harm associated with the administration of alcohol to naive subjects (Wood & Sher, 2000), the National Advisory Council on Alcohol Abuse and Alcoholism recommend that alcohol-naïve subjects not be included in studies that provide alcohol (National Advisory Council on Alcohol Abuse and Alcoholism, 1989) (Box 6.3).

A greater ethical challenge is raised by administering drugs of addiction to drug-dependent people despite compelling evidence that the administration of addictive drugs to addicted participants in the laboratory setting does not exacerbate drug use or cause significant harm (Faillace et al., 1972; Modell et al., 1993). If addiction is a condition which impairs an individual's ability to 'say no' to a drug, can drug-dependent persons provide completely free and uncoerced consent to participate in research that will provide them with that drug? Some bioethicists have expressed doubts about the capacity of addicted individuals to provide completely free or internally uncoerced consent to participate in these studies (Charland, 2002; Cohen, 2002). If their arguments were accepted, they would significantly impair the ability of neuroscientists to conduct this type of research.

As we discussed above, the loss in autonomy in addiction is neither as simple nor absolute as this analysis suggests. While the capacity to make autonomous decisions regarding drug use may be impaired in some individuals in certain circumstances, the majority of drug-dependent individuals possess a degree of autonomous decision-making capacity. Rather than override the autonomy of addicted individuals, researchers need to recruit prospective addicted participants and obtain their consent in ways that facilitate or maximise their autonomy. This could be done by minimising situations that may elicit strong cravings for drugs that may overwhelm the ability to make free decisions about participating in research that administers them, and ensuring that the benefits of participating far outweigh any potential risks (e.g. providing participants access to treatment

---

Box 6.3 Administering drugs to healthy volunteers

Zacny and colleagues (e.g. Zacny et al., 1992; Kirulis & Zacny, 1998) have done extensive work testing the effects of different drugs in healthy volunteers. In 1998, they reported on the results of having tested opioids and nitrous oxide on over 200 healthy volunteers in 24 different laboratory studies (Kirulis & Zacny, 1998). Drugs studied included morphine, fentanyl and buprenorphine. The majority of studies involved intravenous administration. Subjects were followed-up 30 days or later after their participation and asked several questions regarding their drug use; 89% reported no change in any other drug use and 9% reported a decrease. Only 2% reported an increase in any form of drug use. The authors conclude that given the wide range of drugs used and large sample size, there is negligible risk of healthy volunteers initiating or increasing drug use after study participation.

services, health care professionals and medical checkups) (Fitzgerald & Hamilton, 1996; Carter & Hall, 2008). Denying addicted individuals the right to participate in research that may be of benefit to them would not only be a violation of the principle of justice (equal distribution of the benefits of research) but it would, from a utilitarian point of view, lead to poorer outcomes for addicted individuals.

6.4.5 Confidentiality and anonymity

The issue of confidentiality is extremely important when dealing with subgroups in the population, such as heroin users, that are engaging in an illegal and harmful behaviour that marginalises them from the general community. Such marginalisation can lead to discrimination and stigmatisation. Common strategies for ensuring confidentiality include keeping data in locked filing cabinets and/or password-protected electronic data files.

Often when questioning subjects about their participation in crime and illicit drug use, only anonymity can protect them. For instance, it is impossible in Australia for researchers to guarantee that data collected on the criminal activities of drug users will not be subpoenaed by police, despite the best intentions of researchers (Fitzgerald & Hamilton, 1996). In this setting, the only way to ensure research subjects are not harmed via their research participation is to keep the data in an anonymised form. This can be done either at the data collection stage, by asking participants to select a pseudonym, or at the data entry stage, by randomly assigning names or unique code numbers. Anonymising subjects at the data collection stage has the advantage of protecting researchers from ever knowing the participant's real name, preventing this information from being subpoenaed in court, but precludes subject follow-up, which can provide clinically significant information. Longitudinal studies that require storage of personal information for follow-up need to be especially stringent in ensuring the confidentiality of research information (World Health Organization, 2004).

6.5 Writing an ethics application

Writing an ethics application should be viewed as a process of explaining to a group of concerned citizens why the research you propose to do is ethically justified and what you have done to ensure that participants provide free and informed consent and will not be harmed by their participation. ECs can also act as gatekeepers to protect the interests of the institution as well as those of research participants.

The most important thing is to ensure that all questions are answered fully. Your responsibility is to demonstrate that you have engaged in a thorough and exhaustive analysis of the ethical issues that your study raises. The best way to begin an ethics application is to read the background literature from the institution. Once this has been done, it is generally worth contacting the relevant administrative person, often called the **ethics officer**, to answer any questions about the form or issues that you suspect will be of major concern to the committee. Consulting other researchers who have undertaken similar research is also an important step.

6.6 Ethical processes in different countries

Different countries have their own systems for dealing with the ethical review process. For instance, in the United States there is a system of IRBs, whereas Australia and the UK have what are called Ethics Committees. Converging international, research ethical practices mean that the ethical review process is increasingly similar in different countries around the globe (Fitzgerald et al., 2006). ECs in different countries do still have some specific requirements. For instance, many ECs in the UK require validation of statistical methods, whereas this is not required in Australia. Likewise, ECs in New Zealand will almost always have an indigenous representative to protect the rights of indigenous participants (World Health Organization, 2004). Some poorer countries with less of a research tradition may lack procedures for reviewing the protocol and informed consent forms, trained IRB members, knowledge and functions of the IRB, monitoring systems, independence of review and archiving systems (e.g. Hall, 2006; Miller et al., 2006; Adams, 2007). These issues may be worth considering when beginning an ethical review process in the developing world.

6.7 Influence of funding body

Research studies require funding. Success in securing research grants is often seen as a good measure of a scientist's worth to the field. But the successful award of research money can sometimes create problems because of the conditions imposed on researchers by a funding agency. Agencies can have different commercial or other vested interests in setting the research agenda, in the way research is conducted, and if, when and where the results are published (Hall, 2006). Contract conditions which seem reasonable when seeking research funding may prevent studies from being published or result in the selective publication of results that, while acceptable to the funding agency, do not accurately portray the actual findings. These types of issues can rarely be addressed alone but require advice and support from senior colleagues, their institutions, professional associations and academic journals.

Ensuring the integrity and objectivity of scientific evidence requires an awareness of additional stakeholders (i.e. the gambling or alcohol industry) seeking to influence the research findings (Hall, 2006; Miller et al., 2006). This is important for two reasons: (1) keeping true to 'the ideal of science' and (2) adhering to the ethical principle of 'beneficence'. Maintaining the ideal of science is essential, not only in terms of sustaining public trust, but also in terms of ensuring that the field uses the most effective interventions that are available. Adhering to the ideal of beneficence is equally important when considering whether research, which may be censored, partially reported or go unpublished, could truly be said to be in the best interests of the research participants. At the heart of the ethical conversation is an issue of trust for individual's institutions and society. It is vital that researchers consider these ethical issues before deciding to apply for or accept research funding from any source.

6.7.1 PERIL

Peter Adams' (2007) PERIL framework (**purpose, extent, relevant harm, identifiers, link**) provides a useful framework for evaluating individual situations of research funding from an ethical perspective.

Purpose refers to the degree to which purposes between the funder and the recipient agree or diverge. For example, if the primary purpose of the recipient is the advancement of public good, receiving funds from industries that sell dangerous commodities – such as tobacco, alcohol and gambling – will probably conflict with this purpose.

Extent is the degree to which the recipient is reliant on this source of funding. As the proportion of income increases, it becomes more difficult to undertake research that may produce results that adversely affect the interests of the funding source. For example, investigators may find that an award from an industry-sponsored organisation is their sole source of salary support. This could create pressure to obtain industry-favourable results so that funding can continue.

Relevant harm is the degree of harm associated with a particular form of product consumption. The level of harm generated by different forms of drug consumption varies. For example, lower potency products – such as lottery tickets or low-alcohol beer – are on the whole less likely to lead to problems than more potent products – such as electronic gambling machines or injectable heroin (Adams, 2007).

Funders are unlikely to finance research anonymously. The point of their involvement is often to be **identified** with some aim of the project, the researchers or their institution, to form a visible association with public good activities for the purposes of 'positive branding'. The extent of visible association can best be reduced by moving away from high-profile advertisements (such as media releases of findings) to more discreet acknowledgements, such as on plaques or at the end of publications.

Finally, the more direct the **link** between researchers and funders, the stronger the perception of influence and the more visible the association. For example, direct funding by a tobacco company involves more exposure than receiving the funding via an independent intermediary agency, such as a foundation or government funding body. As long as there are no major conflicts of interest for the intermediary agency, the separation reduces the chance that recipients will feel obligations – or perhaps experience coercion – for their activities to serve the interests of the donor.

The overall extent of moral jeopardy on the PERIL framework varies from very high levels, as indicated by high rating on all five dimensions, to very low levels as indicated by consistently low ratings.

6.8   Ethical dissemination

The final part of the research process is the ethical dissemination of your research findings (Babor et al., 2008). Publishing ethics is itself the subject of many books, and we recommend reading *Publishing Addiction Science* by Babor et al. for a more comprehensive discussion of these issues. The responsibilities of authors include, but are not limited to, accurate **authorship credits**, accurate and complete reporting of study findings, study design (including ethical approval of research), complete reporting of potential or perceived **conflicts of interests**, avoiding **redundant publication** and not engaging in **plagiarism**. Authors also have a duty to ensure that press releases or advertising material related to the study are consistent with research findings and faithfully replicate the conclusions which have been approved through the peer review process. It is also important to consider how the research findings will be fed back to participants.

6.9   Conclusion

Ethics should be seen as a way of thinking that informs every part of the research process from ensuring a research question is ethically defensible to guaranteeing that dissemination of results is carried out ethically. The best method of ethical deliberation is to go through a logical, rigorous and transparent process to determine the best possible outcome for your research participants and the wider community. When in doubt seek advice from colleagues and ECs.

Exercises

Exercise 1

Relapse to drug use following periods of abstinence is a common problem in addiction. Stimuli or events associated with drug use (e.g. images of injecting paraphernalia) may elicit strong urges to use drugs (called drug cravings) that can trigger a return to chronic drug use, even months after abstinence has been achieved.

In order to better understand the neural processes that lead to relapse, you plan to conduct a functional magnetic resonance imaging (fMRI) study to identify the brain regions involved in drug cravings. fMRI is a technology that allows researchers to visualise the structure and function of the human brain while subjects perform tasks or witness various images or events. fMRI has the potential to provide information about an individual, such as neuropathology (e.g. brain tumour), mental health, personality and cognitive capacities, that may not otherwise be possible. You are proposing to assess the effects that images of drugs and drug injecting equipment have on brain activation and the subjective experience of drug craving in heroin-dependent individuals. You also propose to study the effect that acute drug use has on cue-induced craving and changes in brain activity. This will be done by administering subjects with a small amount of a prescription opioid (e.g. morphine) to some subjects prior to the neuroimaging study. These studies will also be conducted in a non-dependent control group in order to compare with changes in a heroin-dependent population.

In order to perform this study, you need to obtain approval for the research proposal from your university's ECs. Draft an application for such approval that demonstrates that you are aware of the ethical issues raised by the proposed study, and the measures that you will take to ensure that this study is conducted in an ethically acceptable way. Outline the main issues in the proposed study that raise ethical concerns. What steps will you take to ensure that the study is ethical? In particular, you will need to consider issues that may arise in:

(a) recruiting subjects to the study;
(b) obtaining informed consent; and
(c) conducting the study.

Exercise 2

A university-based school of medicine distributes an email announcing to all faculty and staff the availability of a new research funding opportunity. The announcement reads: 'Please see the link below for an available funding opportunity from the Alcohol and Health Research Grants Scheme – http://www.ahrgs.com.au/How-to-Apply.aspx'. The website invites scientists to submit funding proposals to their independent, peer-reviewed, external research programme, which is willing to support research on the disease mechanisms and health endpoints of alcohol consumption. The scheme is funded by Lion Nathan Limited – a major alcohol producer. The programme's Scientific Advisory Board Members are listed on one of the web pages, an impressive-looking group of academics, including department chairs and distinguished professors. Grants are for medical research only and are capped at $35 000. This announcement raises a number of questions about the moral hazards of industry sponsorship of scientific research.

Assume you are an alcohol researcher at a large academic medical centre whose dissertation was recently completed on a topic related to the announcement. Should you apply for the funds? A PERIL analysis along the lines recommended in Adams' paper would require some independent research and a review of the literature on tobacco industry tactics.

Conduct a PERIL analysis on the above example.

Note

1. Research with prison inmates is an important area of research in addiction. A large percentage of inmates use drugs or are addicted.

References

Adams, P. J. (2007) Assessing whether to receive funding support from tobacco, alcohol, gambling and other dangerous consumption industries. *Addiction*, 102, 1027–1033.

Adler, M. W. (1995) Human subject issues in drug-abuse research. *Drug and Alcohol Dependence*, 37(2), 167–175.

Babor, T. F., Stenius, K., Savva, S. & O'Reilly, J. (eds) (2008) *Publishing Addiction Science: A Guide for the Perplexed*, 2nd edn. Rockville, MD: International Society of Addiction Journal Editors. Available online: http://www.parint.org/isajewebsite/isajebook2.htm (accessed 6 October 2009).

Beauchamp, T. L. & Childress, J. F. (2001) *Principles of Biomedical Ethics*, 5th edn. New York, NY: Oxford University Press.

Callahan, D. (2003) Principlism and communitarianism. *Journal of Medical Ethics*, 29(5), 287–291.

Caplan, A. (2008) Denying autonomy in order to create it: the paradox of forcing treatment upon addicts. *Addiction*, 103(12), 1919–1921.

Carter, A. & Hall, W. (2008) The issue of consent to research that administers drugs of addiction to addicted persons. *Accountability in Research*, 15(4), 209–225.

Charland, L. C. (2002) Cynthia's dilemma: consenting to heroin prescription. *American Journal of Bioethics*, 2(2), 37–47.

Cohen, P. J. (2002) Untreated addiction imposes an ethical bar to recruiting addicts for non-therapeutic studies of addictive drugs. *Journal of Law, Medicine and Ethics*, 30(1), 73–81.

Curran, H. V., Kleckham, J., Bearn, J., Strang, J. & Wanigaratne, S. (2001) Effects of methadone on cognition, mood and craving in detoxifying opiate addicts: a dose-response study. *Psychopharmacology (Berl)*, 154(2), 153–160.

Ebbets, J. (1994) Applicability of the CIWA-A scale. Clinical Institute Withdrawal Assessment for Alcohol. *Journal of Nursing Care Quality*, 8(3), ix–x.

Economic and Social Research Council (2005) *Research Ethics Framework (REF)*. Swindon, UK: Economic and Social Research Council.

Faden, R. R., Beauchamp, T. L. & King, N. M. (1986) *A History and Theory of Informed Consent*. New York, NY: Oxford University Press.

Faillace, L., Flamer, R., Imber, S. & Ward, R. (1972) Giving alcohol to alcoholics. *Quarterly Journal of Studies on Alcohol*, 33, 85–90.

Fitzgerald, J. & Hamilton, M. (1996) The consequences of knowing: ethical and legal liabilities in illicit drug research. *Social Science and Medicine*, 43(11), 1591–1600.

Fitzgerald, M. H., Phillips, P. A. & Yule, E. (2006) The research ethics review process and ethics review narratives. *Ethics and Behavior*, 16(4), 377–395.

Hall, W. (2006) Ensuring that addiction science is deserving of public trust. *Addiction*, 101(9), 1223–1224.

Hall, W., Capps, B. & Carter, A. (2008) The use of depot naltrexone under legal coercion: the case for caution. *Addiction*, 103(12), 1922–1924.

Hando, J. & Darke, S. (1998) *NSW Drug Trends 1997. Findings from the Illicit Drug Reporting System (IDRS) National Drug and Alcohol Research Centre Technical Report 56*. Sydney: National Drug and Alcohol Research Centre, University of NSW.

Keane, H. (2005) Moral frameworks, ethical engagement and harm reduction: commentary on 'ethical challenges and responses in harm reduction research: promoting applied communitarian ethics' by C. L. Fry, C. Treloar & L. Maher. *Drug and Alcohol Review*, 24(6), 551–552.

Kirulis, K. & Zacny, J. (1998) Do healthy volunteers increase drug usage after participation in research involving opioids and nitrous oxide? *Anesthesiology*, 89, A1222.

Levy, N. (2006) Autonomy and addiction. *Canadian Journal of Philosophy*, 36(3), 427–448.

Loff, B. (2006) Ethical challenges and responses in harm reduction research: a critique of applied communitarian ethics. *Drug and Alcohol Review*, 25(4), 371–372.

MacDonald, C. (2002) Nurse autonomy as relational. *Nursing Ethics*, 9(2), 194–201.

Miller, P. G., Moore, D. & Strang, J. (2006) The regulation of research by funding bodies: an emerging ethical issue for the alcohol and other drug sector. *International Journal of Drug Policy*, 17(1), 12–16.

Modell, J. G., Glaser, F. B. & Mountz, J. M. (1993) The ethics and safety of alcohol administration in the experimental setting to individuals who have chronic, severe alcohol problems. *Alcohol and Alcoholism*, 28(2), 189–197.

National Advisory Council on Alcohol Abuse and Alcoholism (1989) *Recommended Council Guidelines on Ethyl Alcohol Administration in Human Experimentation*. Rockville, MD: National Institute on Alcohol Abuse and Alcoholism.

National Health and Medical Research Council (1999) *National Statement on Ethical Conduct in Research Involving Humans*. Canberra: National Health and Medical Research Council, Commonwealth of Australia.

Sherwin, S. (1998) A relational approach to autonomy in health care. In: S. Sherwin (ed.) *The Politics of Women's Health: Exploring Agency and Autonomy*. Philadelphia, PA: Temple University Press.

Smith, K. L., Horton, N. J., Saitz, R. & Samet, J. H. (2006) The use of the mini-mental state examination in recruitment for substance abuse research studies. *Drug and Alcohol Dependence*, 82(3), 231–237.

Solai, S., Dubois-Arber, F., Benninghoff, F. & Benaroyo, L. (2006) Ethical reflections emerging during the activity of a low threshold facility with supervised drug consumption room in Geneva, Switzerland. *International Journal of Drug Policy*, 17(1), 17–22.

Volkow, N. D. & Li, T. K. (2004) Drug addiction: the neurobiology of behaviour gone awry. *Nature Reviews Neuroscience*, 5(12), 963–970.

Wesson, D. R. & Ling, W. (2003) The Clinical Opiate Withdrawal Scale (COWS). *Journal of Psychoactive Drugs*, 35(2), 253–259.

White, W. L. & Popovits, R. M. (2001) *Critical Incidents: Ethical Issues in the Prevention and Treatment of Addiction*, 2nd edn. Bloomington, IL: Chestnut Health Systems.

Wood, M. D. & Sher, K. J. (2000) Risks of alcohol consumption in laboratory studies involving human research participants. *Psychologists in Addictive Behaviors*, 14(4), 328–334.

World Health Organization (2004) Developing the ethical review process. Available online: https://apps.who.int/tdr/publications/tdrnews/news61/ethical.htm (accessed 9 October 2009).

Yucel, M. & Lubman, D. I. (2007) Neurocognitive and neuroimaging evidence of behavioural dysregulation in human drug addiction: implications for diagnosis, treatment and prevention. *Drug and Alcohol Review*, 26(1), 33–39.

Zacny, J. P., Lichtor, J. L., Zaragoza, J. G. & de Wit, H. (1992) Subjective and behavioral responses to intravenous fentanyl in healthy volunteers. *Psychopharmacology (Berl)*, 107(2–3), 319–326.

Recommended readings

Babor, T. F., Stenius, K., Savva, S. & O'Reilly, J. (eds) (2008) *Publishing Addiction Science: A Guide for the Perplexed*, 2nd edn. Rockville, MD: International Society of Addiction Journal Editors. Available online: http://www.parint.org/isajewebsite/isajebook2.htm (accessed 6 October 2009).

Callahan, D. (2003) Principlism and communitarianism. *Journal of Medical Ethics*, 29(5), 287–291.

Dolinsky, Z. S. & Babor, T. F. (1997) Ethical, scientific and clinical issues in ethanol administration research involving alcoholics as human subjects. *Addiction*, 92(9), 1087–1098.

Fitzgerald, M. H., Phillips, P. A. & Yule, E. (2006) The research ethics review process and ethics review narratives. *Ethics and Behavior*, 16(4), 377–395.

Hall, W. & Carter, L. (2004) Ethical issues in using a cocaine vaccine to treat and prevent cocaine abuse and dependence. *Journal of Medical Ethics*, 30(4), 337–340.

Solai, S., Dubois-Arber, F., Benninghoff, F. & Benaroyo, L. (2006) Ethical reflections emerging during the activity of a low threshold facility with supervised drug consumption room in Geneva, Switzerland. *International Journal of Drug Policy*, 17(1), 17–22.

White, W. L. & Popovits, R. M. (2001) *Critical Incidents: Ethical Issues in the Prevention and Treatment of Addiction*, 2nd edn. Bloomington, IL: Chestnut Health Systems.

Section II
Basic Toolbox

Chapter 7

SURVEYS AND QUESTIONNAIRE DESIGN

Lorraine T. Midanik and Krista Drescher-Burke

7.1 Introduction

Survey research has become the principle means by which data are collected from large representative samples in order to estimate the prevalence and incidence of behaviours or conditions and also assess trends over time in large populations. In the alcohol, drug and tobacco fields, surveys are used extensively to monitor use, misuse and dependence for entire populations and important subgroups within them, for example youth and minority groups. Surveys are systematic and standardised ways to obtain data from representative samples of individuals, institutions, organisations and other groups; typically, data are obtained by using questionnaires. The purpose of survey research is not to manipulate a variable, but rather to assess what has been called 'naturally occurring phenomena'. Findings are often generalised from a sample to a larger population, or surveys can be conducted on whole populations. There are three basic components that define sample surveys: (1) sampling, (2) questionnaires and interviews and (3) multivariate data analysis. Unlike experimental designs where threats to internal validity are handled by the study design itself, for example, random assignment to treatment and no treatment groups, potential confounders in survey research analyses are handled through data analysis in which multivariate models are used.

There are six main goals of this chapter: (1) to provide a brief history of surveys and their use in the alcohol, drug and tobacco fields; (2) to present the range of survey research designs, what research questions they can answer and their advantages and disadvantages; (3) to discuss modes of data collection within survey designs; (4) to describe questionnaire designs and pilot testing; (5) to present available software for both qualitative and quantitative analysis of data; and (6) to summarise common challenges to conducting survey research in the substance abuse field. While survey research is widely used in most social science fields, attention is focused on the unique aspects of conducting surveys in the alcohol and drug fields throughout the chapter.

7.2 Brief history

The term 'survey' is both a noun and a verb, and its exact meaning as a research design has been confusing for researchers and the general public. Social scientists in universities and research units conduct surveys, but so do governmental agencies, market researchers, television stations and other non-academic entities. In traditional social science terminology, a survey of a population is often called a 'sample survey', which implies that probability sampling (see Chapter 3) was used so that the sample is representative of a larger population.

This history of survey research is primarily American; its roots are from three arenas: (1) the Census Bureau, (2) commercial polling firms and (3) universities. Mandated by the US constitution, the Census Bureau provides decennial enumeration of the US population; however, it also historically has conducted sample surveys between enumerations for governmental agencies in areas such as crime, housing and urban development. Historically, the Census Bureau has been credited with making major achievements in sampling design and implementation.

Beyond the Census Bureau, there are additional sectors that comprise the federal government sector of the 'survey industry' as termed by Rossi et al. (1983). A wide range of federal agencies conduct or subcontract surveys for policy purposes. In the alcohol field, the US National Institute on Alcohol Abuse and Alcoholism subcontracts the National Alcohol Survey to the Alcohol Research Group, Public Health Institute, and also conducts its own national survey: the National Longitudinal Alcohol Epidemiologic Survey and its follow-up, the National Epidemiologic Survey on Alcohol and Related Conditions. The National Survey on Drug Use and Health is funded by the National Institute on Drug Abuse along with the Monitoring the Future Survey, an ongoing study of the alcohol, tobacco and drug behaviours, attitudes and values of American secondary school students, college students and young adults. These national surveys provide valuable data on the prevalence and predictors of alcohol and drug use and problems in the US population. Moreover, they provide important information on predictors of alcohol or drug-related problems, and, in some of the surveys, need and use of treatment services – all of which are important to policy makers. Other international examples include Australia's National Drug Strategy Household Survey and Illicit Drug Reporting System, and New Zealand's Alcohol and Drug Use Survey and Illicit Drug Monitoring System. The academic sector also conducts sample surveys in conjunction with and separate from governmental funds, as do private organisations, often with subcontracts from academic or governmental funding sources. Finally, surveys are conducted by the mass media and by in-house private agencies.

7.3 Survey research designs

7.3.1 When to use a survey

Essentially, survey research has three separate yet interrelated purposes. First, surveys can be used to describe a population on a wide range of variables, for example demographic or attitudinal. Data on the prevalence or incidence of use of a specific drug, for example, can be important in planning for needed treatment as well as for subsequent policies that can potentially identify, refer and treat its use. Second, large-scale surveys can be used for explanatory purposes. For example, by simultaneously controlling for a large number of variables, researchers can establish whether being alcohol dependent is related to less social support after controlling for demographic variables such as gender, ethnicity and education and alcohol consumption variables such as average volume of alcohol consumed and days of heavier episodic drinking. Finally, the last purpose of survey research is exploratory. Because many sample surveys are robust and include a wide range of variables, researchers have the option to explore relationships among variables without prior hypotheses. Moreover, open-ended questions can be included in surveys to allow for a broader qualitative approach to generate new hypotheses.

7.3.2 Description of designs and questions they can answer

When considering survey research, one way to categorise designs is by time. Surveys that include data collection at *one point in time* are called cross-sectional designs, and they are useful for describing a population or the relationship among variables within a sample at one point in time only. While items within cross-sectional surveys can ask respondents to report behaviours, beliefs, attitudes or conditions that occurred in the past; for example, 3 years ago or within a lifetime, the ability to time-order events is subject to memory errors.

Surveys that assess data *over multiple points in time* are called longitudinal surveys. Within this category of longitudinal designs, there are *trend* studies, *cohort* studies and *panel* studies. Trend studies are a series of cross-sectional studies on the same population with different samples studied at different points in time. In the alcohol field, the National Alcohol Surveys by the Alcohol Research Group have been conducted approximately every 5 years since the 1960s. Thus, research questions concerning changes in alcohol, tobacco and drug use can be assessed for a wide range of demographic subgroups. Cohort studies are based on samples of a specific population over time. For example, a survey based on a sample of individuals who graduated from high school in 1980 may be conducted in 1985, and another sample may be drawn in 1990 from the same population but with different samples. This study might assess use of illicit drugs by this cohort over time given that the use of illicit drugs, primarily cannabis, was higher for younger people during this earlier period. Note that the age of the sample would be approximately 23 years in 1985 and 28 years in 1990. Finally, panel studies involve samples of the same individuals over time. Thus, one can assess change within individuals and can potentially determine factors that may predict the use or misuse of alcohol, drugs or tobacco.

7.4 Advantages and limitations of survey research designs

7.4.1 Advantages

There are several advantages to sample survey designs. When conducted well, sample surveys are parsimonious and allow researchers to generalise findings to a larger population. Surveys give the researcher the ability to examine multiple variables simultaneously because they have the capacity to collect large amounts of data at one time. While surveys cannot determine causality, survey researchers can examine in depth the relationship among variables to determine if primary findings in the total sample, for example, a positive correlation between heavy drinking and gambling, hold for specific subgroups such as women, older people and specific ethnic groups. Finally, if a survey is administered at multiple points in time, a researcher is able to detect trends and assess the relationship among variables over some period.

7.4.2 Limitations

One limitation to using surveys is that they are unable to demonstrate causation between variables. Both cross-sectional and longitudinal designs cannot determine that one variable causes another variable; only associations can be identified. For example, a survey might suggest that heavy alcohol use is associated with family problems in a specific population. We cannot say that the alcohol use caused the family problems, nor can we say that the family problems caused heavy alcohol use. We can only say that these two variables are correlated with each other. Longitudinal survey designs can give us a better idea, but because neither variable is being manipulated, as is the case in experimental designs, we are unable to assert that changes in one variable cause changes in the other.

Surveys are also limited in that they may not be able to capture the complexities of substance use behaviour. For example, if a survey asks the question, 'What factors led you to start using cocaine?', a respondent may give answers provided by the response categories; however, the complexities of the situation may go beyond what is included in the question. Moreover, understanding these complex phenomena becomes more challenging with retrospective reporting, particularly when the time frame of the question is in the distant past.

Survey methods are also generally unable to capture fully the social context of a situation. In-depth qualitative interviews as opposed to survey questionnaires may be a better approach to identifying body language and affect of the respondent. However, just like surveys, qualitative interviews are ultimately limited to what a respondent chooses to divulge.

Questionnaires obtained through surveys are more rigid than other forms of data collection. Unlike in-depth interviews where researchers can often detect themes early and modify questions as necessary, surveys are usually distributed to a large number of potential respondents and data collection is complete before a researcher may realise that additional questions would improve understanding or improve the analysis.

Surveys typically rely on participants' self-report that may be limited by validity and reliability issues. This may be a problem especially among substance-using populations. Although there may be no intent on the part of a respondent to mislead or give intentionally false information, memory can be affected by such factors as the way a question is worded, the time frame of a question, guilt about past behaviours, and also by the substance use itself where, for example, heavy use of alcohol may impede memory. For more detail about self-report validity, see Chapter 2. Similarly, surveys also rely on reports of past behaviour or of a hypothetical action. It is impossible to measure in a survey what a person would actually do in a particular situation. For example, if a survey question inquires about one's course of action if the respondent were to discover his or her daughters were using heroin, respondents could answer the question in several ways, but unless the situation actually arose, there is no way to determine whether that behaviour would occur.

7.5   Modes of data collection

Ways of collecting data for surveys have varied over time from mailed and self-administered questionnaires, to face-to-face and telephone surveys, and finally to computerised and internet surveys using email and websites on the internet. While earlier survey work focused on one method exclusively, increasingly more survey research is being conducted using mixed methods – combining different forms of data collection to ensure a higher response rate. Each method individually and in conjunction with other methods has its strengths and its potential weaknesses. Dillman (2007) argues that there are two factors directly affecting mode differences particularly in comparisons of self-administered versus interview modes: normative/group norms and cognitive processes. Yet, within the research literature on mode effects, there does not appear to be consistent findings concerning which mode is the most effective. Rather, it is assumed that more sensitive or threatening items which are subject to social desirability factors are best asked in more anonymous circumstances.

Recently, more attention has been placed on innovative ways to collect survey data in a computerised form such as web-based surveys, email surveys and interactive voice response (a computerised form of telephone interviews). While email surveys and internet surveys have great potential for ease of administration and appearance, they are hampered by the technological divide that acts as a barrier particularly to lower income individuals. As a result, the ability to generalise from a web-based sample to a larger population is problematic. Moreover, email surveys can be hindered by individuals and households with multiple addresses and no centralised directory from which to sample. However, email and internet surveys can be used well with known populations for which longer-term, inexpensive follow-up data are needed. As internet access increases particularly to those with lower incomes, coverage rates should increase accordingly.

7.6　Questionnaire design

7.6.1　Question development and things to avoid

Developing items for a questionnaire is a process which requires time and effort. Poorly constructed questions can result in invalid or irrelevant findings, whereas a well-written question provides a solid foundation for further analysis and theory testing. This section contains a general guide for developing specific questions as part of a questionnaire.

Remember hypotheses and research questions

When considering which items should be included in a questionnaire, researchers should focus on their hypotheses and research questions. In the process of questionnaire development, it is easy to add items that may not be relevant to the aims of the study. These additional questions may also unnecessarily add to the time and the cost of the survey

Consider analysis

Researchers should consider the level and type of analyses that will be conducted when writing questions. The level of measurement (e.g. nominal and ordinal) needed for the chosen analysis should be reflected in the questions. It is advisable to have the highest level of measurement possible; you can recode the responses to a lower level of measurement, but it is not possible to go in the other direction. For example, consider the following two ways of asking the same question:

How many cigarettes did you smoke yesterday?

a.　0
b.　1–5
c.　6–10
d.　11–15
e.　16–20
f.　21 or more

How many cigarettes did you smoke yesterday? _____ # of cigarettes

Usually, smokers are aware of the number of cigarettes they smoke per day. Thus, by asking the specific number of cigarettes, analysis using interval- or ratio-level variables is possible. If only a range is known, less powerful statistical tests must be used.

Seek input on question development

To strengthen your questionnaire in the development phase, seek input from people who have differing views. Input from insiders and key informants is also invaluable. For example, if researchers are developing a questionnaire about criminal justice involvement and substance use, they should seek input from people who have been involved in both systems such as judges, lawyers and treatment professionals. When considering how to measure concepts, look at existing research and use items and scales that have demonstrated reliability and validity. If a researcher is developing a new instrument, standard scales can be included in the questionnaire along with new items or scales and comparisons can be made a part of the analysis.

Use simple, clear and correct language for questions and answer choices

It is important to use language that is clear, direct, appropriate for your respondents, and written with the reading level of your sample in mind. Questions should also be specific. Some substance users do not consider cannabis or alcohol to be drugs *per se*. When asking about substance use in particular situations, it is advisable to ask about specific substances individually. Researchers should also be familiar with the current terminology of drugs through pilot testing, talking with key informants, and other types of research. Consider whether questions will be asked aloud or if they will be read by respondents on a self-administered questionnaire. A question may be read easily, but when asked aloud, it may sound awkward. When questions are poorly written and do not make sense to respondents, they may not be able to provide answers that accurately reflect their behaviours or their attitudes. Similarly, when answer choices are unclear, or when answer choices do not include all possible responses (answer choices are not *exhaustive*[1]) or seem to overlap (they are not *mutually exclusive*), respondents may not be able to provide valid responses.

Avoid double-barrelled questions

A double-barrelled question includes two or more behaviours or attitudes within one question. They are difficult to answer and should be avoided in survey research. For example, if an item asks, 'Do you smoke cocaine and drink alcohol?', some respondents may have difficulty answering if they drink alcohol but do not smoke cocaine. Similarly, a respondent who snorts cocaine and drinks alcohol may have difficulty answering the question. A better way to obtain this information and eliminate confusion would be to create two distinct questions.

Consider ability to answer

Asking participants about their past behaviours is problematic particularly if the respondents are heavier users of substances. This is true even for people who have never had problems with substances. Asking about recent behaviour may produce more reliable responses.

Similarly, if participants do not have the knowledge to answer a particular question, they may still feel pressured to answer it and thus 'create' an opinion as opposed to reporting their opinion. For example, if a questionnaire includes an inquiry of the respondent's attitude towards the current US laws regarding health care parity for substance abuse treatment, many respondents may be unaware of this law or its specifics. *Consider willingness to answer*. Divulging information about current or past substance use can be embarrassing or potentially dangerous to respondents in some cases because of illegal activity, involvement with child protective services, employment, law enforcement, etc. Even if a researcher guarantees confidentiality to the extent allowed by law, respondents may not feel that their confidentiality is protected. This issue may be mitigated somewhat with anonymous mailed questionnaires, but many people still do not feel that their identities are truly protected. Some of this effect may be mitigated by using language that normalises behaviour. For example, rather than asking, 'What illegal drugs have you used?', a question could read, 'Some people use illegal substances, and some people do not. Have you ever used any illegal substances?'

Avoid negative questions

Including negative language, though not necessarily grammatically incorrect, can be confusing. For example, rather than asking, 'In the month before you came to treatment, about how many days did you not drink alcohol?', you could consider the question, 'In the month before you came to treatment, about how many days did you drink alcohol?'

Some questions that contain negative language can be reworded to be less confusing while still obtaining the same information. For example, consider the following question: 'Do you think that people convicted of drunk driving should not be prohibited from driving again after some specified time period?' The same question could be clearer by removing the negative language: 'Do you think that people convicted of drunk driving should be allowed to drive again after some specified time period?'

7.6.2   Structuring the questionnaire

When developing a questionnaire, a researcher must decide on the types of questions that will be included. For example, should only open-ended questions be used? Should only closed-ended questions be used? Should a combination of both open and closed-ended questions be included? There are benefits and drawbacks to both types of questions. For example, open-ended questions can be beneficial by not limiting respondents to set answer choices. However, particularly on self-administered questionnaires, respondents may give vague or ambiguous answers that may be difficult to code and may not directly pertain to the research questions. In this circumstance, the researcher cannot ask the respondent for clarification. In-person interviews, on the other hand, allow the interviewer to probe more deeply for clarification. Open-ended responses also require coding before they can be entered into a statistical analysis software programme.

Closed-ended questions, sometimes called forced-choice questions, also have benefits and drawbacks. Closed-ended questions are frequently easier for a respondent to answer because they take less time. Closed-ended questions reduce ambiguity in responses and greatly facilitate data processing and analysis. However, closed-ended questions may not be broad enough to capture all possible responses. Frequently, researchers will include a response of 'other', sometimes with space for the respondent to fill in his or her own answer if none of the other answer choices fit. If, during the initial analysis, the researcher finds that the 'other' response category is frequently used, these responses can be coded separately and added to response choices for this item. Because respondents may feel compelled to answer even if they have no knowledge of the issue, it is advisable to include a 'don't know' or 'no opinion' answer category.

The order of items in a questionnaire can also affect responses. In substance use research, some items may be considered sensitive; thus, it is important to place these items later on in a survey after a series of non-threatening questions such as age, gender or education. When conducting a face-to-face interview, this is particularly important. A good rapport between the interviewer and the respondent is essential for respondents to feel comfortable about answering difficult questions in an honest way.

Finally, the questionnaire should include very clear instructions and a brief introduction that describes the study and the types of questions that respondents can expect. For self-administered questionnaires, instructions detailing exactly how responses should be marked (e.g. 'Circle only one answer for each question') should be given. Dividing a lengthy questionnaire into topical subsections that begin with transitional remarks can provide a sense of order and help respondents' transition into different content areas of the questionnaire.

7.6.3   Types of interviews

Survey research can bring to mind an image of mass distribution of self-administered questionnaires with primarily closed-ended questions. Although this is one component of survey research, face-to-face survey or telephone interviews collecting both quantitative and qualitative data are another important means of obtaining data in survey research. Compared with self-administered questionnaires, face-to-face interviews can be less structured, rely more on open-ended questions, and use probes to elicit more information from respondents. There are three main types of survey interviews: unstructured or conversational, semi-structured and standardised.

Unstructured or conversational

This type of interview has little to no predetermined questions and relies on the skill of the interviewer to elicit all necessary information in a conversational, natural style. Typically, the interviewer begins with a topic area and asks a range of questions to elicit relevant narrative comments from the respondent. Unstructured interviews are most useful for exploratory purposes, and their use is preferable in areas in which little prior research has been done. For example, unstructured interviews would be appropriate to find out more about the use of a new drug for which there is limited information available.

Semi-structured

Semi-structured interviews follow a general format, and the interviewer usually has a set of sample questions or topic areas that are to be covered. The order and wording of the questions can be modified as appropriate for a particular respondent. For example, if an interview is about experiences with drug treatment but a respondent first mentions legal problems, the interviewer can follow the lead of the respondent and cover that area, even if it is not the original intended order of questioning. It is very important in this type of interview that the interviewer is familiar and comfortable with the material so that the interview can proceed smoothly.

Standardised

Standardised questionnaires ask the same questions with exactly the same wording and in exactly the same order with all respondents. This type of interview ensures that all topical areas are covered in a consistent and reliable manner; however, it allows for little flexibility.

7.7 Piloting the questionnaire

Pilot testing is crucial in identifying potential problems with the questionnaire. During the first stage of piloting (sometimes referred to as 'pretesting'), participants should be asked to extensively comment on all items in the questionnaire (e.g. identify ambiguities, raise concerns about vocabulary and correct bias). It is critical that the pilot sample feels comfortable offering constructive feedback to the researcher. After feedback is obtained, the questionnaire needs to be revised. If necessary, this stage can be repeated until the questionnaire is sufficiently strengthened and is ready to be used in the next stage of piloting.

The next step would involve actually administering the questionnaire as if it were in its final version. Participants at this stage should not know that they are included in a pilot study. It is not necessary to have a representative sample for pilot testing, but it is important that the pilot group be similar to the sample used for the study. Those participating in the pilot should not be respondents in the actual study. If the researcher cannot use a pilot group that is similar to the study population because of cost and time restraints, it is acceptable to use a group of people knowledgeable about the particular population under study and ask them to participate as if they were a respondent with the characteristics being studied. Like the previous step, after reviewing the questionnaires of the respondents to the pilot, the researcher will need to revise the questionnaire and, if necessary, repeat this stage until the questionnaire is in its final form.

Below, Converse and Presser (1986) outline ten aspects of piloting that present what issues must be considered in developing a questionnaire:

Specific questions

1. Variation: Questions should show variability so that not everyone should answer the question the same way.
2. Meaning: Do researchers and respondents mean the same thing?
3. Task difficulty: Have respondents thought about the questions in the terms asked (e.g. would it be more easily understood to ask about alcohol intake in terms of drinks or in terms of ounces of alcohol)?
4. Respondents' interest and attention: Which questions are boring and which are interesting? Should the questions be reordered, or should the format vary?

Questionnaire as a whole

5. Flow and naturalness of section: Does the questionnaire flow naturally and in a logical order, or does it seem to jump around?
6. Order of questions: Does the order of the questions make sense? Are there interesting questions up front?
7. Skip patterns: Are the skip patterns logical? Do they make sense?
8. Timing: How long does the questionnaire take to complete?
9. Respondents' interest and attention overall: As with individual questions, is the questionnaire interesting? Should the format vary?
10. Respondents' well-being: An interviewer should note effects a questionnaire has on a respondent. Do respondents become overly anxious or uncomfortable? Should questions be reworded to improve respondents' overall experience and to make sure that human subjects are protected?

7.8 Technological assistance

Because of the large datasets and the complexity of analysis used in survey research in which multiple variables are examined at one time, researchers use statistical software to assist with their analysis. When designing questionnaires, it is useful for researchers to enter codes directly onto questionnaires so that when questionnaires are returned, the data can easily be entered into the chosen software programme. Most software programmes allow for numbers to represent answer choices for categorical variables, and putting numbers before answer choices instead of, for example, letters or check boxes, can make the data entry process more efficient.

In the following example, assume the respondent has answered previously that he or she has consumed alcohol on at least one occasion during the last year.

During the last 12 months, which type of alcohol did you drink *most* often? Please circle one response.

(1) Beer or malt liquor
(2) Wine or wine coolers
(3) Distilled spirits
(4) Other (please specify) _____

Because the codes are directly next to the answer choices, a researcher will be able to enter the data into the software programme directly from the questionnaires.

It is important that researchers have a basic knowledge of different software programmes that can assist with their analysis. For example, one of the most commonly used statistical software programmes used by social scientists is SPSS (the Statistical Package for the Social Sciences). With SPSS, and with most other statistical software programmes, researchers can conduct univariate, bivariate and multivariate analysis most commonly used with survey research. Common statistical techniques that are used are t-test, linear regression, chi-square and correlation. Researchers can also conduct basic univariate analyses such as determining frequencies, means and standard deviations (see Chapter 11 for more information). Software is also available to help researchers organise and analyse qualitative data gathered as part of survey research (e.g. Atlas.ti and NVivo). For more information on qualitative analysis, see Chapter 5.

7.9 Common challenges

There are many issues that specifically face researchers in the alcohol, tobacco and drug fields who want to conduct surveys and develop valid and reliable research instruments. Measurement of substance use can be challenging depending on whether the goal is to diagnose dependence and/or abuse or describe a population's use of substances and related consequences of use. In determining which scales to use, researchers need to balance their need to have comparability with previous studies by choosing commonly used instruments to include in their questionnaires with more creative and innovative ways of assessing alcohol, tobacco and drug use. While comparability with prior research is important, researchers should be encouraged to continue to assess the reliability and validity of these scales and to develop new instruments as needed to better assess alcohol, tobacco and drug use and its effects. Self-report validity, while important in all areas of research, is particularly important in surveys of alcohol and drug use. While absolute validity is impossible to determine, factors such as brief, clearly worded items, clear time frames, assured confidentiality of responses and privacy during interviews – all enhance the ability for respondents to answer truthfully. Finally, making repeated efforts to include hard-to-find respondents who are often heavier, more problematic users of substances is critical to surveys on alcohol and drug use. This can be costly, but is important in assuring that the sample is representative of the larger population. In summary, survey research offers tremendous opportunities to conduct research and gain valuable knowledge on use and abuse of alcohol, tobacco and drugs in a population that can be very useful to determine the need for alcohol, tobacco and drug treatment services, to evaluate substance abuse treatment services, to assess existing substance abuse policies, and to develop new policies.

Exercises

I. Design a questionnaire that gathers information about respondents' alcohol use in the last 30 days.
II. Consider the following questions and their response categories. How can each of these questions be strengthened?
   a. What drugs have you ever used?
      i. Crack cocaine
      ii. Heroin
      iii. Marijuana

b. Have you ever stolen money or sold drugs to support your own habit?
    i. Yes
    ii. No
c. How many drinks of alcohol have you had in the last 30 days?
    i. 0
    ii. 1–2
    iii. 3–4
    iv. 5 or more
III. Identify a scale that focuses on alcohol or drug consumption (e.g. the AUDIT) and critique the instrument. How could this instrument be strengthened?

Note

1. A good way to avoid this is to include an answer choice that is something along the lines of 'none of the above' or 'other'.

References

Converse, J. M. & Presser, S. (1986) *Survey Questions: Handcrafting the Standardized Questionnaire*. Sage University Paper series on Quantitative Applications in the Social Sciences, series no. 07-063. Beverly Hills, CA: Sage.

Dillman, D. A. (2007) *Mail and Internet Surveys. The Tailored Design Method*, 2nd edn. New York: John Wiley & Sons, Inc.

Rossi, P.H., Wright, J.D. & Anderson, A. B. (eds) (1983) *Handbook of Survey Research*. New York: Academic Press.

Recommended readings

Aday, L. A. (1996) *Designing and Conducting Health Surveys: A Comprehensive Guide*, 2nd edn. New York: Jossey-Bass.

Babbie, E. R. (1990) *Survey Research Methods*, 2nd edn. Belmont, CA: Wadsworth Publishing Company.

Babbie, E. R. (2007) *The Practice of Social Research*, 11th edn. Belmont, CA: Wadsworth Publishing Company.

Dillman, D.A. (1978) *Mail and Telephone Surveys: The Total Design Method*. New York: John Wiley & Sons, Inc.

Recommended websites

Atlas.ti information
www.atlasti.com
NVivo information
www.qsrinternational.com

Chapter 8

INTERVIEWS

Barbara S. McCrady, Benjamin Ladd, Leah Vermont and Julie Steele

8.1 Introduction

More than 70 years ago, Hartmann (1933) argued for the utility and universal applicability of the interview, calling it a 'conversation with a purpose'. Today, the research interview is an important tool in a research scientist's repertoire. However, the line between an interview and other data-gathering methods may be unclear. An interview is an information-gathering technique in which the defining feature is the presence of an interaction between the interviewer and the interviewee. The interviewer must have the ability to respond differentially based on the interviewee's responses. An interview can be conducted face-to-face, by telephone or computer. Two broad types of information can be collected through interviews: quantitative data, initially collected in numerical form, and qualitative data such as words, pictures, or objects, which require a qualitative judgement that then can be described numerically. Both types of information are used in research, can be statistically analysed and collected effectively and efficiently through an interview (Kvale, 1983). The distinction should also be made between clinical and research interviews. A clinical interview is an assessment technique to collect information about an individual, while a research interview is an information-seeking tool to collect data that will lead to generalisable information about a particular population. However, the aims of clinical and research interviews frequently overlap.

8.2 Why interviews?

Researchers have a variety of tools at their disposal to collect pertinent information (e.g. see Allen & Wilson, 2003). Research data can be collected through numerous methods including face-to-face interviews, self-report questionnaires and biological assays. Reliable and valid data can be collected using research interviews to screen information to identify people with high-risk drinking patterns, establish substance use disorder diagnoses, measure alcohol consumption, measure adverse consequences of drinking and measure biological, psychological and social functioning.

A number of factors are considered when deciding to collect research data through an interview rather than a self-report survey. Interviews are used most commonly when (1) follow-up questions are needed to clarify initial responses to structured questions; (2) clarification of questions, phrases, or words in the interview is needed; (3) future questions are based on responses to initial questions; (4) some respondents may not have sufficient reading skills and automated voice recognition technology is not available; (5) the target population includes individuals who are likely to become inattentive during data collection, which could affect the quality of data provided; (6) sensitive information is being collected and the development of personal rapport might increase trust and comfort; (7) non-verbal behaviours are used to identify inconsistencies in responses to obtain more valid data; or (8) there is judgement required to code responses (see Brown, 2006).

Box 8.1   Advantages and concerns to consider when using interviews

Advantages	Concerns
Probing for additional information	Influence of social desirability concerns
Explanation of questions and words	Decreased standardisation of administration
Expert judgement in coding	Possible systematic biases in coding
Branching	Possible systematic biases in interviewees' responses to certain interviewers
Use of interviewees' non-verbal behaviours	Possible systematic biases in interviewers' responses to certain interviewees
Identification of inconsistencies in responses	Confidentiality concerns
More complete data	Resource intensive
Enhanced rapport of increased study compliance	

Despite the reasons to use interviews, interviews have some drawbacks (George et al., 2003) (see Box 8.1).

Disadvantages include the following:

1. Respondents may provide lower estimates of behaviours perceived as socially undesirable (e.g. substance use, illegal behaviours and certain sexual behaviours) in an intimate interviewing situation.
2. Measures are not fully standardised in administration when interviewers are able to ask follow-up and clarifying questions. If certain categories of respondents (e.g., English is a second language) require additional follow-up questions, then systematic biases might be introduced into the data.
3. Interviewer characteristics may affect the respondent's comfort with providing specific information and therefore skew the data collected in certain interviewer–interviewee combinations.
4. Respondents may also simply not like or are prejudiced against a particular interviewer, and therefore provide less accurate information.
5. Interviewers have biases or personal reactions towards the respondents and may subtly code responses differently.
6. Confidentiality may be an issue if respondents are concerned that their responses may be overheard.
7. Interviews can be time and resource intensive, requiring extensive training and monitoring to assure that they are administered and scored in a consistent and standardised manner.

8.3   Reliability and validity of self-reported information

Historically, self-reported data from substance users were thought to be unreliable and invalid (e.g. Babor et al., 1990). Several driving assumptions have caused clinicians and researchers to be distrustful of self-reported substance use data. The popular fallacy of 'never trust an addict' continues to permeate addiction research, although research consistently has found that substance users provide valid self-report data when accounting for certain variables (Babor et al., 2000; Del Boca & Noll,

2000). Other unsubstantiated heuristics include (1) substance users provide lower estimates of use because they desire to be seen in a positive light (Babor et al., 1990), (2) the 'more is more valid' approach when comparing methods of measuring substance use and (3) independent sources provide data that are superior to self-report measures. Commonly, people place more confidence in reports that indicate larger and more severe substance use quantity and frequency, and also in information provided by 'objective' third parties (Del Boca & Noll, 2000). Although some aspects of these heuristics are true at times, the specific context should always be considered, and they should not result in the belief that self-report data are unreliable and invalid. The literature over the past 30 years suggests that self-reported information obtained from substance users is neither strictly true nor untrue. Rather, these domains fall on a continuum that is contingent on many variables. Thus, the focus has shifted from attempting to find 'truth' in substance users' reported information to understanding the factors that influence the validity of these data (Del Boca & Darkes, 2003).

8.3.1 Interview characteristics

The interview context encompasses real and perceived consequences in relation to the setting and administration of the interview, the interviewer and confidentiality. For example, if the interview is being conducted for the purpose of treatment access, participants may over-report use in an attempt to gain admission or to justify why they are seeking treatment (Midanik, 1982). Conversely, a criminal justice or parole setting may result in lower self-reported substance use due to the potential consequences (Harrison, 1995). In addition, if individuals are in treatment, having non-clinical personnel administer the research interviews may help improve the accuracy of self-reported information as it conveys to participants that their treatment will not be impacted (Ehrman & Robbins, 1994). Also, substance users' self-report data may be more valid when the interviewer self-discloses as a former drug addict or alcoholic and perhaps then is perceived as less judgemental, versus a research professional (Magura et al., 1987).

Since the procedures used to collect data can also affect the consistency and accuracy of responses, a standardised interview protocol should be implemented. For example, the variability between participant responses will be decreased by having a defined procedural sequence that uses a script for instructions, anticipating questions and having a set of responses, in addition to having a defined manual for consistent coding of responses. Also, the protocol should include an explanation regarding anonymity and confidentiality.

Corroborating reports are often utilised both to verify self-report data and to increase participants' motivation to accurately respond to questions (e.g. Babor et al., 2000). The predominant method of validating self-report data is by acquiring collateral reports from individuals (e.g. spouses, partners or concerned significant others) that have direct knowledge of the participant's substance use (Sobell et al., 1997). Biochemical markers, such as blood or urine, can also be used to substantiate information provided by substance users. Although some believe that corroborative data provide only circumstantial evidence instead of a direct validity check of self-reported data, these sources are valuable tools because they may increase accuracy via a 'bogus pipeline effect', provide information about additional aspects of participants' substance use behaviour and detect response biases (Del Boca & Drakes, 1998). The bogus pipeline effect (Jones & Sigall, 1970) occurs when participants are led to believe their responses will be validated by external sources. This method has been effective mainly with socially undesirable behaviours, but since many bogus pipeline studies about drinking have used adolescent samples, the bogus pipeline effect may be minimal if adolescents find heavy drinking socially acceptable.

8.3.2 Respondent characteristics

Respondent characteristics can negatively impact the validity and reliability of self-reports. Other characteristics that may impact reporting include sobriety, physical condition or affective state (Del Boca & Noll, 2000). Participants with comorbidity and symptoms of severe psychopathology, such as bipolar disorder or schizophrenia, may also provide less accurate self-reports (Langenbucher & Merrill, 2001; Stasiewicz et al., 2008).

In addition, the severity of substance use can negatively affect self-report data by decreasing participants' ability to accurately report due to decreased cognitive, emotional and physical functioning (e.g. Stasiewicz et al., 2008). Further, certain substances such as crack and cocaine have a higher probability of being reported inaccurately by participants due in part to the social desirability bias. That is, respondents may provide lower estimates of behaviours that they perceive as socially undesirable (e.g. alcohol or drug use, illegal behaviours and certain sexual behaviours) (Langenbucher & Merrill, 2001).

More state-specific respondent characteristics include level of intoxication at the time of the interview. To increase accuracy and consistency of self-reported data, breath alcohol level should be measured at the start of the interview to verify that the respondent is sober (Sobell & Sobell, 2003). Furthermore, assessing participants' physical and emotional states ensures they are not currently in withdrawal from a substance, as this can also have a negative impact on their ability to respond accurately.

8.4 Interviewing skills

8.4.1 Clinical and research interviewing

Research interviews are distinct from clinical interviews in purpose, structure and the relationship between the interviewer and the interviewee. Typically, clinical interviews are used to establish rapport and motivation for change, increase clients' awareness of their problems, identify problems requiring immediate attention, establish a diagnosis, collect information for case conceptualisation and treatment planning and monitor response to treatment (Johnson, 2003; Hunsley & Mash, 2008). Although clinicians should use assessment approaches that have empirical support for their reliability and validity, they may at times use other interview approaches, or may elect to use only the measures that are most relevant to the client. Clinicians' responsibility is to help their clients achieve changes that improve their lives.

In contrast, the primary purpose of research interviews is to collect consistent, systematic information in a standardised manner from all participants. Because of this goal, research interviewers have a different set of responsibilities that focus on collecting the same information in the same manner from everyone in a research study, and coding and recording the information consistently. Research interviewers using standardised interviews typically test for intoxication before collecting information, and will reschedule an interview if participants show evidence of having alcohol or drugs in their system. In addition, all the questions in a research protocol must be administered consistently, regardless of their applicability to an individual respondent. Research interviewers should also remain neutral and reinforce participation in research rather than any specific outcome. Unstructured and street intercept interviews may use different procedures and may also interview participants when intoxicated.

Regardless of the purpose of an interview, clinicians and researchers have certain shared clinical, ethical and legal responsibilities (see McCrady & Bux, 1999). For example, assuring that participants

---

Box 8.2 Checklist for a successful research interview

Beginning
  Be on time
  Be professional and respectful; thank the people for their participation
  Be positive in your demeanour
  Introduce yourself, the topic under investigation and the purpose of the interview
  Explain the process
  Determine if the individuals are sober enough to provide reliable information; if they appear intoxicated, ask 'When did you have your last drink?'

Conducting
  Follow the structure of the interview as closely as possible
  When asking open-ended questions, avoid asking 'why?' as it can be seen as judgemental
  Reinforce for *providing* information, not for specific content
  Practice 'skilled empathy'
  Express genuine interest and positive regard for the individual
  Recognise and respond to feelings
  Maintain a non-judgemental stance; put your judgements aside
  If part of the protocol, use reflective listening, keep inflection down so that your response does not become a question
  Be culturally sensitive
  Recognise your own biases and prejudices, especially when conducting open interviews
  Redirect when off-track
  Practice interviewing difficult people
  Respond to non-verbal behaviour when appropriate
  Offer your opinion only when allowed within the research protocol
  Provide reassurance that the information being provided is useful and informative
  Be aware of potential risks due to substance use
  When possible, administer urine screens to check for substance use and breathanalysers for alcohol to substantiate self-report

Concluding
  Give the participants an opportunity to ask questions; reassure them that they may contact you after the interview should questions arise later
  Thank the people for their time

---

can get home safely if they are high or intoxicated, responding to situations of imminent danger to self or others, and acting on suspicions of child or elder abuse or neglect are all shared responsibilities. Additionally, all interviewing requires certain skills in building rapport, creating a safe and respectful environment for persons from diverse backgrounds and having skills to handle difficult interviewing situations and persons. Below are some brief comments about the general skill set that underpins all types of interviewing. Key points are summarised in Boxes 8.2 and 8.3.

8.4.2 Rapport building

Rapport is the 'mysterious force' that draws people together. Fortunately, the basic elements of rapport building are not so mysterious. Rapport building is a skill that can be practiced and learnt, and is used throughout the interview. Talented research interviewers learn how to establish rapport with each interviewee and practice these skills extensively as part of their training.

Box 8.3 Factors to be sensitive to in interviewing

Ethnicity/culture
Gender
Age and stage of life
Socioeconomic status
Religious preference
Presenting problems
Comorbidity
Problem severity
And your own biases

There are several elements involved with establishing rapport. One important element is eye contact, which helps to create an interested and warm atmosphere. Eye contact also suggests confidence; the participant will share more if the interviewer is confident in him/herself and in the research, although one should be aware of cultural differences in response to eye contact. A second element is engaging the interviewee with a warm smile to communicate acceptance, comfort and confidence. A third element is to partially mirror the participant's posture and mannerisms.

A fourth element is to join with the research participant. For example, simply saying 'before I became a researcher, I too participated as a research participant, and I remember feeling ...' may help to recognise common ground and help the participant feel as if the interviewer is an ally. An interviewer might also join with the participant by acknowledging that many research participants have found the interviews to be difficult or long, or by recognising the inherent discomfort involved with revealing private information to a stranger (see Zweben et al., 1998).

8.4.3 Setting the stage for research interviews

The research setting should be one of confidentiality and comfort, and researchers need to pay attention to a variety of environmental considerations. A participant must feel safe, especially when sharing sensitive information such as substance use; therefore, a room with a door is a must. Research interviewers should also attend to physical space issues such as the distance between the interviewer and the participant and the lighting in the research setting. Research sites ideally should have beverages and snacks available if an interview is longer than an hour. Finally, interviewers need to limit opportunities for interruption. In essence, a well-designed research setting should be similar to a clinical setting and create an environment that communicates respect for the privacy and comfort of research participants.

8.4.4 Culturally appropriate interviewing

Establishing rapport with clients of diverse identities is complex and requires understanding of diverse communication styles, language preferences and values systems (for detailed information on establishing rapport and demonstrating respect with participants of diverse identities, see Hays, 2008). Members of ethnic minority groups may resist participation in research because they may feel excluded from full participation in society. For example, in the United States, American Indians may be resistant to the 'White man's' authority and hesitant to offer information. Many studies attempt to have interviewers of the population's same ethnic group (e.g. Jansen et al., 2004); however, interviewers from different backgrounds can also conduct successful interviews.

Researchers may consider modifying questionnaires for more sensitive wording and include questions on culture. Interviewers also need to be well trained to understand the different meanings of certain 'symptoms' in different cultures. For example, if a substance user reports visual hallucinations, an interviewer should gather sufficient information to determine if these experiences are culturally normative or signs of a psychiatric disorder. Researchers also need to consider the setting or population from which the sample is drawn and modify the interpretation of the data accordingly. It is important for interviewers to ask participants how they identify culturally and be trained not to ascribe mono-racial models to them or to make assumptions based on their appearance (Pedrotti et al., 2008).

During the design phase, investigators should ask a series of questions about the expected cultures of the sample population, for example: Which cultures might be present? Are there concerns individuals from this culture may have about participating in research? How can the study and procedures be designed to reassure the participants that the study is ethical and proper? Are there questions that may be misinterpreted or insulting? What types of responses could be culturally influenced and misunderstood? Are there any guidelines or culturally sensitive instruments available for this population? Researchers should answer these questions by researching the literature, online resources, and/or consulting others who have personal and professional expertise.

8.4.5 Difficult interviewees

Challenging research interviewing situations exist. A common issue is for a participant to come to an interview intoxicated. When collecting standardised data, routine research procedures might include an alcohol and drug screening test, and to maximise the accuracy of the research data (Sobell & Sobell, 2003), interviews should be rescheduled if the participant is intoxicated. The presence of an intoxicated individual in the research setting can create challenges for the researchers. If the person has a very high blood alcohol level (BAL) or appears dangerously intoxicated, medical intervention on-site or through transport to a hospital emergency room is required. If individuals' BAL is higher than the legal limit for driving, arrangements must be made to ensure that they do not drive – by keeping them on-site until their BAL is below the legal limit, or arranging alternative transportation. Researchers may also need to consult with an attorney, institutional review board/ethics committee or other expert to determine what precautions are required in their locale if an individual insists on leaving the site while intoxicated.

A second interviewing challenge is the reluctant research participant. For instance, a participant may become less enthused about research participation over the life of a longitudinal or treatment research study. Interviewers face two different kinds of challenges in these situations – obtaining agreement from the individual to complete the interview and obtaining accurate information. Obtaining compliance is an art beyond the scope of this chapter, but excellent resources are available to guide researchers (e.g. Zweben et al., 1998). The most valuable strategy for obtaining good-quality data is to treat participants with respect, express empathy for the difficulties a participant is experiencing and express enthusiasm and appreciation for their willingness to participate. Additional strategies include normalising participants' experiences and providing a clear rationale for why their data are important (Zweben et al., 1998). Vouchers or direct financial incentives can at times help encourage a reluctant participant to complete the interview.

Combative participants present another type of challenge. Such participants typically have been strongly encouraged to get treatment by a significant other or employer, or mandated to treatment by the judicial system. Research with these populations is essential to improving services, and special procedures are in place to ensure that they are free to refuse to participate in the study. However, some still reluctantly consent to research but may be angry and verbally combative. Substantial research suggests that motivational interviewing strategies are clinically effective with angry clients (e.g. Project MATCH Research Group, 1997). Research interviewers must keep their role as researchers clearly in the forefront, but several motivational interviewing strategies, such as expressing empathy or rolling with resistance (Miller & Rollnick, 2002), are helpful in defusing participants' anger.

Loquacious interviewees present a different kind of challenge. These participants either are constitutionally talkative or view the research interview as a therapy session in which they can express their concerns. Since research interviewers are trained to establish rapport, communicate respect and interest, and create an environment that is warm and welcoming, it is understandable that participants might confuse research with a clinical session. Research interviewers must make it clear that the interview is about research and that they have a task to complete, which involves the participant responding to a series of questions. Polite interruptions and redirections are often necessary.

A final challenge is the participant with a comorbid psychiatric disorder. Research suggests that actual psychiatric symptomatology is not a major contributor to unreliable reports (e.g. Stasiewicz et al., 2008). However, impaired cognitive functioning, more severe alcohol dependence and a positive drug screen – all can predict less reliable self-reports. Research with persons with comorbid disorders might generally include a brief cognitive screen to detect impairment as a minimum requirement. The use of collateral data from a relative who has regular contact with the participant might also help to obtain valid data.

8.5   Types of interviews

8.5.1   Interview formats

Research interviews follow three formats: structured, semi-structured and unstructured. (See Box 8.4 for a summary of advantages and disadvantages of different formats.) In *structured* interviews, the researcher adheres strictly to a set of questions in a specific order. This format is advantageous as every interview will be conducted exactly the same, thus increasing reliability. The structured interview also ensures that the desired information is always requested. The disadvantage of a structured interview is that there is no opportunity for additional probing or follow-up questioning based on participants' responses. Thus, the potential for a more complete picture of an event or phenomena may be missed.

The advantages and disadvantages of the *unstructured* interview are almost the mirror image of the structured format. Unstructured interviews may be preferable in situations in which the interviewer is looking for a full description of a phenomenon. In this format, the interviewer is encouraged to follow any course of relevance to the ultimate aim(s) of the study. Unstructured interviews are less common in quantitative research because of their inherently unpredictable nature. Due to the flexibility of the interview, the same interviewer may elicit different categories of information from different participants. However, they are particularly valuable in qualitative research studies.

Semi-structured interviews split the difference between structured and unstructured interviews, gaining some of the benefits while sharing some of the negatives. They have the same set of questions for each participant, thus increasing reliability; however, they can probe for additional information. All three of these formats are utilised in research to achieve particular goals.

> **Box 8.4   Factors to consider when selecting an interview format**
>
> Aim(s) of study
> Desired scope of data collection
> Interviewers' skills/training
> Available resources/time for interviews
> Sensitivity level of data
> Literacy level of population of study
> Ability of participants to travel/meet in person
> Participants' familiarity with technological aids/availability of necessary technology

8.5.2   Method of administration

Another issue when evaluating which interview format to use is the method of administration. *Face-to-face interviews* are conducted in person; the interviewer asks the participant questions and records the responses. These interviews lend a personal air to research, and allow the interviewer to intuit additional information from non-verbal responses and clarify the meaning of a question if necessary. However, this direct contact may cause concerns from a research perspective. Face-to-face interviews may introduce additional variables (e.g. interviewer characteristics and skill) and decrease the anonymity of participants, which may be especially problematic with sensitive topics (Del Boca & Noll, 2000).

Less direct methods of administering interviews include telephone interviews and computerised interviews (online, chat room, interactive). Research suggests that information collected by telephone versus face-to-face is not significantly different (Greenfield et al., 2000) and both have a personal element. Telephone interviews eliminate geographical and transportation complications. Also, participants who are unwilling to meet in person may agree to a telephone interview.

Computerised interviews can be conducted using two general methods. In one method the interview is conducted in real time, online via an instant messaging programme or chat room set-up. The pros and cons of this type of interview are similar to those of a telephone interview, with the additional requirements of having access to a computer and the skills to use one and being able to read. Also, there is risk that someone else might pose as the participant (particularly when there is a financial incentive for participation). The second method is to use a computerised interactive interview. The computer is programmed to provide the questions and ask different follow-up questions based on the participant's response. This type of computer interview is well structured and promotes strong reliability, increases data integrity, and may decrease discomfort or embarrassment. However, this type of interview may be viewed as impersonal, wording of questions cannot be clarified, and a computer cannot process non-verbal cues (Williams et al., 2000; Newman et al., 2002).

There are additional methods of interviewing used in research settings. Street intercept interviews are useful to collect data more likely to be representative of a population. In street interviews, trained interviewers are sent to public areas where the targeted population is believed to be present, randomly stop individuals, and ask them to complete surveys or interviews. Potentially, street interviews can recruit a more representative sample than more traditional research methods. However, the randomness or representativeness of the sample cannot be known (Spooner et al., 1993). Focus groups are utilised to gather information from a number of people at the same time. This technique can be useful to gather basic information quickly and easily, but is less useful for collecting sensitive information or asking follow-up questions that may not be applicable to everyone in the group.

8.6   Types of interview data

Not only do interviews vary in format and mode of administration, they also differ in the types of information they are designed to collect.[1] Table 8.1 summarises information on the interviews described in this section.

Screening interviews are relatively brief interviews used to identify individuals with or at risk for alcohol and/or drug problems; however, they do not gather additional information about the nature or extent of the problem. The CAGE[2] (Ewing, 1984) is a 4-item questionnaire developed to detect an alcohol use disorder and is used most commonly in primary care settings. The TWEAK[3] (Russell, 1994) is a 5-item scale developed to detect risky drinking during pregnancy, and now used to detect risky drinking in general. The Fast Alcohol Screening Test (FAST; Hodgson et al., 2002) is a 4-item questionnaire developed to quickly identify hazardous alcohol use. The Rapid Alcohol Problems Screen (RAPS4; Cherpitel, 2000) is a 4-item measure that assesses alcohol dependence in the past year and was developed for emergency rooms and primary care settings. Finally, the Rutgers Alcohol Problem Index (RAPI; White and Labouvie, 1989) is an 18-item screening tool to assess adolescent problem drinking and negative consequences of alcohol use.

Diagnostic interviews determine whether an individual meets classification criteria for a substance use disorder and explicate the severity and manifestation of the problem. The Structured Clinical Interview for the DSM (SCID; First et al., 2002) is a semi-structured diagnostic interview for Axis I and Axis II diagnoses. Other diagnostic interviews include the Psychiatric Research Interview for Substance and Mental Disorders (PRISM) (Hasin et al., 1996), Composite International Diagnostic Interview – Substance Abuse Module (CIDI-SAM) (Cottler, 2000) and the Substance Dependence Severity Scale (SDSS) (Miele et al., 2000a, b).

Alcohol and drug use – a third type of information of interest to researchers is the quantity and frequency of substance use. Such interviews collect data to determine the volume and frequency with which alcohol and/or drugs are used. The Timeline Followback Interview (TLFB; Sobell et al., 1979) assesses daily substance use using a calendar covering a specified period. The Form-90 (Tonigan et al., 1997) assesses past 90 days of substance use in a semi-structured format. The Customary Drinking and Drug Use Record (CDDR; Brown et al., 1998) is a research-focused, structured interview that measures drug and alcohol consumption in the past 3 months and the lifetime and was designed for adolescent populations. Finally, quantity-frequency (QF) interviews are sometimes used in research. These interviews generally ask people to estimate their average pattern of use (i.e. how many days in a typical week a person drank and how much a person typically drank on a drinking day). QF interviews should be used with caution, however, as they often underestimate substance use (Redman et al., 1987). An example of a QF interview is the Lifetime Drinking History (LDH; Skinner & Sheu, 1982), a structured interview that traces the patterns and stages of an individual's lifetime drinking.

Consequences of use – a fourth category of information collected through research interviews is the direct and indirect adverse consequences of substance use. As with QF measures, these interviews are useful as outcome indicators. The Addiction Severity Index (ASI; McLellan et al., 1980) is a semi-structured interview that addresses seven problem areas: (1) medical status, (2) employment and support, (3) drug use, (4) alcohol use, (5) legal status, (6) family/social status and (7) psychiatric status. The Global Appraisal of Individual Needs (GAIN; Allen & Wilson, 2003) is a structured interview designed to assess course of diagnosis, treatment motivation and relapse potential, physical health, risk/protective involvement, mental health, environment and vocational situation.

Collateral interviews such as the collateral version of the Form-90 (Tonigan et al., 1997) are conducted with an individual close to the participant (often a spouse or family member) and ask

Table 8.1 Psychometric properties and indicated populations for interviews

Interview	Type	Reliability			Validity			Indicated populations	Research utility	Training required?
		Test-retest	Inter-rater	Internal consistency	Content	Construct	Criterion			
CAGE	S			✓			✓		A	N
TWEAK	S						✓	Women, pregnant women	A	N
FAST	S				✓	✓			A	N
RAPS4	S				✓		✓	Good across gender, ethnicity (Caucasian, African-American, Hispanic)	A	N
RAPI	S, C	✓		✓	✓	✓	✓	Adolescents	G	N
SCID	D	✓	✓	✓	✓	✓	✓	Comes in adolescent version	E	Y
PRISM	D	✓		✓		✓		Adults and adolescents	E	Y
CIDI-SAM	D	✓			✓	✓		Adults and adolescents	E	Y
SDSS	D	✓		✓		✓	✓	Good across age groups, gender, ethnicity	G	Y
TLFB	F	✓			✓	✓	✓		E	Y
Form-90	F	✓		✓	✓	✓		Adults and adolescents	E	Y
CDDR	F	✓	✓	✓	✓	✓	✓	Adolescents	E	Y
LDH	F	✓	✓		✓	✓		Adults and adolescents	G	Y
ASI	C	✓	✓	✓	✓	✓	✓	Good across many populations, tested in pregnant women, prisoners, homeless	E	Y
GAIN	C	✓	✓	✓	✓	✓	✓	Adults and adolescents	G	Y

Type: S, screening; D, diagnostic; F, frequency/quantity; C, consequences and adverse effects.
Reliability and validity: ✓, scale has been tested.
Research utility: E, excellent; G, good; A, acceptable.
Training required: Y, yes; N, no.

questions comparable to those asked of the participant. Collateral information can be used when primary data collection is not possible, or to validate self-reported substance use.

8.7   Technological resources

8.7.1   Computer-assisted self-interviews

With ever-increasing complexity and technological abilities, computer-assisted self-interviews (CASIs) are becoming more common in addiction-related research. These interviews can be programmed to alter the questions asked based on participant responses (e.g. skip a question if it is not applicable based on a previous answer or ask follow-up questions if a specific response is given). They can also be administered in audio format, eliminating the need for literate participants. Additionally, CASIs can be designed to concurrently enter data, which reduces data transcription errors.

8.7.2   Real-time data entry programmes

With programmes that allow for immediate recording of interview data as the participant provides it, the risk of transcription errors is eliminated. However, improbable answers, for example if the interviewer mis-keys a response, will not be caught until it is too late to correct it. Real-time data entry programmes are available for the ASI and the clinician version of the SCID; programmes can be written for other interviews as well.

8.7.3   Optical scanning systems

Integrated hardware/software systems (e.g. Cardiff TELEform^{TM}) are available to scan completed interview forms and then export the data to a database for analysis. More sophisticated systems can read marks in choice fields (i.e. an 'x' or a filled out bubble) as well as handwritten entries. Such systems give researchers the ability to scan large numbers of completed interviews without the need for manual data entry. Early data analyses suggested that accuracy was comparable to manual data entry for choice fields, but lower for numeric recognition (Jùrgensen & Karlsmose, 1998). Other disadvantages include the extensive time involved with creating the instruments in scannable form, the high cost of the equipment, the additional time required when the company upgrades the software and some difficulties in managing the system within a network (Nies & Hein, 2000).

8.7.4   Digital recordings or digitizing of taped interviews

Converting conventional recording sources to digital files or simply recording an interview via a digital medium can reduce the time and effort spent by researchers in gleaning information, especially for coding purposes. They also reduce the need to physically store audio and videotapes; however, confidentiality and specific destruction dates of the digital files still need to be assured.

8.8   Summary

Interviews are a major approach to collecting data in addiction-related research, and there are clear advantages and disadvantages to their use. There are a wide range of structures for interviews, and interviews with well-established psychometric properties exist for screening and diagnostic purposes and to assess quantity, frequency and consequences of alcohol and drug use. Knowing the best structure and format of interviews to use for specific research purposes is important, as any one may be more appropriate depending on the research question and design.

Exercise

1. Try conducting a structured interview with classmates, family or friends using the World Health Organization's ASSIST Questionnaire to document their current and past substance use. Note how different people respond differently to the questions and whether you use any sorts of prompts or introductory dialogue to make the process easier.

Notes

1. Further information regarding the individual interviews can be found in *Assessing Alcohol Problems: A Guide for Clinicians and Researchers* (NIAAA, 2003) and Green et al. (2008). These sources provide thorough summary descriptions of the psychometric studies and results for many of the interviews commonly encountered in substance use research.
2. CAGE: c, cut down; a, annoyed; g, guilt; e, eye-opener.
3. TWEAK: t, tolerance; w, worried, e, eye-openers; a, amnesia, k (c), cut down.

References

Allen, J. P. & Wilson, V. B. (2003) *Assessing Alcohol Problems: A Guide for Clinicians and Researcher*, 2nd edn. NIH Publication No. 03-3745. Bethesda, MD: National Institute on Alcohol Abuse and Alcoholism.

Babor, T. F., Brown, J. & Del Boca, F. K. (1990) Validity of self-reports in applied research on addictive behaviors: fact or fiction? *Behavioral Assessment*, 12, 5–31.

Babor, T. F., Steinberg, K., Anton, R. & Del Boca, F. (2000) Talk is cheap: measuring drinking outcomes in clinical trials. *Journal on Studies of Alcohol*, 61, 55–63.

Brown, J. H. (2006) Interviewer as instrument: accounting for human factors in evaluation research. *Evaluation Review*, 30, 188–208.

Brown, S. A., Meyer, M. G., Lippke, L., Tapert, S. F., Stewart, D. G. & Vik, P. W. (1998) Psychometric evaluation of the customary drinking and drug use record (CDDR): a measure of adolescent alcohol and drug involvement. *Journal of Studies on Alcohol*, 59, 427–438.

Cherpitel, C. J. (2000) A brief screening instrument for alcohol dependence in the emergency room: the RAPS 4. *Journal of Studies on Alcohol*, 61, 447–449.

Cottler, L. B. (2000) *Composite International Diagnostic Interview – Substance Abuse Module (SAM)*. St Louis, MO: Department of Psychiatry, Washington University School of Medicine.

Del Boca, F. K. & Darkes, J. (2003) The validity of self-reports of alcohol consumption: state of the science and challenges for research. *Addiction*, 98, 1–12.

Del Boca, F. K. & Noll, J. A. (2000) Truth or consequences: the validity of self-report data in health services research on addictions. *Addiction*, 95(Supplement 3), S347–S360.

Ehrman, R. N. & Robbins, S. J. (1994) Reliability and validity of 6-month timeline reports of cocaine and heroin use in a methadone population. *Journal of Consulting and Clinical Psychology*, 62, 843–850.

Ewing, J. A. (1984) Detecting alcoholism: the CAGE questionnaire. *JAMA: Journal of the American Medical Association*, 252, 1905–1907.

First, M. B., Spitzer, R. L., Gibbon, M. & Williams, J. (2002) *Structured Clinical Interview for DSM-IV-TR Axis I Disorders, Research Version, Non-patient Edition (SCID-I/NP)*. New York: Biometrics Research, New York State Psychiatric Institute.

George, W. H., Zawacki, T. M., Simoni, J. M., Stephens, K. A. & Lindgren, K. P. (2003) Assessment of sexually risky behaviors. In: D. M. Donovan & G. A. Marlatt (eds) *Assessment of Addictive Behaviors*, 2nd edn. New York: Guilford Press, pp. 424–443.

Green, K., Worden, B., Menges, D. & McCrady, B. S. (2008) Assessment of alcohol use disorders. In: J. Hunsley & E. Mash (eds) *A Guide to Assessments That Work*. New York: Oxford University Press, pp. 339–369.

Greenfield, T. K., Midanik, L. T. & Rogers, J. D. (2000) Effects of telephone versus face-to-face interview modes on reports of alcohol consumption. *Addiction*, 95, 277–284.

Harrison, L. D. (1995) The validity of self-reported data on drug use. *Journal of Drug Issues*, 25, 91–111.

Hartmann, G. W. (1933) The interview as a research and teaching device. *Journal of Applied Psychology*, 17, 205–211.

Hasin, D., Trautman, K., Miele, G., Samet, S., Smith, M. & Endicott, J. (1996) Psychiatric Research Interview for Substance and Mental Disorders (PRISM): Reliability for substance abusers. *American Journal of Psychiatry*, 153, 1195–1201.

Hays, P. A. (2008) *Addressing Cultural Complexities in Practice: Assessment, Diagnosis, and Therapy*, 2nd edn. Washington, DC: American Psychological Association, pp. 85–101.

Hodgson, R. J., Alwyn, T., John, B., Thom, B. & Smith, A. (2002) The fast alcohol screening test. *Alcohol and Alcoholism*, 37, 61–66.

Hunsley, J. & Mash, E. J. (2008) Developing criteria for evidence-based assessment: an introduction to assessments that work. In: J. Hunsley & E. J. Mash (eds) *A Guide to Assessment That Work*. New York: Oxford University Press, pp. 3–14.

Jansen, H. A. F. M., Watts, C., Ellsberg, M., Heise, L. & García-Moreno, C. (2004) Interviewer training in the WHO multi-country study on women's health and domestic violence. *Violence Against Women*, 10, 831–849.

Johnson, S. L. (2003) *Therapist's Guide to Substance Abuse Intervention*. New York: Academic Press.

Jones, E. E. & Sigall, H. (1970) The bogus pipeline: a new paradigm for measuring affect and attitude. *Psychological Bulletin*, 76, 349–364.

Jùrgensen, C. K. & Karlsmose, B. (1998) Validation of automated forms processing. A comparison of Teleform™ with manual data entry. *Computers in Biology and Medicine*, 28, 659–667.

Kvale, S. (1983) The qualitative research interview: a phenomenological and a hermeneutical mode of understanding. *Journal of Phenomenological Psychology*, 14, 171–196.

Langenbucher, J. & Merrill, J. (2001) The validity of self-reported cost events by substance abusers. *Evaluation Review*, 25, 184–210.

Magura, S. D., Goldsmith, D., Casriel, C., Goldstein, P. J. & Lipton, D. S. (1987) The validity of methadone clients' self-reported drug use. *International Journal of the Addictions*, 22, 727–749.

McCrady, B. S. & Bux, D. (1999) Ethical issues in informed consent with substance abusers. *Journal of Consulting and Clinical Psychology*, 67, 186–193.

McLellan, A. T., Luborsky, L., O'Brien, C. P. & Woody, G. E. (1980) An improved diagnostic instrument for substance abuse patients: The Addiction Severity Index. *Journal of Nervous and Mental Diseases*, 168, 26–33.

Midanik, L. T. (1982) The validity of self-reported alcohol consumption: a literature review. *British Journal of Addiction*, 77, 357–382.

Miele, G. M., Carpenter, K. M., Cockerham, M. S., Trautman, K. D., Blaine, J. & Hasin, D. S. (2000a) Concurrent and predictive validity of the Substance Dependence Severity Scale (SDSS). *Drug and Alcohol Dependence*, 59, 77–88.

Miele, G. M., Carpenter, K. M., Cockerham, M. S., Trautman, K. D., Blaine, J. & Hasin, D. S. (2000b) Substance Dependence Severity Scale (SDSS): reliability and validity of a clinician-administered interview for DSM-IV substance use disorders. *Drug and Alcohol Dependence*, 59, 63–75.

Miller, W. R. & Rollnick, S. (2002) *Motivational Interviewing: Preparing People for Change*, 2nd edn. New York: Guilford Press.

Newman, J. S., Des Jarlais, D. C., Turner, C. F., Gribble, J., Cooley, P. & Paone, D. (2002) The differential effects of face-to-face and computer interview modes. *American Journal of Public Health*, 92, 294–297.

NIAAA. (2003) *Assessing Alcohol Problems: A Guide for Clinicians and Researchers*, 2nd edn. NIH publication no. 03-3745.

Nies, M. A. & Hein, L. (2000) Teleform: a blessing or burden? *Public Health Nursing*, 17, 143–145.

Pedrotti, J. T., Edwards, L. M. & Lopez, S. J. (2008) Working with multiracial clients in therapy: bridging theory, research and practice. *Professional Psychology: Research and Practice*, 39, 192–201

Project MATCH Research Group (1997) Project MATCH secondary a priori hypotheses. *Addiction*, 92, 1671–1698.

Redman, S., Sanson-Fisher, R. W. & Wilkinson, C. (1987) Agreement between two measures of alcohol consumption. *Journal of Studies on Alcohol*, 48, 104–108.

Riskind, J. H., Beck, A. T., Berchick, R. J., Brown, G. & Steer, R. A. (1987) Reliability of DSM-III diagnoses for major depression and generalized anxiety disorder using the structured clinical interview for DSM-III. *Archives of General Psychiatry*, 44, 817–820.

Russell, M. (1994) New assessment tools for drinking in pregnancy: T-ACE, TWEAK, and others. *Alcohol Health and Research World*, 18, 55–61.

Skinner, H. A. & Sheu, W. J. (1982) Reliability of alcohol use indices: the lifetime drinking history and the MAST. *Journal of Studies on Alcohol*, 43, 1157–1170.

Sobell, L. C., Agrawal, S. & Sobell, M. B. (1997) Factors affecting agreement between alcohol abusers' and their collaterals' reports. *Journal of Studies on Alcohol*, 58, 405–413.

Sobell, L. C., Maisto, S. A., Sobell, M. B. & Cooper, A. M. (1979) Reliability of alcohol abusers' self-reports of drinking behavior. *Behavior Research and Therapy*, 17, 157–160.

Sobell, L. C. & Sobell, M. B. (2003) Alcohol consumption measures. In: J. P. Allen & V. B. Wilson (eds) *Assessing Alcohol Problems: A Guide for Clinicians and Researcher*, 2nd edn. NIH Publication No. 03-3745. Bethesda, MD: National Institute on Alcohol Abuse and Alcoholism.

Spooner, C. J., Flaherty, B. J. & Homel, P. J. (1993) Illicit drug use by young people in Sydney: results of a street intercept survey. *Drug and Alcohol Review*, 12, 159–168.

Stasiewicz, P. R., Vincent, P. C., Bradizza, C. M., Connors, G. J., Maisto, S. A. & Mercer, N. D. (2008) Factors affecting agreement between severely mentally ill alcohol abusers' and collaterals' reports of alcohol and other substance use. *Psychology of Addictive Behaviors*, 22, 78–87.

Tonigan, J. S., Miller, W. R. & Brown, J. M. (1997) The reliability of Form 90: an instrument for assessing alcohol treatment outcome. *Journal of Studies on Alcohol*, 58, 358–364.

White, H. R. & Labouvie, E. W. (1989) Towards the assessment of adolescent problem drinking. *Journal of Studies on Alcohol*, 50, 30–37.

Williams, M. L., Freeman, R. C., Bowen, A. M., Zhao, Z., Elwood, W. N., Gordon, C., Young, P., Rusek, R. & Signes, C.-A. (2000) A comparison of the reliability of self-reported drug use and sexual behaviors using computer-assisted versus face-to-face interviewing. *AIDS Education and Prevention*, 12, 199–213.

Zweben, A., Barrett, D., Carty, K., McRee, B., Morse, P. & Rice, C. (1998) *Strategies for Facilitating Protocol Compliance in Alcoholism Treatment Research*. Project MATCH monograph series, Volume 7. Bethesda, MD: US Department of Health and Human Services.

Recommended readings

Allen, J. P. & Wilson, V. B. (2003) *Assessing Alcohol Problems: A Guide for Clinicians and Researcher*, 2nd edn. NIH Publication No. 03-3745. Bethesda, MD: National Institute on Alcohol Abuse and Alcoholism.

Donovan, D. M. & Marlatt, G. A. (2005) *Assessment of Addictive Behaviors*, 2nd edn. New York: Guilford Press.

Green, K., Worden, B., Menges, D. & McCrady, B. S. (2008) Assessment of alcohol use disorders. In: J. Hunsley & E. Mash (eds) *A Guide to Assessments That Work*. New York: Oxford University Press, pp. 339–369.

Miller, W. R. & Rollnick, S. (2002) *Motivational Interviewing: Preparing People for Change*, 2nd edn. New York: Guilford Press.

Rohsenow, D. J. (2008) Substance use disorders. In: J. Hunsley & E. Mash (eds) *A Guide to Assessments That Work*. New York: Oxford University Press, pp. 319–338.

Zweben, A., Barrett, D., Carty, K., McRee, B., Morse, P. & Rice, C. (1998) *Strategies for Facilitating Protocol Compliance in Alcoholism Treatment Research*. Project MATCH monograph series, Volume 7. Bethesda, MD: US Department of Health and Human Services.

Recommended resources for developing interviewing skills

Developing research interviewing skills requires several steps:

1. Sufficient knowledge about the topics being assessed. For example, interviewers using the SCID must have knowledge about psychopathology and the specifics of diagnosing Axis I and Axis II disorders. Interviewers assessing drug use need to know what drugs are in each drug class; interviewers assessing alcohol use need to recognise various alcoholic beverages to determine the amount of alcohol per drink.
2. Acquisition of general interviewing skills. These are best learnt through a formal interviewing training programme or course in microcounseling skills.
3. Acquisition of knowledge about how to administer specific interviews. This knowledge is available in the manuals for the administration of each interview, training tapes, articles describing the measures and observing experienced interviewers.
4. Practice conducting the interview to become proficient in the mechanics of administering the interview. Many of the interviews described in this chapter are complex, and the interviewer needs to become proficient with the mechanics – reading the questions exactly as written, coding responses properly and putting the codes in the correct place, following branching programmes (where relevant) exactly. Probing and follow-up questions are easier when the interviewer does not have to fumble to find the next question. This step in learning an interview can be done with any willing respondent since the focus is on learning the mechanics.
5. Observed practice and review of coding, with feedback. Once an interviewer feels comfortable with the mechanics, observed practice is crucial to learning the nuances of an interview. At this point, the interviewer also needs feedback about the accuracy of his or her coding of responses.
6. Knowledge of guidelines and procedures within a specific study for the management of difficult participants and handling of emergency situations. Interviewers should be certain that they know in advance what to do should a difficult or emergency situation arise. Being confronted with a highly intoxicated participant at 7 PM is not the time to find out what to do.
7. Certification as competent in each specific interview. For more complex interviews, there is often a formal process, either from the developer of the instrument or through the individual research study, to certify that the interview has sufficient competence to administer and score the interview correctly.
8. Regular review and feedback to maintain skills. Ongoing supervision and discussion is important – participants rarely adhere perfectly to the protocols that researchers lay out, and ongoing discussion of challenging situations is necessary to maintain consistency across interviewers.

The guidelines listed above are relevant to learning any complex interview. The interested reader is referred to the following sites for specific training materials:

1. Websites for general information about assessment measures:
    *   Center on Alcoholism, Substance Abuse, and Addictions, University of New Mexico: http://casaa.unm.edu
    *   University of Washington: http://depts.washington.edu/adai/
    *   National Institute on Alcohol Abuse and Alcoholism: http://pubs.niaaa.nih.gov/publications/Assesing%20Alcohol/index.htm

2. Online resources for selected interviews:
    - Addiction Severity Index: http://www.tresearch.org/resources/instruments.htm
    - Form 90: http://pubs.niaaa.nih.gov/publications/match.htm; also http://casaa.unm.edu/inst.html
    - PRISM: http://www.columbia.edu/˜dsh2/prism/
    - SCID: http://www.scid4.org/index.html
    - Timeline Followback Interview: Training materials available through the author Linda Sobell, Ph.D.; http://www.cps.nova.edu/˜sobelll/

Chapter 9

SCALES FOR RESEARCH IN THE ADDICTIONS

Shane Darke

9.1 Introduction

One of the most common questions to be asked when planning a research project concerns the choice of research instruments. An appropriate choice of instruments is crucial to the success of any good research project. In this chapter, we examine the major domains of relevance to drug and alcohol research, and the instruments most relevant to these domains. Of course, there is no 'correct' choice of instrument for studies. The choice of instrumentation will be determined by the research questions being asked and the logistical realities of the research situation, particularly in relation to available time. We are fortunate in this field that a wide range of instrumentation is now available for clinical and research use. The range of instruments is far too vast to be covered in any one chapter (or book). This chapter thus should not be seen as an exhaustive list of instruments, but a brief guide to the most widely used instruments. Readers are directed to Dawe et al. (2002) for a more comprehensive analysis of diagnostic instruments. This is not a review of psychometrics, but of what to use and when. All instruments presented here have been tested for reliability and validity. Those interested in the psychometric properties of particular scales should examine the key references and manuals for these instruments.

9.1.1 Self-report

Before proceeding, however, we need to briefly mention the issue of self-report among substance users, as there are misconceptions that plague the field. Scales by definition rely upon self-report. Concern is often raised about the accuracy of such self-report, particularly amongst illicit drug users. In this field, however, self-report is often the only feasible methodology that can address the research questions of interest to the investigators. Investigations of drug use, criminal behaviours, needle sharing, etc., by their very nature, involve a reliance on self-report from respondents. Two major concerns are often raised. First, there is the commonly held view that drug users are pathological liars by nature. Second, the nature of the activities being investigated is frequently illegal and socially undesirable. Respondents may be reluctant to admit to socially undesirable behaviours because of the stigma attached to these behaviours. There is no evidence for either of these assertions. This is an area that has been extensively researched, and the self-report of drug users in research settings has repeatedly been demonstrated to have high levels of reliability and validity (Darke, 1998; Welp et al., 2003; Jackson et al., 2004). This has been found to be true for substance use, crime, risk-taking, etc. Given accurate instrumentation, the researcher in the drug and alcohol field should have confidence in the data that are produced.

9.2   Screening instruments

Screening instrument refers to a range of scales that are used to determine the presence or absence of a substance use problem by means of specified cut-off scores. They are, by definition, not diagnostic of clinical problems. Rather, they are used to indicate whether diagnostic testing is required.

9.2.1   Alcohol use disorders identification test

What is it?

The alcohol use disorders identification test (AUDIT) is a ten-item screener for problem drinking. The ten items cover quantity and frequency of alcohol use, binge drinking and a range of alcohol-related problems (e.g. others being injured due to the person drinking and blackouts). As such, it can be used to examine levels of drinking, to determine whether drinking levels are harmful and to screen for a presumptive diagnosis of dependence.

When would I use it?

The AUDIT is an excellent instrument for both clinical and research applications. While its major utility is to screen for the presence of alcohol-related problems, it can also be used as a continuous measure in research. Thus, AUDIT scores might be used a covariate in multivariate analyses in which levels of alcohol-related problems need to be statistically controlled for.

How is it administered?

The AUDIT is self-completed by the interviewee. It can, of course, be administered by the clinician or researcher if literacy is a problem. Scores of 8 or more is indicative of harmful alcohol consumption. Scores of 13 or more are indicative of possible alcohol dependence. The AUDIT is in the public domain, may be used without cost, with appropriate acknowledgement of the source.

Key reference

Saunders et al. (1993).

9.2.2   CAGE

What is it?

The CAGE is a brief four-item screener for lifetime alcohol abuse and dependence. Questions refer to whether behaviours have ever occurred. As such, it is not a specific screener for current alcohol problems. The title is an acronym of the first letters of the four symptoms of alcohol dependence that are addressed in the four questions: cutdown, annoyed, guilty, eyeopener. Answers of 'yes' to two or more questions are indicative of a need to further clinical testing for abuse and dependence.

When would I use it?

The CAGE is not by definition a diagnostic test. Rather it is used to determine whether further testing for alcohol dependence is necessary. It can also be used as a continuous measure in studies that wish to have a quick measure of levels of alcohol problems.

How is it administered?

The CAGE can be administered by the clinician or researcher, and takes less than a minute to administer. It can also be self-completed by the interviewee. The CAGE is in the public domain, may be used without cost, with appropriate acknowledgement of the source.

Key reference

Ewing (1984).

9.2.3 Drug Abuse Screening Test

What is it?

The Drug Abuse Screening Test (DAST) is a 20-item scale for measuring the presence of drug abuse problems over the preceding 12 months, and specifically relates to substances other than alcohol. It specifically covers both licit and illicit substances other than alcohol. The scale addresses aspects of substance dependence such as withdrawal as well as social and emotional problems related to substance use.

When would I use it?

The DAST is primarily a clinical tool used to screen for the presence of substance use problems. There is no reason, however, that it could not be used as a continuous measure of problem severity for research purposes.

How is it administered?

The DAST can be self-completed, or administered by the interviewer, and takes approximately 5 minutes to complete. Higher scores indicate greater problem severity. A cut-off of 5/6 is recommended as indicative of the presence of substance use disorders. The DAST is in the public domain, may be used without cost, with appropriate acknowledgement of the source.

Key reference

Gavin et al. (1989).

9.2.4 Michigan Alcohol Screening Test

What is it?

The Michigan Alcohol Screening Test (MAST) is a 24-item screening instrument to detect the presence of lifetime alcohol abuse or dependence. It does not measure the quantity of frequency of drinking, but addresses a range of social and personal problems associated with alcohol use. There is no time frame on the occurrence of alcohol-related problems, and no onset or recency data.

When would I use it?

The MAST is essentially a clinical tool used to screen for the presence of lifetime alcohol abuse or dependence. The absence of a time frame for the scale severely limits its utility as a research instrument. It would not be an appropriate instrument to examine change over time, for instance. Total score could be used for research purposes, however, if lifetime severity is the variable of interest.

How is it administered?

The MAST is self-administered and takes approximately 5–10 minutes to complete. It could be administered by the interviewer if necessary. A cut-off score of 13 is recommended as indicative of the presence of alcohol abuse or dependence. The MAST is in the public domain, may be used without cost, with appropriate acknowledgement of the source.

Key reference

Selzer (1971).

9.3 Frequency of substance use

The core business of any drug and alcohol researcher, or clinician, is to obtain accurate measures of current consumption. This is not a simple task, as use patterns vary, and a variety of methods have been employed.

9.3.1 Addiction Severity Index

What is it?

The alcohol and drug information section of the Addiction Severity Index (ASI). The section measures consumption in the preceding 30 days, lifetime years of regular use and route of administration. For recent consumption, for each substance the number of use days over the preceding 30 days is obtained. Substances measured are alcohol, heroin, methadone, other opiates/analgesics, barbiturates, benzodiazepine, cocaine, methamphetamine, cannabis, hallucinogens, inhalants and polydrug use. Alcohol is recorded as number of use days and number of days upon which the person drank to intoxication.

When would I use it?

Clearly, such a measure has both clinical and research uses. The section would be of use in any study where a quick assessment of use across a range of drug classes is required, and where the amount used on any day is not of critical importance. The 1-month window period makes the ASI ideal for longitudinal research.

How is it administered?

The ASI is interviewer-administered and the alcohol and drug use section and takes approximately 10 minutes to administer. The ASI is in the public domain, may be used without cost, with appropriate acknowledgement of the source.

Key reference

McLellan et al. (1980).

9.3.2   Opiate Treatment Index

What is it?

The drug use section of the Opiate Treatment Index (OTI), a multi-dimensional instrument for measuring drug use and drug-related problems (see below). The section measures consumption over the preceding month of heroin, other opiates, alcohol, cannabis, amphetamines, cocaine, benzodiazepines, barbiturates, hallucinogens, inhalants and tobacco. For each substance, participants are asked about their three most recent use days. Data are collected on the number of 'use episodes' on each day (e.g. number of heroin injections), and the interval between the use days is recorded. A measure of consumption across the month is made on the basis of consumption on the two most recent days and the two most recent intervals between use days.

When would I use it?

The drug use section is an ideal instrument in any study that requires measures of recent consumption across a range of substances. The 1-month recall period means that it has both cross-sectional and longitudinal utility. The recent used episode of methodology also provides data on actual consumption on the most recent episodes of use across a range of substances.

How is it administered?

The drug use scale is interviewer administered, and may be used independently of the rest of the OTI. It takes approximately 10 minutes to complete. The OTI is available from the National Drug and Alcohol Research Centre (University of New South Wales) for a nominal fee.

Key reference

Darke et al. (1991).

9.3.3   Quantity frequency measures

What is it?

Quantity frequency (QF) measures are used to obtain 'average' levels of consumption, and were developed in relation to alcohol. They typically ask about (a) the average number of days in a specified period upon which alcohol was consumed and (b) the number of drinks that are consumed on an average use day. The QF methodology thus does not measure actual consumption on any one day, and is not sensitive to binge use (although this presents a major problem for all consumption measures). The method relies upon the individual being able to make estimates of what is 'average' for them in terms of frequency, and level, of consumption.

When would I use it?

The QF method can be used by clinicians or researchers who wish to obtain very quick measures of recent average consumption. Whilst developed for alcohol, there is no reason why the method cannot be applied to the use of other drugs. The specification of a recall period makes the methodology suitable for longitudinal research.

How is it administered?

QF measures may be administered by the interviewer or self-administered. Essentially, QF measures consist of the two questions presented above that give average interval and average consumption on use days. The administration time is less than a minute for a single substance. QF measures are in the public domain, may be used without cost, with appropriate acknowledgement of the source.

Key reference

Allen and Wilson (2003).

9.3.4 Timeline Follow-Back Method

What is it?

The Timeline Follow-Back Method (TFBM) is a means of obtaining detailed information on drinking across a specified period, usually the preceding 3 months. The methodology is based on a calendar that is used by the interviewer and participant to estimate the amount of alcohol consumed on each drinking occasion over the specified study period. In order to assist memory for these events, a series of key markers are identified over the study period, for example birthdays, and holidays that serve as anchor points for recall.

When would I use it?

The TFBM has both clinical and research utility. The major use of the methodology is when particularly 'fine-grained' detail of drinking patterns is required. Thus, the methodology has the potential to measure drinking patterns and triggers for drinking. The fact that the TFBM examines a specified period means that it can be used in longitudinal research such as alcohol treatment outcome research.

How is it administered?

The TFBM is interviewer-administered as a paper and pen version, or can be administered as a self-completed computer interview. The TFBM takes approximately 30 minutes to administer. The TFBM is available from Centre for Addiction and Mental Health, 33 Russell St, Ontario, Canada, M5S 2S1.

Key reference

Sobell and Sobell (1995).

9.4 Multi-dimensional scales

It is rare in addictions research (or in clinical practice) that a single measure is required. Generally, and particularly in treatment outcome studies, a range of different domains need to be measured. In response to this need, a number of multi-dimensional scales have been developed that cover consumption and a range of drug-related problems. Such scales are typically designed so that subsections of the parent instrument can be independently administered, if all the outcome domains are not of relevance.

9.4.1 Addiction Severity Index

What is it?

The Addiction Severity Index (ASI) is a multi-dimensional structured interview that examines recent substance use and a range of drug-related outcome domains: alcohol use, drug use, medical problems, psychiatric problems, family/social problems, employment and legal problems. All domains measure problem severity over the month preceding interview. The ASI is not substance specific, so it can be used to obtain a clinical picture with users of any psychoactive substance.

When would I use it?

The ASI has excellent clinical and research utility. It provides a comprehensive clinical profile of problem severity, using continuous measures, across a range of outcome domains. The fact that it has a 30-day time frame makes it an ideal tool for longitudinal research, such as treatment outcome trials. It is not necessary to administer the entire ASI if it is not required, as the individual subscales stand alone, and they may be administered separately.

How is it administered?

The ASI is interviewer-administered and takes approximately 30–60 minutes to administer. Higher scores in any domain are indicative of higher levels of problem severity within that domain. The ASI is in the public domain, may be used without cost, with appropriate acknowledgement of the source.

Key reference

McLellan et al. (1980).

9.4.2 Comprehensive Drinker Profile

What is it?

The Comprehensive Drinker Profile (CDP) is a structured interview that measures lifetime drinking histories, drinking patterns and alcohol-related problems and motivation for treatment.

When would I use it?

The CDP is an excellent clinical and research tool. It provides comprehensive data on the history of drinking, patterns of alcohol consumption and alcohol-related problems. It can be used in both cross-sectional and longitudinal studies. The current consumption measure examines drinking in the preceding 3 months. It is particularly relevant to studies that require a detailed picture of lifetime drinking history.

How is it administered?

The CDP is interviewer-administered and takes approximately 2 hours to complete.

Key reference

Miller and Marlett (1984).

9.4.3 Maudsley Addiction Profile

What is it?

The Maudsley Addiction Profile (MAP) is a brief, structured interview for treatment outcome research. The MAP measures problems in four domains: substance use, health risk behaviour, physical/psychological health and personal/social functioning. Questions relate to the 30 days preceding interview.

When would I use it?

The MAP was designed as a tool for longitudinal research, with 30-day recall periods. Like the ASI and OTI, it thus presents a 'snapshot' of the individual over the preceding month. It is ideal for treatment outcome research, its original purpose. It can also be used, however, to provide a comprehensive measure of current drug use and related problems in cross-sectional studies.

How is it administered?

The MAP is interviewer-administered and takes approximately 15 minutes to complete. Higher scores indicate higher levels of problem severity. The MAP is in the public domain, may be used without cost, with appropriate acknowledgement of the source.

Key reference

Marsden et al. (1998).

9.4.4 Opiate Treatment Index

What is it?

The Opiate Treatment Index (OTI) is a multi-dimensional structured interview that examines recent substance use and a range of drug-related outcome domains. The OTI examines recent drug use, needle and sexual risk-taking behaviours, crime, social functioning, physical health and psychological distress. Psychological distress is measured using the General Health Questionnaire 28-item version (Goldberg & Williams, 1988). As with the ASI, domains measure problem severity over the month preceding interview. The exception to this is the social functioning scale, which addresses the preceding 6 months, as changes in this domain are substantially slower than in other domains. While the OTI was originally designed, as the name suggests, for opiate users, it is not drug specific and can be used for all substances, although its greatest utility is for illicits.

When would I use it?

The primary use of the OTI is as a research tool, although it has been used clinically. It may be used for both cross-sectional and longitudinal research. In terms of cross-sectional research, the OTI gives a broad 'snapshot' of the current drug use and drug-related problems of the interviewee. The 1-month time frame means that it is sensitive to changes in behaviour over time, and may be used as a pre-post measure of treatment effectiveness.

How is it administered?

The OTI is interviewer-administered and takes approximately 30–40 minutes to administer. Higher scores in any domain are indicative of higher levels of problem severity within that domain. Individual subscales may be independently administered. The OTI is available from the National Drug and Alcohol Research Centre (University of New South Wales) for a nominal fee.

Key reference

Darke et al. (1992).

9.5 Dependence

The concept of a dependence syndrome was first postulated in relation to alcohol by Edwards and Gross (1976). Dependence was conceptualised as a cluster of symptoms derived for a single syndrome relating to the 'drive' for alcohol. The success of the concept led to the expansion of the dependence syndrome to substances other than alcohol (Edwards et al. 1981). Substance dependence is defined by DSM IV (American Psychiatric Association, 2000) as a maladaptive pattern of substance use, leading to clinically significant impairment or distress, as manifested by three (or more) of the following symptoms, occurring at any time in the same 12-month period: (1) tolerance; (2) withdrawal; (3) the substance is often taken in larger amounts or over a longer period than was intended; (4) there is a persistent desire or unsuccessful efforts to cut down or control substance use; (5) a great deal of time is spent in activities necessary to obtain the substance, use the substance or recover from its effects; (6) important social, occupational or recreational activities are given up or reduced because of substance use; (7) substance use is continued despite knowledge of having a persistent or recurrent physical or psychological problem that is likely to have been caused or exacerbated by the substance. Dependence scales typically address all, or components, of the symptomatology of the dependence syndrome.

9.5.1 Short Alcohol Dependence data

What is it?

The Short Alcohol Dependence Data (SADD) is a 15-item scale that measures the severity of alcohol dependence. The scale focuses on attitudes and behaviours surrounding alcohol use, such as the salience of alcohol to the individual, loss of control and an inability to cut down on consumption. Questions specifically refer to the person's *most recent* drinking habits, so it is a measure of current alcohol dependence.

When would I use it?

The SADD has both clinical and research applications. Clinical utility relates to cut-off scores for low, medium and high dependence. The SADD also provides a continuous measure of levels of dependence that can be used in research as either an outcome or predictor variable. The fact that the scale focuses on the most recent drinking habits indicates that the scale could be used in longitudinal research to measure changes in levels of dependence over time.

How is it administered?

The SADD is typically self-administered and takes approximately 5 minutes to complete. It can also be interviewer-administered if necessary. Higher scores indicate higher levels of dependence. Scores of 10–19 indicate medium levels of dependence and 20 or more of severe dependence. The SADD is in the public domain, may be used without cost, with appropriate acknowledgement of the source.

Key reference

Raistraick et al. (1983).

9.5.2   Composite International Diagnostic Instrument – Substance Abuse Module

What is it?

The Composite International Diagnostic Instrument – Substance Abuse Module (CIDI-SAM) is a structured psychiatric interview developed by the World Health Organization (WHO), and is used to obtain DSM IV and ICD 10 diagnoses of substance abuse and dependence, the diagnoses including onset and recency data. Diagnoses may be obtained for alcohol, opioids, psychostimulants, cannabis and benzodiazepines.

When would I use it?

The CIDI-SAM has obvious uses as a clinical tool to obtain formal psychiatric diagnoses of abuse and dependence. It is also an excellent research tool, as trained research staff who are not psychiatrists may administer it to obtain formal diagnoses. It is useful in any study of dependence and of multiple substance dependence in particular. Onset data mean that studies can examine the age of onset of dependence, and recency data enable current and lifetime diagnosis to be made. Recency data mean that it can be used in longitudinal studies of substance dependence, onset and recency data

How is it administered?

The CIDI is exclusively interviewer-administered and requires training from a WHO-accredited centre in order to be permitted to administer the instrument. It can be administered either by paper and pencil or by computer. The complete CIDI-SAM takes approximately 20 minutes to complete.

One of the major advantages of the CIDI-SAM is that it does not have to be administered by a psychiatrist, but provides formal psychiatric diagnoses. The CIDI is not in the public domain. It must be obtained through a WHO-accredited training centre.

Key reference

Cottler et al. (1989).

9.5.3 Leeds Dependence Questionnaire

What is it?

The Leeds Dependence Questionnaire (LDQ) is a ten-item measure of current psychological substance dependence that measures dependence over the preceding week. It is a non-specific measure that can be used to examine current levels of dependence upon any psychoactive substance. While it was originally designed for use with alcohol and opioids, the scale could be used for any substance.

When would I use it?

The LDQ is a quickly administered research tool. It can be used in any study that requires a continuous measure of levels of substance dependence. The LDQ, with its focus on dependence over the preceding week, is particularly well suited to examining changes in levels of dependence across time. It is thus ideally suited to treatment outcome studies.

How is it administered?

The LDQ is generally self-completed, although interviewer administration is possible. Scores are continuous, with higher scores indicating higher levels of dependence. To date, there are no cut-off scores derived from studies to indicate dependence on any particular substance. The LDQ is in the public domain, may be used without cost, with appropriate acknowledgement of the source.

Key reference

Raistrick et al. (1994).

9.5.4 Severity of Dependence Scale

What is it?

The Severity of Dependence Scale (SDS) is a five-item scale that measures levels of current psychological dependence on psychoactive substances, that measures dependence over the preceding 12 months. The scale was originally a component of the Severity of Opiate Dependence Questionnaire (SODQ; Sutherland et al., 1986). The questions address issues of control over substance use. There are no questions relating to psychological dependence. One of the major advantages of the SDS is that is non-specific test. While it was originally designed to form a component of the SODQ, it can be used to measure dependence on any substance. Thus, in addition to heroin dependence, it has been used to measure current dependence on methamphetamine, cocaine, alcohol and benzodiazepines.

When would I use it?

The primary use of the SDS has been in research. It provides a continuous measure of dependence that can be used as an outcome measure or as a predictor variable. It can also be used to screen for probable clinical dependence using cut-offs specific to a particular substance determined through receiver operating characteristic analyses. The fact that the SDS is time anchored means that it can be used to measure change over time in levels of dependence (e.g. to examine the efficacy of treatment in reducing levels of dependence).

How is it administered?

The SDS takes approximately 1–2 minutes to complete. It can be self-completed by the interviewee or administered by the interviewer. Higher scores are indicative of higher levels of dependence. Cut-off scores indicative of dependence have been determined for methamphetamine (Topp & Mattick, 1997), cocaine (Kaye & Darke, 2002) and benzodiazepines (Ross & Darke, 2000). The SDS is in the public domain, may be used without cost, with appropriate acknowledgement of the source.

Key reference

Gossop et al. (1995).

9.5.5 Severity of Alcohol Dependence Questionnaire

What is it?

The Severity of Alcohol Dependence Questionnaire (SADQ) is a 20-item scale that measures the severity of alcohol dependence over the preceding 6 months. The scale has subscales that address physical withdrawal, affective withdrawal symptoms, craving and withdrawal relief drinking, consumption and reinstatement. The scale has also items that address heavy consumption.

When would I use it?

The scale has clinical and research utility. As a clinical scale it provides a measure of dependence severity and a clinical profile of symptom presentation. As a research tool, it provides a continuous measure of severity that can be used as an outcome or predictor variable. The 6-month time frame means that the instrument is appropriate for longitudinal research examining changes in dependence severity over time, such as treatment outcome studies.

How is it administered?

The SADQ is generally self-competed and takes 5–10 minutes to complete. It can also be interviewer administered. A cut-off of 30 is recommended as indicative of severe dependence. The SADQ is in the public domain, may be used without cost, with appropriate acknowledgement of the source.

Key reference

Stockwell et al. (1994).

9.5.6   Severity of Opiate Dependence Questionnaire

What is it?

The SODQ was developed as an analogue of the SADQ, and is a measure of the degree of opiate dependence. It is a five-section, 21-item scale that measures dependence in '*a recent month when you were using opiate heavily …*'. Its structure is similar to the SADQ, with sections that address physical withdrawal, affective withdrawal symptoms, craving and withdrawal relief drug taking, consumption and reinstatement.

When would I use it?

The SODQ provides a clinical profile of patients in their heavy periods of opiate use. As a research tool, it provides a continuous measure of severity that can be used as an outcome or predictor variable, if a typical heavy-use period is the period of interest. The absence of a specific time restricts research utility, as it is essentially a measure of a 'heavy period'. It is thus not appropriate for longitudinal research, as it cannot examine changes in dependence severity over time. The absence of a time frame also means that cross-sectional studies that require measures of current dependence could not use the instrument.

How is it administered?

The SODQ is generally self-competed and takes 5–10 minutes to complete. It can also be interviewer-administered. To date, there is no formal cut-off score indicative of dependence. It is thus solely a continuous measure of dependence. The SODQ is in the public domain, may be used without cost, with appropriate acknowledgement of the source.

Key reference

Sutherland et al. (1986).

9.6   Psychopathology

Rates of psychopathology are high amongst dependent substance users across the board (cf. Wilcox et al., 2004; Darke et al., 2008). One of the major aims of substance treatment programmes is to reduce the levels of psychological distress experienced by patients. A large number of well-validated tools exist that address specific types of pathology, such as depression or anxiety, or provide global measures of distress.

9.6.1   Beck Depression Inventory

What is it?

The most commonly used self-report measure of current depression. It is composed of 21 items that address symptoms of depression as defined by DSM IV (American Psychiatric Association, 2000), such as pessimism, suicide ideation and guilt. The window period for the scale is the preceding 2 weeks.

When would I use it?

The Beck Depression Inventory (BDI) is an excellent clinical and research tool in any study where depression is of interest. It gives classifications of depression severity, which may be of clinical or research interest. The fact that the window period is 2 weeks means that the scale is ideal for longitudinal research tracking changes in levels of depression across time.

How is it administered?

The BDI is a self-completion tool that takes approximately 5 minutes to complete. It may also be interviewer-administered, but this will increase the time to administer, as response options must be read out. Scores of 10–18 indicate mild–moderate depression, 19–29 moderate–severe depression and 30 or more extremely severe depression. The BDI is copyright protected and is available from the Psychological Corporation.

Key reference

Beck et al. (1996).

9.6.2   Brief Symptom Inventory

What is it?

The Brief Symptom Inventory (BSI) is the short version of the Symptom Checklist 90-Revised (SCL-R-90). The BSI consists of 53 items covering nine symptom dimensions: somatisation, obsession-compulsion, interpersonal sensitivity, depression, anxiety, hostility, phobic anxiety, paranoid ideation and psychoticism. In addition to scores on individual dimensions, the BSI generates three global indices of distress: Global Severity Index, Positive Symptom Distress Index, and Positive Symptom Total. The recall period is the week preceding interview.

When would I use it?

The number of dimensions covered by the BSI makes it an ideal instrument for researchers wishing to obtain measures over a range of different forms of psychopathology in a short period. The 1-week recall period means that it is suitable for longitudinal research.

How is it administered?

The BSI is generally self-completed, but may be interviewer administered. It takes approximately 10 minutes to complete. Higher scores in any dimension indicate higher levels of pathology. The BSI is copyright protected, and may be purchased from National Computer Systems, Inc., Minneapolis, USA.

Key reference

Derogatis (1993).

9.6.3   Composite International Diagnostic Instrument (CIDI)

The Composite International Diagnostic Instrument (CIDI) is a structured psychiatric interview developed by the WHO, and is used to obtain DSM IV and ICD 10 psychiatric diagnoses, for example major depression and social phobia. All diagnoses include onset and recency data.

When would I use it?

The CIDI has obvious uses as a clinical tool to obtain formal psychiatric diagnoses of abuse and dependence. It is also an excellent research tool, as trained research staff who are not psychiatrists may administer it to obtain formal diagnoses. It is useful in any study where formal diagnoses are required, rather than continuous measures. Onset data mean that studies can examine the age of onset of pathology, and recency data enable current and lifetime diagnosis to be made. Recency data mean that it can be used in longitudinal studies.

How is it administered?

The CIDI is exclusively interviewer-administered, and requires training from a WHO-accredited centre in order to be permitted to administer the instrument. It can be administered either by paper and pencil or by computer. The complete CIDI takes approximately several hours to complete. One of the major advantages of the CIDI is that it does not have to be administered by a psychiatrist, but provides formal psychiatric diagnoses. The CIDI is not in the public domain. It must be obtained through a WHO-accredited training centre.

Key reference

World Health Organization (1993).

9.6.4   General Health Questionnaire

What is it?

The General Health Questionnaire (GHQ) is a global measure of current, non-psychotic, psychological distress. It comes in a variety of forms, including 60, 30, 28 and 12-item versions. The GHQ-28 provides a total score and four subscales: somatic symptoms, anxiety, social dysfunction and depression. The window period is 'the past few weeks'.

When would I use it?

The GHQ is an ideal instrument for providing a continuous measure of current global distress. The 28-item version has the advantage that it also provides data on 4 subscales of distress that may be of clinical interest. The GHQ is also ideal if 'caseness' is required, in addition to the continuous measure. The recent recall focus of the GHQ makes it ideal for longitudinal research on psychiatric distress.

How is it administered?

The GHQ is generally self-completed, but may be interviewer-administered. Administration time is approximately 5–10 minutes. Higher scores are indicative of higher levels of current distress in all forms of the instrument. GHQ items are typically scored dichotomously, but may also be scored as Likert scales. For the GHQ-28, dichotomous scores range from 0 to 28, with 4/5 being the most commonly used cut-off point to determine 'cases' of psychopathology. As noted before, the GHQ-28 provides 4 subtotals in addition to the overall total.

Key reference

Goldberg and Williams (1988).

9.6.5   Social Functioning 12

What is it?

The Social Functioning 12 (SF12) is a 12-item global measure of current psychological and physical health. It is derived from the original version of the scale, the 36-item SF36. The scale addresses health over the 4 weeks preceding interview. One of the advantages of the SF12 is that sample scores may be compared to population norms.

When would I use it?

The SF12 is a quick, reliable instrument of use in any study that is examining global distress. The fact that both physical and psychological health scores are generated makes it a scale of choice in large-scale study measuring a large number of variables. The 4-week recall period makes it an ideal instrument for longitudinal research. The fact that scores may be compared to population norms means that the comparative profile of substance using samples may be compared to that of the general population.

How is it administered?

The SF12 is typically self-completed, but may be interviewer-administered. The SF12 takes less than 5 minutes to complete. Each of the two subscales has a mean of 50 and a standard deviation of 10, with lower scores indicating poorer health. Scores of less than 30 (i.e. more than two standard deviations below the mean) are indicative of severe disability.

Key reference

Ware et al. (1996).

9.6.6   State Trait Anxiety Index Inventory

What is it?

The State Trait Anxiety Index Inventory (STAI) is a continuous measure of current (state) and enduring (trait) anxiety. State anxiety questions refer to anxiety at the time of testing, whilst trait items refer to the general predisposition to anxiety. It is a 40-item scale, with half the items measure state anxiety and half trait anxiety. Separate scores are given for levels of state and trait anxiety. The most recent version of the STAI is the STAI-Form Y.

When would I use it?

The scale is a well-validated instrument for measuring anxiety. The scale would be of use in any study that requires a continuous measure of current anxiety levels and of the general predisposition to anxiety. The state anxiety subscale would be of utility in longitudinal research, although the fact that it refers to anxiety at the time of testing limits its applicability.

How is it administered?

The STAI is typically self-completed and administration time is approximately 5–10 minutes. The STAI is copyright protected and must be purchased.

Key reference

Speilberger et al. (1983).

9.7 Summary

In the preceding sections, we have examined a range of instruments that address screening, drug use, multi-dimensional outcomes and psychopathology. As noted above, the choice of instrumentation will be determined by the research questions being asked and the logistical realities of the research situation. Thus, investigators must decide what domains they wish to measure, whether they want categorical or continuous measures, whether they require formal diagnoses or scale scores, etc. The time available to the researcher to interview will have a major impact upon what it measured. As a general rule, whether in clinical practice or research, it is preferable to use published, validated scales. It is only then that we may have confidence in the data itself. We are fortunate that the field now has an abundance of such instruments from which to choose.

References

Allen, J. P. & Wilson, V. B. (2003) *Assessing Alcohol Problems. A Guide for Clinicians and Researchers*, 2nd edn. Maryland: National Institute on Alcohol Abuse and Alcoholism.

American Psychiatric Association (2000) *Diagnostic and Statistical Manual of Mental Disorders*, 4th edn. Text Revision. Washington, DC: American Psychiatric Association.

Beck, A. T., Steer, R. A. & Brown, G. K. (1996) *Beck Depression Inventory II Manual*. San Antonio: The Psychological Corporation.

Cottler, L. B., Robins, L. N. & Helzer, J. E. (1989) The reliability of the CIDI-SAM: a comprehensive substance abuse interview. *British Journal of Addiction*, 84, 801–814.

Darke, S. (1998) Self-report among injecting drug users: a review. *Drug and Alcohol Dependence*, 51(3), 253–263.

Darke, S., Hall, W., Heather, N., Wodak, A. & Ward, J. (1992) Development and validation of a multi-dimensional instrument for assessing outcome of treatment among opioid users: The Opiate Treatment Index. *British Journal of Addiction*, 87, 593–602.

Darke, S., Heather, N., Hall, W., Ward, J. & Wodak, A. (1991) Estimating drug consumption in opioid users: reliability and validity of a 'recent use' episodes method. *British Journal of Addiction*, 86, 1311–1316.

Darke, S., Kaye, S., McKetin, R. & Duflou, J. (2008) The major physical and psychological harms of methamphetamine use. *Drug and Alcohol Review*, 27, 253–262.

Dawe, S., Loxton, N., Hides, L., Kavanagh, D. & Mattick, R. (2002) *Review of Diagnostic Screening Instruments for Alcohol and Other Drug Use and Other Psychiatric Disorders*. Canberra: Commonwealth of Australia.

Derogatis, L. R. (1993) *BSI Brief Symptom Inventory. Administration, Scoring, and Procedures Manual*, 4th edn. Minneapolis: National Computer Systems.

Edwards, G., Arif, A. & Hodgson, R. (1981) Nomenclature and classification of drug- and alcohol-related problems: a WHO memorandum. *Bulletin of the World Health Organization*, 59, 225–242.

Edwards, G. & Gross, M. M. (1976) Alcohol dependence: provisional description of a clinical syndrome. *BMJ*, 1(6017), 1058–1061.

Ewing, J. A. (1984) Detecting alcoholism. The CAGE questionnaire. *JAMA: The Journal of the American Medical Association*, 252, 1905–1907.

Gavin, D. R., Ross, H. E. & Skinner, H. A. (1989) Diagnostic validity of the drug abuse screening test in the assessment of DSM-III drug disorders. *British Journal of Addiction*, 84, 301–307.

Goldberg, D. & Williams, P. (1988) *A User's Guide to the General Health Questionnaire*. Berkshire: NFER-Nelson.

Gossop, M., Darke, S., Griffiths, P., Hando, J., Powis, B., Hall, W. & Strang, J. (1995) Psychometric properties of the SDS in English and Australian samples of heroin, cocaine and amphetamine users. *Addiction*, 90, 607–614.

Jackson, C. T., Covell, N. H., Frisman, L. K. & Essock, S. M. (2004) Validity of self-reported drug use among people with co-occurring mental health and substance use disorders. *Journal of Dual Diagnosis*, 1, 49–63.

Kaye, S. & Darke, S. (2002) Determining a diagnostic cut-off on the Severity of Dependence Scale (SDS) for cocaine dependence. *Addiction*, 97, 727–731.

Marsden, J., Gossop, M., Stewart, D., Best, D., Farrell, M., Lehmann, P., Edwards, C. & Strang, J. (1998) The Maudsley Addiction Profile (MAP): A brief instrument for assessing treatment outcome. *Addiction*, 93, 1857–1867.

McLellan, T., Luborsky, L., Woody, G. E. & O'Brien, C. P. (1980) An improved diagnostic instrument for substance abuse patients the Addiction Severity Index. *Journal of Nervous and Mental Disease*, 168, 26–33.

Miller, W. R. & Marlett, A. (1984) *Manual for the Comprehensive Drinker Profile, Brief Drinker Profile and Follow-up Drinker Profile*. Florida: Psychological Assessment Resources.

Raistrick, D., Bradshaw, J., Tober, G., Weiner, J., Allison, J. & Healey, C. (1994) Development of the Leeds Dependence Questionnaire (LDQ): a questionnaire to measure alcohol and opiate dependence in the context of a treatment package. *Addiction*, 89, 563–572.

Raistraick, D., Dunbar, G. & Davidson, R. (1983) Development of a questionnaire to measure alcohol dependence. *British Journal of Addiction*, 78, 89–95.

Ross, J. & Darke, S. (2000) The nature of benzodiazepine dependence among heroin users in Sydney, Australia. *Addiction*, 95, 1785–1793.

Saunders, J. B., Aasland, O. G., Babor, T. F., de la Fuente, J. R. & Grant, M. (1993) Development of the alcohol use disorders identification test (AUDIT). WHO collaborative project on early detection of persons with harmful alcohol consumption. *Addiction*, 88, 791–804.

Selzer, M. L. (1971) The Michigan Alcohol Screening Test: the quest for a new diagnostic instrument. *American Journal of Psychiatry*, 127, 1653–1658.

Sobell, L. C. & Sobell, M. B. (1995) *Alcohol Timeline Follow-Back Users' Manual*. Toronto: Addiction Research Foundation.

Speilberger, C. D., Gorusch, R. L., Lushene, R., Vagg, P. R. & Jacobs, G. A. (1983) *Manual for the State Trait Anxiety Index Inventory (Form Y)*. Palo Alto, CA: Consulting Psychologist Press, Inc.

Stockwell, T., Sitharthan, T., McGrath, D. & Lang, E. (1994) The measurement of alcohol dependence and impaired control in community samples. *Addiction*, 89, 167–174.

Sutherland, G., Edwards, G., Taylor, C., Phillips, G., Gossop, M. & Brady, R. (1986) The measurement of opiate dependence. *British Journal of Addiction*, 81, 479–484.

Topp, L. & Mattick, R. P. (1997) Choosing a cut-off on the severity of dependence scale (SDS) for amphetamine users. *Addiction*, 92(7), 839–846.

Ware, J. E., Kosinski, M. & Keller, S. D. (1996) A 12-Item Short-Form Health Survey: construction of scales, and preliminary tests of reliability and validity. *Medical Care* 34, 220–233.

Welp, E. A. E., Bosman, I., Langedam, M. W., Totte, M., Maes, R. A. A. & van Ameijden, E. J. C. (2003) Amount of self-reported illicit drug use compared to quantitative hair test results in community-recruited young drug users in Amsterdam. *Addiction*, 98, 987–994.

Wilcox, H. C., Connor, K. R. & Caine, E. D. (2004) Association of alcohol and drug use disorders and completed suicide: an empirical review of cohort studies. *Drug and Alcohol Dependence*, 76S, S11–S19.

World Health Organization (1993) *Composite International Diagnostic Interview (version 1.1)*. Geneva: World Health Organization.

Chapter 10

BIOMARKERS OF ALCOHOL AND OTHER DRUG USE

Scott H. Stewart, Anton Goldmann, Tim Neumann and Claudia Spies

10.1   Introduction

This chapter reviews the use of state markers for the consumption of alcohol and other drugs in research protocols. State markers are used to estimate substance involvement, regardless of the presence or absence of a substance use disorder. The chapter begins with a discussion of how such biomarkers are used in clinical research involving human subjects, followed by an overview of general considerations pertinent to their validity and interpretation. The latter sections of the chapter are devoted to a discussion of specific state markers for alcohol and commonly abused drugs, which is a dynamic field. We do not review trait markers that indicate susceptibility to drug use (Farren & Tipton, 1999), physiologic markers such as level of response to drug cues (Drummond, 2000), functional magnetic resonance imaging or positron emission tomography (Lindsey et al., 2003), issues that are particularly germane to the clinical use of biomarkers (such as laboratory certification and chain of custody) (Center for Substance Abuse Treatment, 2005), or studies specifically designed to evaluate biomarker validity.

10.2   Uses of state biomarkers in research

As a component of research protocols, biomarkers have been used to describe the study sample, determine study eligibility, assess drug safety, increase confidence in self-report and serve as a primary or secondary outcome measure (Allen et al., 2003). The latter two uses are particularly relevant for epidemiologic or treatment studies, and merit additional consideration.

10.2.1   Increasing confidence in accuracy of reported substance use

In general, the most compelling reason for including biomarkers in addiction research is to increase confidence in other means for measuring substance use, mainly self-report or collateral report. This is a vital role, as estimating the relationship of alcohol and drug use to specific events or the success of substance abuse treatment is prone to several sources of reporting error (Del Boca & Darkes, 2003). These include the specific method of obtaining self-report (e.g. being asked to recall substance use over days vs months), subject characteristics including personal attitudes about the desirability or stigmatisation of continued alcohol and drug use, secondary gains from reporting abstinence such as eligibility for liver transplantation, and the quality of interaction with research staff. This can substantially bias estimates of treatment effects or associations of substance use with outcomes of interest. For example, some evidence suggests that the lower threshold of alcohol consumption

---

Box 10.1 COMBINE study

In the COMBINE study (Anton et al., 2006), a large alcoholism treatment trial, percentage of carbohydrate-deficient transferrin (%CDT) was used to support the validity of alcohol self-report and change in alcohol consumption over time (Miller et al., 2006). Specifically, persons who reported abstinence during the study averaged a 15% reduction in %CDT, while those reporting any drinking had an average increase of 5%. However, since approximately 40% of chronic heavy drinkers do not develop an elevated %CDT, the biomarker itself cannot be used as a sole outcome in alcoholism treatment trials.

---

associated with high blood pressure has been underestimated in population-based epidemiologic studies (Klatsky et al., 2006). Unfortunately, due to inherent limitations in any laboratory test (e.g. limited detection window, less-than-perfect specificity for the outcome of interest), biomarkers usually cannot be used to replace self-report in measuring substance involvement.

When used to increase confidence in self-report, a common approach is to correlate quantitative biomarker results with the reported quantity and frequency of substance use at discrete time points. While this method does not confirm an individual's substance use, it at least demonstrates that those who report heavier use tend to have higher biomarker values. Another similar approach is to compare the amount of self-reported substance use between groups of individuals above or below a certain threshold biomarker value. A statistically significant difference in substance use between these groups increases confidence in self-report (Box 10.1).

10.2.2   Surrogate for reported substance use

State biomarkers for alcohol consumption are typically not adequately sensitive and specific enough to replace self-reported drinking in outcome assessment. However, urine screening for specific drug metabolites is often incorporated into drug treatment studies for this purpose. In some instances, urine screens are performed frequently enough (e.g. three times weekly for a marker with a 24-hour half-life) to trump self-report. However, the period of detection (qualitatively) and the concentration of drug or drug metabolite over time (quantitatively) are not consistent across individuals because the amount of drug used and drug metabolism varies among individuals. Because this renders it difficult to estimate an outcome such as drug use frequency, self-reported amount or frequency of use is still the typical outcome measure. In addition, intentionally diluted urine can provide falsely negative results, although this may be less important in research involving treatment-seeking subjects. When biomarkers are used to overrule self-report, a detailed set of rules must be specified in the study protocol. A good example of this are the rules suggested for cocaine monitoring with urine benzoylecgonine (the major metabolite of cocaine) during treatment studies (Preston et al., 1997). These include the concentration and changes in concentration of the metabolite, as well as urine creatinine to account for the effects of specimen dilution, as summarised in Table 10.1.

Similar rules based on the elimination of other drugs would also be feasible as long as their elimination has been well characterised. The potential also exists to monitor alcohol consumption in this manner (i.e. frequent measurement of minor ethanol metabolites such as ethyl glucuronide). For example, urine ethyl glucuronide has been studied in monitoring impaired professionals use of alcohol (Skipper et al., 2004). Other reports suggest that additional validation is needed before urinary ethanol metabolites are used in this manner (Costantino et al., 2006; Wojcik & Hawthorne, 2007).

Table 10.1 Rules for determining new cocaine use based on urine benzoylecgonine concentration and urine creatinine

Rule	Determining if 'new' cocaine use occurred
Increase in concentration to over 300 ng/mL compared to previous sample >48 hours ago	Concentration exceeds cut-off for positive screen *and* previous specimen >48 hours was less than the cut-off
[a]Concentration decreased to less than one-fourth of concentration in previous sample >48 hours ago	Concentration exceeds cut-off for positive screen *and* is greater than 25% of the prior specimen
Concentration >300 ng/mL in the first urine specimen	If initial specimen exceeds cut-off value, it is considered to represent 'new' use
If previous sample missing, any specimen with concentration >300 ng/mL	If a scheduled urine specimen was not collected, 'new' use has occurred if concentration exceeds cut-off
Creatinine <20 mg/dL is higher compared to the previous specimen	Assume 'new' use if urine creatinine <20 mg/dL *and* the cocaine metabolite/creatinine ratio exceeds that of the prior specimen

[a]Adapted from 'Use of Quantitative Urinalysis in Monitoring Cocaine Use', NIDA Research Monograph 175, National Institutes of Health, 1998.

10.3 General principles when considering biomarkers

Careful consideration of biomarker characteristics and characteristics of the assay employed should be an important component in the research design. Some of these characteristics are listed in Table 10.2.

Knowledge of biomarker characteristics will allow the research team to anticipate the probability of falsely positive or falsely negative test results at a specific cut-off concentration (e.g. to estimate if test results can reasonably invalidate self-report or serve as main outcome variables). As sensitivity decreases, falsely negative biomarker results will increase. Thus, treatment effects may be overestimated, or drug associations with important outcomes underestimated. As specificity decreases, falsely positive biomarker results will increase. At established cut-off concentrations, specificity for substance exposure is generally high for direct measurement of drugs or drug metabolites (i.e. a positive biomarker result is very likely a true exposure). However, many alcohol markers are influenced by other processes (e.g. gamma-glutamyltransferase is often elevated from factors unrelated to alcohol drinking). Sensitivity and specificity must be provided for a defined detection period, which is dependent on the half-life of the marker. In general, the half-life should approximate the desired window of detection. For example, %CDT, with a half-life of about 2 weeks, is useful for detecting heavy drinking in the past 2–4 weeks. Conversely, benzoylecgonine, the major metabolite of cocaine, has a half-life of about 24 hours. As a result, this marker will only detect use in the past 2–3 days.

If a research sample includes subjects with no exposure as well as a wide range of substance exposure at baseline, the concepts of positive predictive value (i.e. the probability that a positive biomarker result indicates real substance use) and negative predictive value (i.e. the probability that a negative biomarker result indicates real lack of substance exposure) should also be considered.

Table 10.2 Factors to consider in choice of biomarkers

Factor	Importance
Characteristics of the marker	
Sensitivity	Probability that the test will be positive in those with the targeted condition. What are the chances of a falsely negative biomarker result?
Specificity	Probability that the test will be negative in those without the targeted condition. What are the chances of a falsely positive biomarker result?
Positive predictive value	Probability that a positive biomarker result indicates actual substance exposure. Increases with the prevalence of substance use.
Negative predictive value	Probability that a negative biomarker result indicates actual lack of substance exposure. Inversely related to prevalence.
Cut-off concentration	In general, higher cut-offs increase specificity and decrease sensitivity. Lower cut-offs increase sensitivity and decrease specificity.
Biomarker half-life	The time required to eliminate 50% of the biomarker. A biomarker is typically detectable for two to three half-lives.
Stability of the sample	Under what conditions is the specimen collected and stored? Under these conditions, for how long will the assay be valid?
Characteristics of the assay method	
Accuracy	The accuracy is the proportion of true results (both true-positives and true-negatives) in the population. An accuracy of 100% means that the test identifies all sick and well people correctly.
Specificity	Is the assay result influenced by other substances that may reasonably be present in the sample?
Precision	Was the assay result stable between different batches in the same laboratory or between different laboratories?
Robustness	Is the result sensitive to slight variations in the conduct of the assay that might occur with routine use?

Positive and negative predictive values are functions of sensitivity, specificity and prevalence of the targeted condition. In relatively low-prevalence populations (e.g. an epidemiologic study involving a general population sample), a positive result is more likely to be a false-positive and a negative result is more likely to be a true-negative. The converse is true for high-prevalence populations (e.g. persons with known substance use disorders such as subjects in a substance abuse treatment trial). The importance of positive and negative predictive value is solely due to the less-than-perfect sensitivity and specificity for virtually all substance use biomarkers (i.e. there is always some probability of misclassification).

Finally, the stability of the sample will dictate how the specimens are collected, stored and shipped to the laboratory. For example, if a biomarker is stable in sera frozen at −30°C for 6 months, it will be less expensive to store samples at the collection sites and send batches to the laboratory at specified intervals.

Characteristics of the assay and assay validation are also important considerations (Peters et al., 2007). Confirmatory tests for substance use generally consist of a gas or liquid chromatography separation phase with mass spectrometry for detection and quantification. These assays are typically validated by analysis of 'spiked' samples containing a known concentration of marker, in animals, or, if not too risky, volunteers consuming a specified amount of substance. Chromatographic and mass spectrometry-based assays may be all that is available for novel biomarkers, but they are often labour-intensive and expensive. However, antibodies are often developed for promising markers, and the confirmatory tests provide the basis for validating less expensive and more generalisable immunoassays. Immunoassays are generally very sensitive but less specific than confirmatory methods, and their use to rule in substance exposure is thus not defensible in medico-legal settings. Validated immunoassays can be used as a screening test to confirm negative self-report, and, if sufficiently specific, their use in ruling in substance use might be considered in research settings. A preferable approach however would be to mirror the medico-legal procedures in performing a confirmatory assay following a positive immunoassay (DuPont & Selavka, 2003).

10.3.1 Laboratory markers of drug use

For detection of drug use, the following body fluids and tissues can be used: blood, urine, saliva, sweat and hair. Urine or hair specimens are often used due to ease of collection (urine) or longer detection windows (hair) relative to blood. In urine, suspected drug use in the previous several days can be detected, while hair, with a growth rate of 1–2 cm/month, provides a much longer window of detection (months to years). The long detection window conferred by hair analysis may be desirable for some epidemiologic studies, but less desirable for shorter-term treatment studies. Conversely, frequent urine testing is useful for assessing treatment outcomes, but the disadvantage of urine analysis is that the sample can be exchanged or manipulated. Drug screening in saliva has been suggested as a preferred alternative (Lillsunde, 2008), but measurement and elimination of drug metabolites from saliva have in general not been well characterised. Sweat analysis is complicated by the sample collection method. Sweat patches are available (Pharmchem, Menlo Park, CA, USA), but they have to be worn at least 7 days on the skin, which may be impractical in most settings. The following section provides a brief overview of the major drug classes and their detection time in blood, urine and hair.

Opiates

Heroin is mostly injected or smoked. The typical start dose is approximately 10 mg and up to 1–2 g in heavy users. Heroin and its metabolites 6-acetylmorphine and morphine can be detected in blood for about 20 hours (Jenkins et al., 1994), and in urine for approximately 11–54 hours (Smith et al., 2001). Heroin and its metabolites are also measurable in hair (Musshoff et al., 2005; Moore et al., 2006).

Cocaine

Cocaine is a crystalline tropane alkaloid that is obtained from the leaves of the coca plant. It can be used through the nose, injected or smoked (as crack). A typical single dose is 20–100 mg. Cocaine and its major metabolite benzoylecgonine can be detected in blood 12–48 hours and in urine 48–72 hours (Hamilton et al., 1977). By hair analysis, a single dose of 25–35 mg administered intravenously is detectable for 2–6 months (Henderson et al., 1996).

Cannabinoids

Most users smoke cannabis as a 'joint', which equals an absorbed dose of 5–30 mg. Tetrahydrocannabinol (THC) has a short half-life and can be detected in blood only 5 hours, while the metabolite 11-nor-9-carboxy-delta-9-tetrahydrocannabinol is detectable up to 36 hours in blood and 87 hours in urine (dose depending) (Huestis et al., 1996). Although hair analysis is also possible for the detection of cannabis consumption, there are some problems, including environmental contamination of hair (e.g. in subjects without THC abuse but who are exposed to the smoke) and a low sensitivity due to a very low incorporation of THC and its metabolites in hair (Musshoff et al., 2006).

Amphetamines

Methamphetamines, amphetamines and methylenedioxymethamphetamine (MDMA) (ecstasy) are usually smoked or ingested as pills. Detection times in blood range from 24 hours for MDMA (Pacifici et al., 2001) to 40–48 hours for amphetamines and methamphetamines (Cook et al., 1993). New testing methods have been described for hair analysis, but methamphetamine detection is difficult due to low incorporation into the hair matrix (Kim et al., 2005). The detection time window in urine is approximately 48 hours for MDMA (Pacifici et al., 2001) and 87 hours for methamphetamine and its metabolite amphetamine (Oyler et al., 2002).

Lysergic acid diethlyamide

The typical dose of lysergic acid diethlyamide (LSD) is quite small (50–100 µg). The detection time in urine is approximately 36 hours, but up to 96 hours for its metabolite 2-oxo-3OH-LSD (Foltz & Reuschel, 1998). Hair analysis for LSD is not currently feasible (Nakahara et al., 1996; Rohrich et al., 2000).

10.3.2   Laboratory markers of alcohol use

While the outcome of interest for drug research is often substance use, interests in alcohol research fall along a spectrum from exposure to chronic heavy use. Accordingly, state markers can be differentiated as acute markers (e.g. direct detection of alcohol and its metabolites) and markers of chronic consumption. These latter markers are often not specific for heavy alcohol use, but can be influenced by other subject characteristics or disease processes. Ideally, markers should show high sensitivity and specificity and discriminate between safe social drinking and heavy, hazardous drinking. Additionally, there are markers of organ damage (e.g. liver enzymes, indices of immune system function, acid–base status or electrolytes). The following sections include a discussion of traditional and novel alcohol biomarkers based on their window of detection. Those with a short detection window are typically markers of recent use, while those with longer detection windows are typically markers of chronic use.

Very recent use (i.e. hours to days)

Ethanol
Ethanol is highly water soluble and is detectable in most body fluids including blood, urine, sweat and saliva. Uniquely, blood ethanol concentration can also be estimated from the breath ethanol concentration. Measuring alcohol in breath and body fluids can be used to detect recent alcohol

intake (Swift, 2003), but cannot discriminate between acute and chronic consumption. The detection time window is limited, with ethanol usually dropping below detectable levels within 8–12 hours of drinking cessation. However, due to its specificity and ease of measurement, blood alcohol concentration (BAC) is often estimated by breathalyser in research settings as a means of confirming reported abstinence in the preceding hours.

Non-oxidative ethanol metabolites

In addition to ethanol, several non-oxidative direct ethanol metabolites are known and each of them has a characteristic detection period in blood and urine after alcohol intake. Whereas ethanol is quickly removed from the body within hours, certain ethanol metabolites can be found in blood or urine up to 5 days after drinking cessation. Thus, they can be used to detect recent alcohol consumption for some time after the BAC itself becomes undetectable. The main metabolites in this class are fatty acid ethyl esters, ethyl glucuronide (EtG), ethyl sulfate (EtS) and ethyl phosphate (EtP).

Fatty acid ethyl esters

Fatty acid ethyl esters (FAEEs) are a group of more than 20 substances which are esterification products of ethanol and fatty acids. Measurement of FAEE in blood plasma is performed by gas chromatography with mass spectrometry (Kulig et al., 2006). The detection period of FAEE after alcohol intake ranges between 24 hours (Doyle et al., 1994) and up to 99 hours in heavy drinkers (Borucki et al., 2007). In addition, FAEEs are also detectable in meconium (the earliest stools of an infant resulting from nutrients ingested in utero) and can be used to detect fetal alcohol exposure. It has also been suggested that FAEEs are involved in ethanol-induced organ damage (Laposata & Lange, 1986).

Although the use of FAEE in blood has been suggested as a short-term marker for alcohol consumption (Doyle et al., 1996), its use is limited by the shorter detection window relative to other non-oxidative metabolites that are primarily analysed in urine.

EtG, EtS and EtP

EtG results from a conjugation of glucuronic acid with ethanol in the presence of membrane-bound mitochondrial uridine diphosphate glucuronyl transferase (Foti & Fisher, 2005). There are diverse methods validated for measurement of EtG in serum or urine: gas chromatography with mass spectrometry, liquid chromatography with mass spectrometry, and liquid chromatography with pulsed electrochemical detection and capillary zone electrophoresis. For urine samples, an enzyme immunoassay is also available (Bottcher et al., 2008). EtG has been receiving increased interest as a short-term marker for alcohol consumption. While EtG in serum is detectable only for about 8 hours (Schmitt et al., 1997), EtG in urine can persist for up to 75–80 hours (Wurst et al., 2000). EtG in urine was shown to be sensitive and specific for recent alcohol intake and is correlated with the amount of alcohol consumed (Halter et al., 2008).

EtS is a newer marker (Helander & Beck, 2004) that has similarities to EtG. However, there are currently fewer validation studies related to EtS. EtS is formed by sulfate conjugation through the action of cytosolic sulfotransferase. Determination of EtS is performed by liquid chromatography with mass spectrometry. The detection window is similar to EtG (Hoiseth et al., 2008).

EtG and EtS are influenced by urine dilution and therefore should be assessed together with urine creatinine concentration. Furthermore, it has been shown that wine contains some EtS and to a lesser extent EtG (Politi et al., 2005). In consequence, the concentration of EtS in urine might be influenced by the type of alcoholic beverage.

For EtP, another direct ethanol metabolite, a detection method by liquid chromatography–tandem mass spectrometry has been published (Bicker et al., 2006). This marker seems to be less sensitive than EtG and EtS, and so far insufficient data are available for estimating its validity.

5-HTOL/5-HIAA ratio

The serotonin metabolites 5-hydroxytryptophol (5-HTOL) and 5-hydroxyindole-3-acetic acid (5-HIAA) are products of serotonin degradation and can be measured in urine. During ethanol metabolism the ratio of these metabolites is shifted towards 5-HTOL, and after alcohol intake the 5-HTOL/5-HIAA ratio increases. The sensitivity of the 5-HTOL/5-HIAA as a short-term alcohol marker is comparable to EtG and EtS in urine, but the time window for detection is shorter (8–12 hours), which is a relative limitation for this marker (Hoiseth et al., 2008).

Recent use (i.e. days to weeks)

Traditional markers

The traditional alcohol markers include gamma-glutamyltransferase (GGT), aspartate aminotransferase (AST), alanine aminotransferase (ALT), carbohydrate-deficient transferrin (CDT) and mean corpuscular erythrocyte volume (MCV). These markers (except for the relatively newer marker, CDT) reflect effects of chronic alcohol abuse on the liver (GGT, AST, ALT) and red blood cells (MCV). They generally require regular heavy alcohol use for a long period (at least 4 weeks and even longer for MCV). The sensitivity and specificity of each of these markers is insufficiently low and ranges between 34–89% and 26–91%, respectively, for MCV, and for GGT 34–85% and 11–85%, respectively (Neumann & Spies, 2003). The aminotransferases (AST and ALT) do not provide further information compared to GGT and are less specific for chronic heavy drinking. The major problem is that these alcohol markers can be influenced by concomitant diseases or medication. For example, hematological conditions such as hemolysis (breakage of red blood cell membranes causing a release of hemoglobin into the bloodstream), bleeding, folate or B_{12} deficiency can influence MCV. GGT can be increased in people with acute liver diseases, obesity, or using certain medications. The aminotransferases are also influenced by liver or muscle diseases. However, one advantage of these markers is their widespread availability in clinical laboratories. They might be used to compare average marker levels in persons exceeding and not exceeding a certain consumption threshold, or as a correlate of reported consumption. In this way they can increase confidence in reported alcohol involvement. Changes in GGT may also correlate with drinking changes during the course of a treatment study.

The relatively newer marker, CDT, results from alterations of the normal glycosylation of plasma transferrin in the presence of chronic heavy ethanol use. Transferrin is a glycoprotein synthesised by the liver and involved in iron transport between sites of absorption and delivery (Flahaut et al., 2003). The necessary amount of ethanol intake to increase CDT plasma levels is about 1000 g over 2 weeks (equivalent to about five to six standard alcoholic drinks per day). The specificity of this marker is higher than that of the other traditional markers, although CDT alone is not sufficient to detect chronic heavy alcohol consumption due to sensitivity of approximately 60%. Although specificity is high, CDT is affected by end-stage liver disease, inherited disorders of glycosylation and female sex hormones (Heinemann et al., 1998; Sillanaukee et al., 2001; Whitfield et al., 2001; Fleming et al., 2004).

The traditional alcohol markers can be used in combination to increase sensitivity and specificity for heavy drinking. In men the combination of three markers (MCV, GGT and CDT) seems to have the best potential, while in women a combination of MCV and CDT is recommended (Rinck et al., 2007). Such combinations can be useful for detecting regular heavy drinking, but are unlikely to detect infrequent binge drinking.

Newer markers
Phosphatidylethanol
The newer marker phosphatidylethanol (PEth) offers the opportunity to detect moderate-to-heavy alcohol consumption during the prior 2–3 weeks. PEth is an abnormal phospholipid (a class of lipids that are a major component of all biological membranes), which is formed only in the presence of ethanol as a product of a phospholipase D-catalysed reaction between phosphatidylcholine and ethanol (Gustavsson, 1995). It was discovered in 1983 in alcohol-treated rats (Alling et al., 1983) and bovine lymphocytes (Wrighton et al., 1983). Measurement of PEth is performed by high-performance liquid chromatography in whole blood (Varga et al., 1998). BAC ideally should have reached zero at the sampling time point.

Several studies have been completed that examined the validity of PEth in differentiating known alcoholics from known abstainers or social drinkers, and evaluated the correlation of PEth with alcohol consumption in heavy drinkers (Aradottir et al., 2006; Hartmann et al., 2006). A daily amount of about 40–60 g ethanol intake (about three to five standard alcohol drinks) over a period of several days seems to be required to increase PEth concentration in blood above the detection limit (Varga et al., 1998). A single intake of even high amounts of ethanol does not lead to elevated PEth concentrations. Depending on the cut-off value, the sensitivity of PEth can reach up to 94%. PEth has also had extremely high specificity in early validity studies (Hartmann et al., 2006), but additional validation in broadly representative samples is needed.

Sialic acids
Sialic acids are small aminosaccharides, which can be found in many human tissues and body fluids. The concentration of total sialic acid is elevated in serum and urine of heavy alcohol drinkers (Sillanaukee et al., 1999). Currently, the diagnostic value of total sialic acid as an alcohol marker remains unclear and further investigation is needed.

Acetaldehyde adducts
Acetaldehyde is the major oxidative metabolite formed during alcohol metabolism. Acetaldehyde–protein adducts (a product of the addition of two or more molecules) are formed from circulating acetaldehyde reacting with plasma and cell proteins. In heavy drinkers, IgA antibodies against aldehyde adducts of erythrocyte proteins were found (Hietala et al., 2006). While few validation studies have been completed, they appear to distinguish chronic heavy alcohol users from abstainers with high sensitivity and specificity.

Use in past weeks to months

Hair analysis has been shown to be a very promising tool for detection of long-term alcohol consumption. Ethanol itself is not suitable for hair analysis due to its high volatility and the possibility of contamination from external sources. However, direct ethanol metabolites are incorporated into the hair matrix. Their detection in hair can be used as a marker of heavy consumption during the prior weeks to several months.

FAEE in hair

Four FAEEs have been identified as the most characteristic in hair: ethyl myristate, ethyl palmitate, ethyl oleate and ethyl stearate (Pragst et al., 2001). Incorporation of FAEE into the hair occurs mainly through sebum, an oily substance which is continuously produced by sebaceous glands in the hair root. Hence, there is a typical increase in FAEE concentration in hair from the proximal to distal shaft (Auwarter et al., 2001). Although during periods of abstinence, no FAEEs are deposited in newly grown hair, it is not possible to make a time-resolved drinking evaluation by segmental hair analysis. Therefore, hair FAEE concentration can only be used as an indicator of general drinking behaviour. Total hair FAEE concentration can be used to distinguish between heavy drinking, moderate social drinking and abstinence (Auwarter et al., 2001). A cut-off value of 1.0 ng/mL has been suggested for detecting heavy alcohol use (Hartwig et al., 2003). In the hair of teetotallers, low concentrations of FAEE can be found, possibly due to external use of alcohol-containing hair care products. Therefore, hair FAEE concentrations up to 0.4 ng/mg do not contradict reported abstinence.

EtG in hair

Like FAEEs, EtG is incorporated into the hair matrix and can be used to detect heavy alcohol consumption during the prior several months. The mechanism of incorporation is not yet clear. A recent study suggested that the major advantage of EtG analysis in hair might be that segmental hair analysis may provide information about time course of drinking behaviour (Appenzeller et al., 2007). Although time resolution is low due to inter-individual differences in hair growth, it is possible to give an overview of the drinking history using an assumed growth rate of 1 cm/month. Furthermore, in this study, EtG concentration was correlated with the amount of alcohol consumption. As this was not found in previous investigations (Yegles et al., 2004), further studies are needed to confirm these findings.

10.4 Summary

Biomarkers can improve confidence in reported treatment effects or the strength of epidemiologic associations with any outcome of interest. Drug metabolites and a wide variety of alcohol consumption markers are available to support self-reported use of substances or, less commonly, to serve as the primary measure of substance use. If biomarker results are used to supersede self-report, the rules for establishing this should be explicit in the study protocol. Drug metabolites in urine are generally useful for determining substance exposure in the past few days, and are a strong complement to self-reported use with frequent monitoring. Hair can be analysed to detect use of many addictive drugs in the past several months, but the detection window is too long for monitoring treatment outcomes in most intervention studies. The choice of alcohol markers depends on research needs such as period of detection and pattern of consumption, and sensitivity or specificity is typically suboptimal for replacing self-reported drinking. Nevertheless, urine testing for non-oxidative metabolites of ethanol may be quite sensitive and specific for estimating any use in the past 1 to 2 days, and markers of moderate to heavy consumption in blood and hair have a role for detecting and monitoring these patterns within the past days to months. The choice of a biomarker should also be influenced by the validation results for the analytical method that will be used for the study – a particularly relevant point for newer markers that are not in general use. For novel markers of any condition or disease process, early validity studies tend to include extreme cases, and initial estimates of sensitivity and specificity are often too optimistic (Sackett & Haynes, 2002). Preferably, markers should be well validated in large populations that include persons with a wide range of exposure and no exposure to the targeted substance.

Excercises

1. Which of these characteristics of a marker or laboratory test is *false*:
   A. Sensitivity = Probability that the test will be positive in those with the targeted condition
   B. Specificity = Probability that the test will be negative in those without the targeted condition
   C. Cut-off concentration = Higher cut-offs decrease specificity and increase sensitivity; lower cut-offs decrease sensitivity and increase specificity
   D. Negative predictive value = Probability that a negative biomarker result indicates actual lack of substance exposure
   E. Positive predictive value = Probability that a positive biomarker result indicates actual substance exposure
2. Which of these alcohol markers is a non-oxidative ethanol metabolite:
   A. GGT
   B. PEth
   C. CDT
   D. MCV
3. Which characteristic detection windows do the following markers have (H = several hours, D = several days, W = several weeks, M = several months):
   PEth in blood
   EtG in urine
   BAC in blood
   EtG in hair
   %CDT in blood
4. Which of the markers listed in question 3 would be most appropriate to compare alcohol treatment interventions in the following settings?
   A. Follow-up on a brief motivational intervention vs. a booklet about alcohol problems in emergency room trauma patients (infrequent, binge drinking)
   B. Monitoring liver transplant recipients for alcohol relapse with frequent vs. infrequent clinical follow-up.
   C. Short-term follow-up on the effects of a pharmacologic stress axis intervention vs. usual care in a pre-operative clinic aimed at minimizing post-operative alcohol complications.
5. Which tissues/fluids can be used to detect recent drug consumption?

References

Allen, J. P., Sillanaukee, P., Strid, N. & Litten, R. Z. (2003) Biomarkers of heavy drinking. In: J. P. Allen & V. B. Wilson (eds) *Assessing Alcohol Problems: A Guide for Clinicians and Researchers*, 2nd edn. Bethesda, MD: US Department of Health and Human Services, National Institutes of Health.

Alling, C., Gustavsson, L. & Anggard, E. (1983) An abnormal phospholipid in rat organs after ethanol treatment. *FEBS Letters*, 152(1), 24–28.

Anton, R. F., O'Malley, S. S., Ciraulo, D. A., Cisler, R. A., Couper, D., Donovan, D. M., Gastfriend, D. R., Hosking, J. D., Johnson, B. A., LoCastro, J. S., Longabaugh, R., Mason, B. J., Mattson, M. E., Miller, W. R., Pettinati, H. M., Randall, C. L., Swift, R., Weiss, R. D., Williams, L. D. & Zweben, A. (2006) Combined pharmacotherapies and behavioral interventions for alcohol dependence: the COMBINE study: a randomized controlled trial. *JAMA: The Journal of the American Medical Association*, 295(17), 2003–2017.

Appenzeller, B. M., Agirman, R., Neuberg, P., Yegles, M. & Wennig, R. (2007) Segmental determination of ethyl glucuronide in hair: a pilot study. *Forensic Science International*, 173(2–3), 87–92.

Aradottir, S., Asanovska, G., Gjerss, S., Hansson, P. & Alling, C. (2006) Phosphatidylethanol (PEth) concentrations in blood are correlated to reported alcohol intake in alcohol-dependent patients. *Alcohol and Alcoholism*, 41(4), 431–437.

Auwarter, V., Sporkert, F., Hartwig, S., Pragst, F., Vater, H. & Diefenbacher, A. (2001) Fatty acid ethyl esters in hair as markers of alcohol consumption. Segmental hair analysis of alcoholics, social drinkers, and teetotalers. *Clinical Chemistry*, 47(12), 2114–2123.

Bicker, W., Lammerhofer, M., Keller, T., Schuhmacher, R., Krska, R. & Lindner, W. (2006) Validated method for the determination of the ethanol consumption markers ethyl glucuronide, ethyl phosphate, and ethyl sulfate in human urine by reversed-phase/weak anion exchange liquid chromatography-tandem mass spectrometry. *Analytical Chemistry*, 78(16), 5884–5892.

Borucki, K., Dierkes, J., Wartberg, J., Westphal, S., Genz, A. & Luley, C. (2007) In heavy drinkers, fatty acid ethyl esters remain elevated for up to 99 hours. *Alcoholism Clinical Experimental Research*, 31(3), 423–427.

Bottcher, M., Beck, O. & Helander, A. (2008) Evaluation of a new immunoassay for urinary ethyl glucuronide testing. *Alcohol Alcohol*, 43(1), 46–48.

Center for Substance Abuse Treatment (2005) *Drug Testing as a Tool Medication-Assisted Treatment for Opioid Addiction in Opioid Treatment Programs*. Rockville, MD: US Department of Health and Human Services.

Cook, C. E., Jeffcoat, A. R., Hill, J. M., Pugh, D. E., Patetta, P. K., Sadler, B. M., White, W. R. & Perez-Reyes, M. (1993) Pharmacokinetics of methamphetamine self-administered to human subjects by smoking S-(+)-methamphetamine hydrochloride. *Drug Metabolism and Disposition*, 21(4), 717–723.

Costantino, A., Digregorio, E. J., Korn, W., Spayd, S. & Rieders, F. (2006) The effect of the use of mouthwash on ethylglucuronide concentrations in urine. *Journal of Analytical Toxicology*, 30(9), 659–662.

Del Boca, F. K. & Darkes, J. (2003) The validity of self-reports of alcohol consumption: state of the science and challenges for research. *Addiction*, 98(Suppl 2), 1–12.

Doyle, K. M., Bird, D. A., al-Salihi, S., Hallaq, Y., Cluette-Brown, J. E., Goss, K. A. & Laposata, M. (1994) Fatty acid ethyl esters are present in human serum after ethanol ingestion. *Journal of Lipid Research*, 35(3), 428–437.

Doyle, K. M., Cluette-Brown, J. E., Dube, D. M., Bernhardt, T. G., Morse, C. R. & Laposata, M. (1996) Fatty acid ethyl esters in the blood as markers for ethanol intake. *JAMA: The Journal of the American Medical Association*, 276(14), 1152–1156.

Drummond, D. C. (2000) What does cue-reactivity have to offer clinical research? *Addiction*, 95(Suppl 2), S129–S144.

DuPont, R. & Selavka, C. (2003) Drug testing in addiction treatment and criminal justice settings. In: A. W. Graham, T. K. Schultz, M. F. Mayo-Smith, R. K. Ries & B. B. Wilford (eds) *Principles of Addiction Medicine*, 3rd edn. Chevy Chase, MD: American Society of Addiction Medicine, pp. 1001–1008.

Farren, C. K. & Tipton, K. F. (1999) Trait markers for alcoholism: clinical utility. *Alcohol and Alcoholism*, 34(5), 649–665.

Flahaut, C., Michalski, J. C., Danel, T., Humbert, M. H. & Klein, A. (2003) The effects of ethanol on the glycosylation of human transferrin. *Glycobiology*, 13(3), 191–198.

Fleming, M. F., Anton, R. F. & Spies, C. D. (2004) A review of genetic, biological, pharmacological, and clinical factors that affect carbohydrate-deficient transferrin levels. *Alcoholism Clinical and Experimental Research*, 28(9), 1347–1355.

Foltz, R. L. & Reuschel, S. A. (1998) Investigation of the metabolism of LSD and the development of methods for detecting LSD use. *NWBR*, 98, 1–29.

Foti, R. S. & Fisher, M. B. (2005) Assessment of UDP-glucuronosyltransferase catalyzed formation of ethyl glucuronide in human liver microsomes and recombinant UGTs. *Forensic Science International*, 153(2–3), 109–116.

Gustavsson, L. (1995) Phosphatidylethanol formation: specific effects of ethanol mediated via phospholipase D. [ESBRA 1994 Award Lecture]. *Alcohol and Alcoholism*, 30(4), 391–406.

Halter, C. C., Dresen, S., Auwaerter, V., Wurst, F. M. & Weinmann, W. (2008) Kinetics in serum and urinary excretion of ethyl sulfate and ethyl glucuronide after medium dose ethanol intake. *International Journal of Legal Medicine*, 122(2), 123–128.

Hamilton, H. E., Wallace, J. E., Shimek, E. L., Jr, Land, P., Harris, S. C. & Christenson, J. G. (1977) Cocaine and benzoylecgonine excretion in humans. *Journal of Forensic Sciences*, 22(4), 697–707.

Hartmann, S., Aradottir, S., Graf, M., Wiesbeck, G., Lesch, O., Ramskogler, K., Wolfersdorf, M., Alling, C. & Wurst, F. M. (2006) Phosphatidylethanol as a sensitive and specific biomarker: comparison with gamma-glutamyl transpeptidase, mean corpuscular volume and carbohydrate-deficient transferrin. *Addiction Biology*, 12(1), 81–84.

Hartwig, S., Auwarter, V. & Pragst, F. (2003) Fatty acid ethyl esters in scalp, pubic, axillary, beard and body hair as markers for alcohol misuse. *Alcohol and Alcoholism*, 38(2), 163–167.

Heinemann, A., Sterneck, M., Kuhlencordt, R., Rogiers, X., Schulz, K. H., Queen, B., Wischhusen, F. & Puschel, K. (1998) Carbohydrate-deficient transferrin: diagnostic efficiency among patients with end-stage liver disease before and after liver transplantation. *Alcoholism: Clinical and Experimental Research*, 22(8), 1806–1812.

Helander, A. & Beck, O. (2004) Mass spectrometric identification of ethyl sulfate as an ethanol metabolite in humans. *Clinical Chemistry*, 50(5), 936–937.

Henderson, G. L., Harkey, M. R., Zhou, C., Jones, R. T. & Jacob, P., III (1996) Incorporation of isotopically labeled cocaine and metabolites into human hair: 1. dose-response relationships. *Journal of Analytical Toxicology*, 20(1), 1–12.

Hietala, J., Koivisto, H., Latvala, J., Anttila, P. & Niemela, O. (2006) IgAs against acetaldehyde-modified red cell protein as a marker of ethanol consumption in male alcoholic subjects, moderate drinkers, and abstainers. *Alcoholism, Clinical and Experimental Research*, 30(10), 1693–1698.

Hoiseth, G., Bernard, J. P., Stephanson, N., Normann, P. T., Christophersen, A. S., Morland, J. & Helander, A. (2008) Comparison between the urinary alcohol markers EtG, EtS, and GTOL/5-HIAA in a controlled drinking experiment. *Alcohol and Alcoholism*, 43(2), 187–191.

Huestis, M. A., Mitchell, J. M. & Cone, E. J. (1996) Urinary excretion profiles of 11-nor-9-carboxy-delta 9-tetrahydrocannabinol in humans after single smoked doses of marijuana. *Journal of Analytical Toxicology*, 20(6), 441–452.

Jenkins, A. J., Keenan, R. M., Henningfield, J. E. & Cone, E. J. (1994) Pharmacokinetics and pharmacodynamics of smoked heroin. *Journal of Analytical Toxicology*, 18(6), 317–330.

Kim, J. Y., Suh, S. I., In, M. K. & Chung, B. C. (2005) Gas chromatography-high-resolution mass spectrometric method for determination of methamphetamine and its major metabolite amphetamine in human hair. *Journal of Analytical Toxicology*, 29(5), 370–375.

Klatsky, A. L., Gunderson, E. P., Kipp, H., Udaltsova, N. & Friedman, G. D. (2006) Higher prevalence of systemic hypertension among moderate alcohol drinkers: an exploration of the role of underreporting. *Journal of Studies on Alcohol*, 67(3), 421–428.

Kulig, C. C., Beresford, T. P. & Everson, G. T. (2006) Rapid, accurate, and sensitive fatty acid ethyl ester determination by gas chromatography-mass spectrometry. *Journal of Laboratory and Clinical Medicine*, 147(3), 133–138.

Laposata, E. A. & Lange, L. G. (1986) Presence of nonoxidative ethanol metabolism in human organs commonly damaged by ethanol abuse. *Science*, 231(4737), 497–499.

Lillsunde, P. (2008) Analytical techniques for drug detection in oral fluid. *Therapeutic Drug Monitoring*, 30(2), 181–187.

Lindsey, K. P., Gatley, S. J. & Volkow, N. D. (2003) Neuroimaging in drug abuse. *Current Psychiatry Reports*, 5(5), 355–361.

Miller, P. M., Spies, C., Neumann, T., Javors, M. A., Hoyumpa, A. M., Roache, J., Webb, A., Kashi, M., Sharkey, F. E., Anton, R. F., Egan, B. M., Basile, J., Nguyen, S., Fleming, M. F. & Dillie, K. S. (2006) Alcohol biomarker screening in medical and surgical settings. *Alcoholism: Clinical and Experimental Research*, 30(2), 185–193.

Moore, C., Feldman, M., Harrison, E., Rana, S., Coulter, C., Kuntz, D., Agrawal, A., Vincent, M. & Soares, J. (2006). Disposition of hydrocodone in hair. *Journal of Analytical Toxicology*, 30(6), 353–359.

Musshoff, F., Driever, F., Lachenmeier, K., Lachenmeier, D. W., Banger, M. & Madea, B. (2006) Results of hair analyses for drugs of abuse and comparison with self-reports and urine tests. *Forensic Science International*, 156(2–3), 118–123.

Musshoff, F., Lachenmeier, K., Wollersen, H., Lichtermann, D. & Madea, B. (2005) Opiate concentrations in hair from subjects in a controlled heroin-maintenance program and from opiate-associated fatalities. *Journal of Analytical Toxicology*, 29(5), 345–352.

Nakahara, Y., Kikura, R., Takahashi, K., Foltz, R. L. & Mieczkowski, T. (1996) Detection of LSD and metabolite in rat hair and human hair. *Journal of Analytical Toxicology*, 20(5), 323–329.

Neumann, T. & Spies, C. (2003) Use of biomarkers for alcohol use disorders in clinical practice. *Addiction*, 98(Suppl 2), 81–91.

Oyler, J. M., Cone, E. J., Joseph, R. E., Jr, Moolchan, E. T. & Huestis, M. A. (2002) Duration of detectable methamphetamine and amphetamine excretion in urine after controlled oral administration of methamphetamine to humans. *Clinical Chemistry*, 48(10), 1703–1714.

Pacifici, R., Farre, M., Pichini, S., Ortuno, J., Roset, P. N., Zuccaro, P., Segura, J. & de la Torre, R. (2001) Sweat testing of MDMA with the Drugwipe analytical device: a controlled study with two volunteers. *Journal of Analytical Toxicology*, 25(2), 144–146.

Peters, F. T., Drummer, O. H. & Musshoff, F. (2007) Validation of new methods. *Forensic Science International*, 165(2–3), 216–224.

Politi, L., Morini, L., Groppi, A., Poloni, V., Pozzi, F. & Polettini, A. (2005) Direct determination of the ethanol metabolites ethyl glucuronide and ethyl sulfate in urine by liquid chromatography/electrospray tandem mass spectrometry. *Rapid Communications in Mass Spectrometry*, 19(10), 1321–1331.

Pragst, F., Auwaerter, V., Sporkert, F. & Spiegel, K. (2001) Analysis of fatty acid ethyl esters in hair as possible markers of chronically elevated alcohol consumption by headspace solid-phase microextraction (HS-SPME) and gas chromatography-mass spectrometry (GC-MS). *Forensic Science International*, 121(1–2), 76–88.

Preston, K. L., Silverman, K., Schuster, C. R. & Cone, E. J. (1997) Assessment of cocaine use with quantitative urinalysis and estimation of new uses. *Addiction*, 92(6), 717–727.

Rinck, D., Frieling, H., Freitag, A., Hillemacher, T., Bayerlein, K., Kornhuber, J. & Bleich, S. (2007) Combinations of carbohydrate-deficient transferrin, mean corpuscular erythrocyte volume, gamma-glutamyltransferase, homocysteine and folate increase the significance of biological markers in alcohol dependent patients. *Drug and Alcohol Dependence*, 89(1), 60–65.

Rohrich, J., Zorntlein, S. & Becker, J. (2000) Analysis of LSD in human body fluids and hair samples applying ImmunElute columns. *Forensic Science International*, 107(1–3), 181–190.

Sackett, D. L. & Haynes, R. B. (2002) The architecture of diagnostic research. *BMJ*, 324(7336), 539–541.

Schmitt, G., Droenner, P., Skopp, G. & Aderjan, R. (1997) Ethyl glucuronide concentration in serum of human volunteers, teetotalers, and suspected drinking drivers. *Journal of Forensic Science*, 42(6), 1099–1102.

Sillanaukee, P., Ponnio, M. & Seppa, K. (1999) Sialic acid: new potential marker of alcohol abuse. *Alcoholism: Clinical and Experimental Research*, 23(6), 1039–1043.

Sillanaukee, P., Strid, N., Jousilahti, P., Vartiainen, E., Poikolainen, K., Nikkari, S., Allen, J. P. & Alho, H. (2001) Association of self-reported diseases and health care use with commonly used laboratory markers for alcohol consumption. *Alcohol and Alcoholism*, 36(4), 339–345.

Skipper, G. E., Weinmann, W., Thierauf, A., Schaefer, P., Wiesbeck, G., Allen, J. P., Miller, M. & Wurst, F. M. (2004) Ethyl glucuronide: a biomarker to identify alcohol use by health professionals recovering from substance use disorders. *Alcohol and Alcoholism*, 39(5), 445–449.

Smith, M. L., Shimomura, E. T., Summers, J., Paul, B. D., Jenkins, A. J., Darwin, W. D. & Cone, E. J. (2001) Urinary excretion profiles for total morphine, free morphine, and 6-acetylmorphine following smoked and intravenous heroin. *Journal of Analytical Toxicology*, 25(7), 504–514.

Swift, R. (2003) Direct measurement of alcohol and its metabolites. *Addiction*, 98(Suppl. 2), 73–80.

Varga, A., Hansson, P., Lundqvist, C. & Alling, C. (1998) Phosphatidylethanol in blood as a marker of ethanol consumption in healthy volunteers: comparison with other markers. *Alcoholism: Clinical and Experimental Research*, 22(8), 1832–1837.

Whitfield, J. B., Zhu, G., Heath, A. C., Powell And, L. W. & Martin, N. G. (2001) Effects of alcohol consumption on indices of iron stores and of iron stores on alcohol intake markers. *Alcoholism: Clinical Experimental Research*, 25(7), 1037–1045.

Wojcik, M. H. & Hawthorne, J. S. (2007) Sensitivity of commercial ethyl glucuronide (ETG) testing in screening for alcohol abstinence. *Alcohol and Alcoholism*, 42(4), 317–320.

Wrighton, S. A., Pai, J. K. & Mueller, G. C. (1983) Demonstration of two unique metabolites of arachidonic acid from phorbol ester-stimulated bovine lymphocytes. *Carcinogenesis*, 4(10), 1247–1251.

Wurst, F. M., Kempter, C., Metzger, J., Seidl, S. & Alt, A. (2000) Ethyl glucuronide: a marker of recent alcohol consumption with clinical and forensic implications. *Alcohol*, 20(2), 111–116.

Yegles, M., Labarthe, A., Auwarter, V., Hartwig, S., Vater, H., Wennig, R. & Pragst, F. (2004) Comparison of ethyl glucuronide and fatty acid ethyl ester concentrations in hair of alcoholics, social drinkers and teetotallers. *Forensic Science International*, 145(2–3), 167–173.

Recommended readings

Neumann, T. & Spies, C. (2003) Use of biomarkers for alcohol use disorders in clinical practice. *Addiction*, 98(Suppl. 2), 81–91.

Fleming, M. F., Anton, R. F. & Spies, C. D. (2004) A review of genetic, biological, pharmacological, and clinical factors that affect carbohydrate-deficient transferrin levels. *Alcoholism, Clinical and Experimental Research*, 28(9), 1347–1355.

Anton, R. F., O'Malley, S. S., Ciraulo, D. A., Cisler, R. A., Couper, D., Donovan, D. M., Gastfriend, D. R., Hosking, J. D., Johnson, B. A., LoCastro, J. S., Longabaugh, R., Mason, B. J., Mattson, M. E., Miller, W. R., Pettinati, H. M., Randall, C. L., Swift, R., Weiss, R. D., Williams, L. D. & Zweben, A. (2006) Combined pharmacotherapies and behavioral interventions for alcohol dependence: the COMBINE study: a randomized controlled trial. *JAMA: The Journal of the American Medical Association*, 295(17), 2003–2017.

Allen, J. P., Litten, R. Z., Fertig, J. B. & Sillanaukee, P. (2000) Carbohydrate-deficient transferrin, gamma-glutamyltransferase, and macrocytic volume as biomarkers of alcohol problems in women. *Alcoholism, Clinical and Experimental Research*, 24(4), 492–496

Chapter 11

QUANTITATIVE DATA ANALYSIS

Jim Lemon, Louisa Degenhardt, Tim Slade and Katherine Mills

11.1 Introduction

This chapter describes quantitative data analysis in an imaginary chronology from planning a study to interpreting the results of the analyses. First is a general look at how quantitative analysis differs from qualitative analysis. We then move through selecting the attributes that are to be measured and the methods of measurement to gathering the data, arranging that data into a format suitable for analysis, cleaning and manipulating it, selecting and performing analyses and finally avoiding some common errors in the interpretation of analyses. It is expected that the aspiring quantitative researcher will not emerge with a detailed knowledge of statistical methods, but rather with the ability to know when to consult statistical references or experts and what questions to ask.

Many of the statistical techniques are illustrated with data from a recent study by Copeland et al. (2007), on taste preferences for beverages in adolescents and young adults. We thank the authors for providing access to the original data. The data simulation in the examples and exercises at the end of the chapter were written in the R statistical language (R Development Core Team, 2008) and SPSS© 'syntax'. R is a free version of the S language and can be downloaded from the internet (http://cran.r-project.org), allowing readers to run some of the examples and experiment with them.

11.1.1 Quantitative data analysis

The quantification of information involves no more than agreeing on techniques for mapping observations onto numeric scales. This can be as simple as defining a standard unit of extent like the meter and applying it to the major axis of the human body, yielding height. Such apparently straightforward data are often misunderstood. People may feel that they understand their own heights, and perhaps summaries like the average height of the population. When faced with the variability of height or its relationship to other measures, the reduction in confidence is obvious. Where quantitative research would objectively measure height, or ask for a self-report, qualitative research might inquire how respondents felt about their height. In the former, a single value is obtained that tells us nothing about the personal meaning of that value, and in the latter a rich account of that meaning may emerge that conveys little about how tall the respondent is. The best place to start thinking about quantitative data analysis is before any data have been collected.

11.2 Imagining data – planning the study

Deciding what to measure and how to measure is one of the most important steps in planning a quantitative study. Not only what is measured, but the observations that are collected determine what questions might be answered in the eventual analyses. A common mistake is to attempt to measure everything. The consequent participant burden can result in poor response rates and unreliable data due to researchers and participants' fatigue. It is best to limit the measures to the smallest number that will answer the relevant questions. If too many questions are being asked, perhaps the research problem can be divided into more manageable stages. If a 'pilot study' (run with a small number of participants to test the procedures and estimate the effect sizes) is necessary, the time and resources are usually well spent.

A pilot study can also provide information about the power of the design. 'Power analysis' is often mandatory when applying for funding, as funding bodies are understandably reluctant to allocate resources to projects that have little chance of achieving their stated aims. Using the same mathematical tools that underlie statistical analyses, power analysis calculates how likely it is that a hypothetical model will survive statistical analysis, given the sample size, estimated size of effect and criteria for significance. In practice, the researcher usually knows (or guesses) the last two and uses power analysis to determine the sample size necessary to achieve a specified power (usually set at 0.8–0.9). In the Copeland et al. (2007) study, 350 adolescents and young adults aged 12–30 were asked to rate how much they liked various beverages on a seven-point scale. In one of the examples, sex differences in the liking for white (made with white spirits like vodka) and brown (made with dark spirits like bourbon) 'ready to drink' (RTD) beverages are examined.

Using the observed differences in means and standard deviations, power analyses showed that the study was unlikely to find any sex difference in preference for white RTDs (0.05), but very likely for brown RTDs (0.9). Most power analyses are much more complex than this, requiring detailed knowledge of the model to be tested, but even a simplified power analysis can indicate that the planned design is inadequate. While the computational formulae for comparing two sets of observations are fairly simple, determining the power of the comparison is more complex, requiring the solution of the function for the model distribution given the constraints of sample sizes, means and variances. Interested readers might wish to consult a comprehensive reference such as Cohen (1988).

Having decided what things to measure, the question of how to measure them arises. An attribute like height is easily quantified, while other attributes like hair colour present more of a challenge. The extent to which observations can be quantified determines whether they can be analysed with different statistical techniques. Most researchers recognise four levels of measurement, each successive level having greater quantitative utility (Stevens, 1946).

11.2.1 Levels of measurement

'**Nominal**' variables carry no quantitative information except that each possible value can be distinguished from the others. Males are different from females, but that difference is not inherently numeric. Nominal variables are usually useful if there are not too many possible values. They are typically used to record categories like male/female.

'**Ordinal**' variables include information about order. In the rating of liking for different beverages, the order of ratings is known, but not the exact intervals between ratings. Ordinal variables can have many values and still remain useful. Rankings like the placings in a sporting event are ordinal variables.

'**Interval**' variables add information about the spacing of the values. If a standard scale of liking was available that had measurable, equally spaced values, not simply indifferent or strongly like, it could measure at the interval level. True interval scales, like the commonly used centigrade scale of temperature, are uncommon.

Finally, a measure like age has not only equal intervals (years) but a well-defined zero (birth in most cultures). Such 'ratio' scales allow the statement that A is twice as old as B. Notice how this rigorous definition has excluded aspects of age like mental development.

It would be simpler if there were ratio scales for all the attributes to be measured in a study, but this is rarely the case. Subjective judgements like preference or craving are typically of ordinal level, and entering the resulting data into analyses that are appropriate for interval or ratio level should be done with caution.

Questions to ask when planning a study:

Will the measures planned answer the questions asked?
Will enough participants be recruited to give a reasonable chance of a reliable result?

11.3 Collecting data – gathering the measurements

A good way to avoid many problems is to have a comprehensive description of the dataset, including the elements shown in Table 11.1. This will allow rapid identification of questionable data. Note that sex is a nominal level measure, while age can be considered ratio. Whenever possible, use values that are easily interpreted, like F for female or Y for yes. It is much easier to spot a Y that has crept into the sex field than the same mistake made with female = 2 and yes = 1. It was once necessary to use numeric coding for categorical measures, but modern statistical applications can automatically convert alphabetic coding and order the categories as the researcher desires. Even if the statistical software requires numeric coding, it is preferable to enter the data in an interpretable format and recode it in the analyses. It is not uncommon for the statistical analyses to be performed by a person who has had nothing to do with the collection or recording of the dataset, and interpretable codes with a good description can spare the statistician much grief.

While on the topic of grief, proper planning of simple things like categories and their codes can avoid subsequent catastrophes in analysis. It does not require years of experience to encounter categories that are not exclusive (0–10, 10–20, ...), not exhaustive (weekly, almost daily, daily) or of inadequate range. The order of codes may not make numerical sense (1 = one or two meals/day, 2 = three or four meals/day, 3 = other) and should be recoded or considered as nominal level measures.

Once the description of the dataset is in hand, stick to it. If modifications must be made during data collection, make sure that this information is added to the description.

Table 11.1 A description of the first few measures of a dataset

Label	Type	Values	Other values
subno (participant ID)	Integer	1–350	—
dob (date of birth)	Date	1978-01-01 – 1996-01-01	Blank = not given; 1997 or later = underage for study
sex	Factor	Male Female	NA = not recorded, not given
age	Numeric	12–29	NA = missing

11.3.1   What application should I use?

Many statistical packages have a data entry mode, much like a spreadsheet, built-in. It is often easiest to use one application throughout the study, although this may not be possible. Web-based surveys, for example, typically collect the data in an online database, and the results must be downloaded and imported into the application used for analysis. Whenever transferring data from one application to another, make sure that the transfer preserves the necessary aspects of the data. This is particularly important when a measure contains values that may be interpreted in more than one way. Missing values may be coded as '.', 'NA' or just '' (a blank field). It is often necessary to specify how such values should be interpreted when importing data. If there is any doubt, create a small 'toy' dataset (see Example 2, Appendix), import it and print it out again. The input and output should match. The dataset used for the examples was initially in the SPSS© format, but required minimal processing to import into R. We have included the code for two of the analyses that were performed for this chapter, and for two examples that illustrate common problems in data analysis. The original R code has been translated into equivalent code for SPSS© and both are included.

Some statistical packages are oriented towards 'point and click' use, allowing the user to select options from a menu structure. The results of the analyses selected are displayed, and may be saved. Others, such as the application used for the examples, are oriented towards 'programming' or writing code that is interpreted to produce the results. The difference is not as great as it first appears, for most 'point and click' applications have a 'programming' mode, and there are 'point and click' front ends for applications such as R. The users should select an application with which they can feel confident in conducting the necessary analyses. It is a good idea to save the 'programming' code for an analysis, as it can be very difficult to recall exactly how some complex analyses were carried out. If the code is available, it will show what was done, and can be modified if necessary.

Another consideration is the ease of performing calculations on the data, such as combining test items into total scores. Only experience with the application will reveal if it is suited to the particular requirements of an analysis. The size of the dataset can make a difference, although the power of modern desktop computers means that any statistical application can deal with thousands of records and hundreds of measures. Finally, there are statistical packages that deal with specialised methods like structural equation modeling. Unless the researcher is familiar with these techniques, it is best to ask for assistance in selecting the analysis and application before proceeding.

11.4   Organising data – structuring the measurements

The complexity of the data collected for any study varies enormously. In the example used to illustrate the description of the measures planned (Table 11.1), only three measurements (preceded by a participant identifier) were included. The dataset from Copeland et al. (2007) included a total of 644 measured and calculated variables. These measures were gathered with different methods in different metrics and often by different researchers. Combining all the measurements together in a structure that will facilitate analysis is not a trivial undertaking.

A typical dataset contains one or more records for each participant. If a participant has more than one record, each of these records may be stored in a separate file. Ideally, each record in a file contains the same sequence of information so that each datum can be identified by its position in a record. If the data are held in a database table, this structure is more obvious, but many datasets are recorded in less structured applications like spreadsheets, where it is easy for individual values to change their position. The importance of this will become clear in the next section.

Attributes (measurements or other observations) form horizontal rows for each instance (participant or case) in the conventional dataset layout. So in the example dataset, the attributes of age, sex, date of testing and so on form a row of values for each participant. The result should be one or more 'rectangles' of data in which each column contains the observations for a single attribute.

11.4.1   Cleaning data – trapping errors before they cause trouble

Converting the information collected in a research study into a format suitable for analysis typically requires processing both electronic and hard copy records. Errors may have occurred in the measurement and recording stages, and these may be compounded with data processing errors. The first step in any analysis should be identifying and rectifying such errors. Hardly any substantial dataset is created without the inclusion of impossible, improbable or suspicious values. Initial descriptions of the dataset that include such summaries as the range of values can quickly identify these values.

Impossible values fall outside the range of values defined for an attribute. An example is a negative height. While impossible values are sometimes used to indicate that a datum is missing, such as a −1 for height, it is much better to use a code or a blank field that cannot produce an apparently valid result in a calculation. For instance, if one of the authors calculates his body mass index with a height of −1, it results in a body mass index of 70, a very obese, but not impossible, value. Dates are usually calculated by transforming a calendar representation to an integer representing time units from an arbitrary zero point such as 01/01/1970. Wildly inaccurate or impossible ages are often produced from mistakes in such calculations.

Improbable values may be harder to recognise, but can lead to the same result. A height of 2.4 m does not appear impossible, but a quick check of a popular reference on such topics (Guinness World Records, 2008) reveals that the current record is 2.36 m, and that particular value should be checked. Suspicious values like a height of 1 m should also warrant a check, although the aforementioned reference informs us that the shortest currently known adult is only 0.746 m tall.

Being within the allowable range is not the only criterion applied in data cleaning. Categorical variables that are coded as integers, but contain non-integer values, may signal misalignment in the data. Misalignment occurs when data values are not in the correct column of the dataset. Assume that two adjacent columns in a dataset contain the age and weight of the participants. A value of 70 would be plausible in either column. The example of a Y in the field that should contain only M or F should prompt an examination of the entire row of data, as one of the more common entry errors is to skip a field, shifting all subsequent fields in that record by one cell.

Questions to ask when preparing a dataset

Are all the values in the dataset plausible?
Have derived measures been correctly calculated?
Could someone not on the research team look at the dataset and understand it?

11.5   Describing data – what do the data look like?

As discussed above, the range of each measure taken can help to identify erroneous values that should be corrected or discarded before any analysis is performed. Most analyses make some assumptions about the measurement levels of the values to be analysed, and this is covered in the sections on types of analyses. Another common assumption is that the values are distributed in a particular way that allows particular statistical techniques to be applied with confidence. Both summary statistics of the parameters of the sample distribution and methods to check how well that distribution approximates the model distribution (the distribution used to analytically develop the statistical method – often the normal distribution) is now discussed.

11.5.1 What is the most probable value? (mean, median and mode)

The **mean** is perhaps the best understood of the summary distributional statistics, and is the estimate of the most probable value for a particular measure. Because the mean is sensitive to extreme values, it may not always be the ideal measure of central tendency. With measures of an ordinal level, the **median**, the value in the middle of the ordered values, is usually preferred as it is less sensitive to extreme values and does not make the assumption that the intervals between numeric values are equal. For nominal variables, the **mode** (most commonly observed value) is appropriate. To see why, consider what would happen if the mean is taken of the numbers representing sex (often coded 1 = male, 2 = female). In Copeland et al. (2007), the mean sex would have been 1.5.

11.5.2 How much does the average observation deviate from the most probable value? (variance)

Once the most probable value has been estimated, attention turns to how the observations deviate from that value. The **standard deviation**, the square root of the **variance**, is probably more useful as a description, but the variance is a fundamental measure in statistical analysis. The **F ratio** is a ratio of variances, and the great majority of statistics and the underlying theories depend on variance and how to allocate it to different subsets of the data. Consider the familiar '**repeated measures**' design in which measurements are made at four separate time points. The observations made over time cannot be treated as independent, for whatever personal factors influence those observations will apply to all time points for any given participant. This typically results in the '**within participant**' observations, having lower variance than equivalent '**between participant**' observations (i.e. in the comparisons between participants in the active treatment vs the placebo groups). A common way to deal with this is to treat the repeated time points as separate variables and assign each one components of the within participant variance. The method by which this is accomplished is somewhat mathematically complex, and the interested reader may consult a text such as Pinheiro and Bates (2000, section 1.3). If the observations seem to be distributed in a way that makes variance inappropriate as a description of dispersion, other measures like the median absolute deviation or the interquartile range may produce a more reliable estimate. As with the mean, samples that are not conveniently distributed call for more robust descriptive statistics.

11.5.3 Are deviations from the most probable value symmetric? (skew)

The distribution of ratings of liking for white RTDs in Figure 11.1 is negatively skewed, meaning that negative deviations from the most common rating tend to be larger and more numerous than positive ones. Skewed distributions often result from restrictions on the values that can be observed. In this case, the negative skew is because liking for white RTDs was generally high, a 'ceiling effect'. Positive skew usually occurs when there is a lower limit, as in the number of standard drinks consumed per drinking session. Many observations are close to zero and the frequency of observations gradually decreases at higher values. Figure 11.2 shows the percentage of 4193 male and female police officers consuming different average numbers of standard drinks per drinking session (Davey et al., 2000).

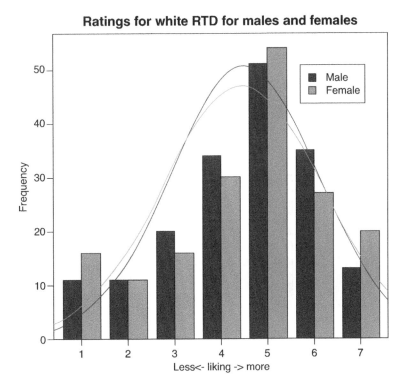

Figure 11.1 Frequency of white RTD ratings.

The normal distribution curves with the approximate means and standard deviations suggest that neither measure is normally distributed. A test of the white RTD ratings showed that they were not normally distributed (Shapiro–Francia $W = 0.9252$, $P < 0.0001$), but the variances of the male and female participant groups were not significantly different (Bartlett's K-squared $= 1.276$, $P = 0.26$).

11.5.4 Are small or large deviations more frequent than expected? (kurtosis)

The final summary distributional statistic to be discussed is kurtosis, a measure of whether large deviations tend to be more (leptokurtic) or less (platykurtic) frequent than in a model distribution having the same mean and variance. Both distributions are somewhat leptokurtic, peaked at the most frequent values and with more observations at large deviations. As with the variance and skew, the kurtosis statistic indicates how well the sample distribution approximates the model distribution. This is an important consideration in deciding what methods of inferential analysis to use. The mean, variance, skew and kurtosis are also known as parameters of the distribution and help to determine whether the sample parameters are close enough to those of the model distribution assumed in a parametric analysis.

11.5.5 Goodness of fit

How well the sample distribution approximates the normal distribution is probably the most commonly sought test of goodness of fit. There are a number of tests and most will be adequate. Recommendations for choosing the most appropriate method for a particular set of values are

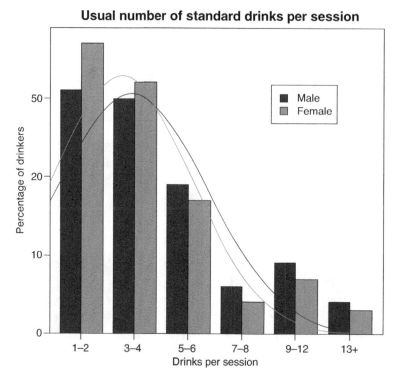

Figure 11.2 Drinks per session.

included in the documentation for most statistical packages and are beyond the scope of this chapter (see Thode, 2002).

The proliferation of statistical methods over the past half-century has reduced the need to use methods based on the normal distribution. Tests based on a number of model distributions are now available, as are methods to check that the sample distribution approximates those distributions. For instance, if a measure is thought to be Poisson distributed, as are certain types of count measures, the sample distribution can be checked and the analysis can be performed in a manner appropriate for that distribution.

If the Copeland et al. (2007) study was intended to be generalised to the entire population of Australia (which it was not), checks would be made that the sample was representative of that population. For example, was the age distribution the same (Figure 11.3)?

Looking at only the age range represented, it is clear that the distribution is far from that of the Australian population ($\chi^2[5] = 60.5$, $P < 0.0001$).

11.5.6 Confidence intervals

When describing summary statistics of a dataset, particularly the measures of central tendency, it is often helpful to include confidence intervals. A confidence interval is an estimate of the range of values that would cover a percentage (usually 95%) of all the obtained summary statistics if every possible sample were taken from the population. The calculation of confidence intervals is very similar to that of inferential statistics like the *t*-test. For example, the confidence interval for the

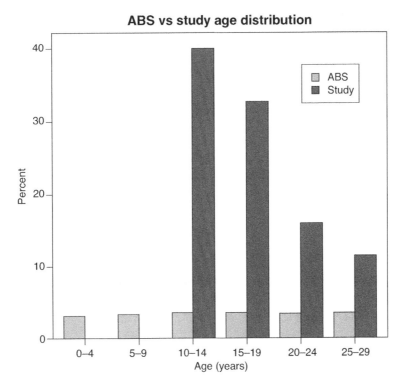

Figure 11.3 Age distribution of the sample.

mean age of the sample in Copeland et al. (2007) is as follows:

$$\langle sample\,mean \rangle \pm 1.96 \times \langle standard\,deviation \rangle / \langle sample\,n \rangle^\wedge 0.5$$
$$18.03 \pm 1.96 \times 5.102/18.708 = 17.5\,to\,18.56$$

This assumes that the sample is normally distributed, which we know it is not. Performing a similar calculation using the actual quantiles of the sample produces the confidence interval:

$$17.7\,to\,18.64$$

Questions to ask when describing a dataset

Are the summary statistics appropriate for the level of the data?
Do the distributions of the data fit the model distributions well enough?
Are the sample summaries concordant with the population that is being studied?

11.6   Manipulating data

The discovery that the obtained data are not ideal for answering the research questions is not a rare event. Fortunately, there are a variety of ways in which the data can be manipulated to be more suitable. The common problem of too many variables will be addressed first.

11.6.1   Data reduction

It is often suspected that an underlying factor influences a number of observed measures. To the extent that this is true, techniques like principal component analysis or factor analysis will show that the measures co-vary, and some combination may be a valid indicator of an interpretable attribute or characteristic of a particular participant. If so, a single component or factor score can be used in the subsequent analyses rather than a number of related scores, improving the power of the analyses.

The analysis in Box 11.1 shows that wine, bourbon, beer and the brown RTD (cola and bourbon) were the most likely to be disliked (PC1), while raspberry soda, chocolate milk and vodka mudshake (chocolate milk and vodka) were most likely to be liked. A possible interpretation would be that PC1 represented the bitterness/strong component of the taste, while PC2 represented the sweetness/light component.

Box 11.1   Principal component analysis of beverage 'liking' ratings

```
R
likenames<-c("cola","white rum","vodka","raspberry soda",
  "chocolate milk","chardonnay","white RTD","wintermelon",
  "bourbon","vodka mudshake","beer","brown RTD")
likelabels<-c("bd1_like","bd2_like","bd3_like","bd4_like","bd5_like",
  "bd6_like","bd7_like","bd8_like","bd9_like","bd10_like","bd11_like",
  "bd12_like")
# use only complete cases for principal components analysis
rtdptlike<-rtdpt[complete.cases(rtdpt[,likelabels]),likelabels]
names(rtdptlike)<-likenames
prcomp(rtdptlike)
                      PC1           PC2            (further components omitted)
cola              -0.1570084     0.22788228
white rum         -0.2764696     0.02747729
vodka             -0.1623065     0.02083041
raspberry soda    -0.1215957     0.42474711
chocolate milk    -0.1983182     0.44657268
chardonnay        -0.3385254    -0.35362899
white RTD         -0.2959564     0.15382449
wintermelon       -0.2811642     0.27005719
bourbon           -0.3803841    -0.13119991
vodka mudshake    -0.2210101     0.35871728
beer              -0.4007043    -0.43472541
brown RTD         -0.4279129    -0.10256455
SPSS
FACTOR
 /VARIABLES bd1_like bd2_like bd3_like bd4_like bd5_like bd6_like
 bd7_like bd8_like bd9_like bd10_like bd11_like bd12_like
 /PRINT extraction
 /EXTRACTION pc
 /METHOD = CORRELATE.
EXECUTE.
```

11.6.2   Calculated variables

Other derived variables can be calculated at this stage. The example of body mass index used above is typical of measures that are calculated from other measures. In the following discussion, a number of variables are calculated to test different hypotheses about the data.

11.6.3   Changing the shape of the distribution

The best way to analyse data that are not normally distributed is to find a model distribution that is approximated and has appropriate test methods. In the absence of such a distribution, the researcher can turn to non-parametric methods that do not make assumptions about the distribution of the values. Failing this, transformations of the observed values may approximate a normal distribution. The most common transformations are based on exponentiation, raising the values themselves to some power (which may be less than one as in a square root transformation) or calculating the logarithms of the values, usually to the natural log base e, or base 10. The disadvantage of such transformations is that any models developed relate to the transformed values. It may be difficult or impossible to translate the interpretation of such models back into the original scale.

11.7   Relationships within the data

The two most common questions in addiction research, and the social sciences in general, are (1) ask whether meaningful differences exist between sets of measurements and (2) the precision of estimates. We can use the simple and intuitive measure of height to illustrate both. Is there a meaningful difference between the heights of men and women? What level of precision may be assumed in the estimate of the mean heights of these two groups, or populations in the technical usage? These two questions are closely related, for the meaningfulness of any apparent difference depends on the precision of the estimates.

11.7.1   Methods for testing relationships between different types of measures

Recalling the discussion of different levels of measurement above, different statistical methods are appropriate for the various types of measures, number of measures to be related, and number of observations in a group of measures.

11.7.2   Relationships between nominal level measures

Strictly speaking, there is no quantitative information provided by the values of a nominal level variable like sex. The attributes of the sexes may have quantitative differences, but male and female are simply categories into which we can place almost all individuals with certainty. A question like, 'Is there a sex difference in the proportion of participants who smoke?' can be answered by testing the two-way classification (or contingency table) of sex and a measure of smoking.

   The answer in the Copeland et al. study was no ($\chi^2[1] = 0.65$, $P = 0.42$). Small counts (less than five) in some cells of the contingency table can be a problem. Fisher's exact test should be substituted for the Pearson chi-squared test in such cases.

11.7.3 Relationships between nominal and ordinal measures

As an ordinal measure contains information about relative magnitude, it is often of interest if the contingency is related to those magnitudes. Here, the question might be, 'Is there a sex difference in the frequency of smoking among the smokers?'

Using a test for trend in the proportions of males and females in each smoking frequency category, it appears that there is no sex difference in smoking frequency ($\chi^2[1] = 0.57, P = 0.45$). The response categories only gave information about the relative order of smoking frequencies, so attempting to assign numeric smoking frequencies was not attempted.

11.7.4 Relationships between nominal or ordinal and interval or ratio measures

Analysis of variance (ANOVA) often tests whether the means of possibly ordered categories are different in the populations from which the samples were drawn. It is known that females prefer white RTDs, while males prefer brown RTDs (White & Hayman, 2006). There was a clear preference by males for the brown RTD in the Copeland et al. (2007) study ($F[1348] = 11.09, P < 0.001$). However, there was no sex difference in the preference for white RTDs. This may indicate that the female preference is due to a relative dislike of the characteristics of brown RTDs rather than a positive preference for the white RTDs.

One possibility is that liking for brown RTDs changes differently over time among males and females. To examine this notion, we can first look at plots of the mean liking by age group and sex (Figures 11.4 and 11.5).

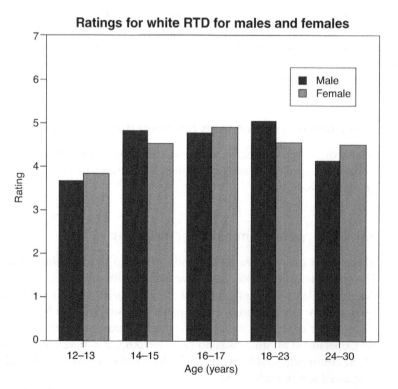

Figure 11.4 Liking for white RTDs.

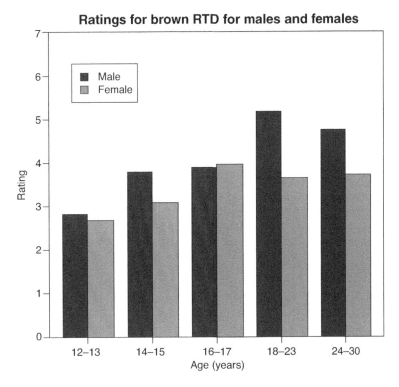

Figure 11.5 Liking for brown RTDs.

The ratings for white RTDs do not show any consistent pattern between the sexes, but males appear to increase their liking for brown RTDs across the age groups more than females ($F[2347] = 17.25, P < 0.0001$).

A topical question is whether the palatability of RTDs is connected with the tendency to drink more heavily (Huckle et al., 2008). As drinking above the recommended limits is often used as a criterion for heavy drinking, logistic regression can be used to determine if liking for a particular type of beverage is associated with this measure of heavy drinking. Copeland et al. (2007) requested an estimate of the number of alcoholic drinks consumed on the last occasion of drinking, so a dichotomous (two-valued) variable can be created, indicating whether males drank more than four and females drank more than two. This will be the response variable indicating heavy drinking. As Box 11.2 shows, liking for RTDs is not associated with drinking beyond the recommended limits ($z = 1.91, P = 0.057$), but liking for spirits is ($z = -3.82, P = 0.00077$).

11.7.5 Relationships between multiple interval and ratio measures

Descriptive analyses of the relationships between interval and ratio measures are often performed with correlation analysis. Use of methods like the Pearson correlation coefficient or t-test should be restricted to measures having a normal distribution. The relationship between sex and beverage preferences mentioned above could have been tested using a non-parametric method. For almost any parametric test like the ANOVA, there is an equivalent test that does not require that the data are distributed in a particular way. Having said this, remember that most parametric test procedures are

---

Box 11.2   Preference for RTDs and spirits and heavy drinking

```
R
# create the "heavy drinking" variable
rtdpt$overlimit<-ifelse(rtdpt$sex=="male",
 as.numeric(rtdpt$lastocc_number) > 4,
 as.numeric(rtdpt$lastocc_number) > 2)
# calculate liking for RTDs by averaging the three ratings
rtdpt$likertd<-(rtdpt$bd7_like+rtdpt$bd10_like+rtdpt$bd12_like)/3
summary(glm(overlimit~likertd,rtdpt,family="binomial"))
Deviance Residuals:
  Min         1Q        Median    3Q       Max
 -1.2729    -1.0682    -0.9107   1.2555   1.6154
Coefficients: Estimate Std. Error z value Pr(>|z|)
(Intercept)  -1.4725   0.6339    -2.323   0.0202
likertd       0.2420   0.1270    1.906    0.0567
SPSS
COMPUTE overlimit = 0.
IF sex = ''male'' AND lastocc GT 4 THEN overlimit = 1.
IF sex = ''female'' AND lastocc GT 2 THEN overlimit = 1.
COMPUTE likertd = (bd7_like + bd10_like + bd12_like)/3.
LOGISTIC REGRESSION overlimit with likertd.
R
# calculate liking for spirits by averaging the three ratings
rtdpt$likespr<-(rtdpt$bd2_like+rtdpt$bd3_like+rtdpt$bd9_like)/3
Deviance Residuals:
Min          1Q        Median    3Q       Max
-1.3279     -1.0411    -0.8364   1.2025   1.7449
Coefficients: Estimate Std. Error z value Pr(>|z|)
(Intercept)  -1.6821   0.4403    -3.821   0.000133
likespr       0.4058   0.1206    3.365    0.000767
SPSS
COMPUTE likespr = (bd2_like + bd3_like + bd9_like)/3.
LOGISTIC REGRESSION overlimit with likespr.
EXECUTE.
```

---

fairly robust, and very large effects will rarely be abolished by using non-parametric test procedures. Applying the Wilcoxon rank sum test to the sex difference in liking for brown RTDs produces much the same result as the ANOVA ($W = 18435$, $P = 0.0008$).

Another important consideration in testing groups of measurements is whether the measurements are independent. Testing the relationship of beverage preference and age as Copeland and colleagues did by employing participants of different ages in a cross-sectional design satisfies the criterion of independence. Testing the same participants as they grow up would not, for beverage preferences persist over time. In a longitudinal cohort design, statistics appropriate for repeated measures should be used.

Questions to ask when examining relationships within data

Have all the defined levels of the measures been sampled (fixed effects) or are there possible levels that were not sampled (random effects)?

Are the observations between different levels of an effect independent or dependent (usually observations made on the same participant across time)?

11.8   Interpreting relationships within the data

Humans have a natural interest in causation as it can afford some degree of prediction of, and control over, events important for our well-being and survival. Thus, we strive to understand causal relationships for our own benefit. It is well known that this can lead to incorrect causal explanations, and so we employ methods to rein in our overenthusiastic causation detectors. The Pearson correlation coefficient is a measure of the extent to which pairs of numeric observations are related. Its minimum value of -1 indicates that each numerically high observation is paired with an equally low one. Its maximum of $+1$ shows that each high observation is paired with one proportionately high. Zero tells us that the pairs have no consistent relationship. Suppose we were to measure the heights and arm spans of a sample of people. The correlation coefficient for these paired measurements is likely to be close to $+1$. Does this mean that height causes arm span or vice versa? Most people immediately realise that this is not so. The growth of the diaphysis (medial shaft) of the long bones in the legs and arms, controlled by human growth hormone, is the major determinant of both. This unmeasured causal factor is responsible for the correlation. Height and arm span are significantly related, but the relationship is not causal (Box 11.3).

11.8.1   Avoiding errors in significance testing

Statistical tests only tell us how unlikely a set of observations are given certain conditions. Null hypotheses almost invariably state that there are no differences between groups, no associations between specified sets of observations or no changes over time. If these hypotheses are sufficiently unlikely given our sample, as in the example of the RTD preferences of males and females, we can accept the alternative that their preferences are different. Research is rarely that simple, and the unexamined application of conventional statistical tests can lead to errors.

It is not uncommon for erroneous conclusions to be made that an association exists, when in fact it does not. This erroneous conclusion has been given the formal title of a **Type I error**. The usual path to this mistake is to perform a large number of statistical tests without adjustment for the number of tests. The ubiquity of personal computers allows most readers to see this first-hand by running Example 1 at the end of the chapter.

Using the conventional critical P of 0.05, two significant differences between the sample means emerged in addition to the one difference that was intentionally created between samples 1 and 6. A variety of procedures have been devised to correct for Type I errors due to simultaneous multiple comparisons. Perhaps the simplest is based on the Bonferroni inequality and involves

---

Box 11.3   Does hair colour influence height?

Measure the heights and arm spans of at least 20 people and calculate the Pearson correlation coefficient. The result will almost always be close to $+1$ and highly significant. As we have seen, this relationship is due to an unmeasured factor that influences both. To gain a better appreciation of the subtlety of unmeasured influences, also record hair colour as blonde/red = 1, brown = 2 and black = 3. In a country like Australia, it is quite likely that you will discover that hair colour is related to height using polyserial correlation (Drasgow, 1986), as one variable is ordinal. Why this is so is usually due to the relationship of hair colour to ethnic background. Australians of northern European ancestry are usually taller and have lighter hair colour than those of southern Asian ancestry. This is an example of confounding. Confounding factors like this must often be controlled in drug and alcohol research to avoid spurious associations.

defining a critical probability by dividing the acceptable probability of error by the number of simultaneous comparisons to be made. This guarantees that the chance of a Type I error is acceptable for that set of comparisons. To see how this works, divide the usual critical probability by the number of comparisons (15) that were made in the example in Box 11.2. This yields a Bonferroni-adjusted critical probability of 0.0033. Using this criterion, the Type I errors produced by multiple comparisons disappear. The Bonferroni correction is quite conservative and can produce Type II errors, or not recognising a relationship that does exist. The only time that the Bonferroni correction is a good choice is when the comparisons have been limited by specifying them before the data are gathered, or when the effect size is so large that it will still produce a significant result, and it is essential to avoid Type I errors. The choice of correction procedure will usually require consulting a comprehensive reference like Toothaker (1993).

The results of a well-conducted quantitative study will survive that most significant test of reliability, replication. Try rerunning Example 1 in Appendix without the set.seed() command that gives the same set of pseudorandom numbers every time. The true result of group 1 differing from group 6 will almost always emerge, but the chance of Type I errors, if they occur, will be between different groups. The simulated replication has identified the reliable difference, just as the adjustment for simultaneous comparisons did. Repeated simulations are the basis for 'Monte Carlo' methods of estimating parameters or statistics when they cannot be calculated analytically.

Questions to ask when formulating conclusions

Can causation be inferred from the relationships in the data?
Have corrections been made for multiple comparisons across the entire study or within related parts?
If this study were replicated, would the same conclusions emerge?

11.9 Conclusion and exercises

To illustrate the major points of this chapter and give the reader some experience with the techniques described, a very simple simulated analysis is presented. Working through this analysis may ease the transition from absorbing the principles of quantitative analysis to actually performing it. As the dataset will be simulated, the outcome cannot be predicted. To allow the same data to be generated repeatedly, set the seed value of the random number generator at the beginning of the simulation, as done in Example 1.

First, simulate a dataset using the code in Example 2. If the reader does not wish to use the R or SPSS code, simply perform the actions in the comment lines (starting with a # character) in the application of your choice. Save the file in a format that can be used in your preferred application.

1. Using summary measures such as checking the range of the data, find the two deliberate mistakes in the data file and correct them (remember, the correct values have been saved).
2. Check that the ages of the participants are not different between the sexes.
3. Test the hypotheses that males prefer beer and females prefer wine, using both parametric and non-parametric tests.
4. Test the hypothesis that those who prefer beer are more likely to have been drunk in the past week.
5. Test the same hypothesis controlling for sex of drinker.

Appendix

Example 1: A demonstration of Type I errors caused by multiple comparisons

```
R
# create an empty list for the simulated data
testdat<-vector("list",6)
# this will get the same values as the original simulation
set.seed(12345)
# sample 50 values from the normal distribution with mean = -0.5 and
sd = 1
testdat[[1]]<-rnorm(50,-0.5,1)
# draw four samples with a mean = 0 and sd = 1
for(variable in 2:5) testdat[[variable]]<-rnorm(50,0,1)
# draw the final sample with a mean = 0.5 and sd = 1
# so it is different from sample 1
testdat[[6]]<-rnorm(50,0.5,1)
# get a matrix of the indices of all pairs of the elements of testdat
allpairs<-combn(1:6,2)
# create a vector to step through all the tests
alltests<-1:dim(allpairs)[2]
# print out the "t" and "p" values of the respective t-tests
# use paired tests to be consistent with the SPSS code below
for(variable in alltests) {
 thistest<-t.test(testdat[[allpairs[1,variable]]],
  testdat[[allpairs[2,variable]]],paired=TRUE)
 cat("testdat[",allpairs[1,variable],"] vs
testdat[",allpairs[2,variable],
  "] t = ",thistest$statistic,", p = ",thistest$p.value,"\n")
}
SPSS
COMMENT You will not get exactly the same results from SPSS
COMMENT as the values were rounded to make the data more compact.
DATA LIST FREE /V1 V2 V3 V4 V5 V6 (F5.4).
BEGIN DATA.
  0.0855    -0.5404     0.2239    -1.6193    -1.4361    -0.3087
  0.2095     1.9477    -1.1562     0.5484    -0.6293     1.5011
 -0.6093     0.0536     0.4224     0.1953     0.2435     0.9561
 -0.9535     0.3517    -1.3248    -0.8065     1.0584    -0.9343
  0.1059    -0.6710     0.1411    -0.1086     0.8313     0.2347
 -2.3180     0.2780    -0.5360    -0.2509     0.1052     1.1418
  0.1301     0.6912    -0.3116     1.6993    -1.7417     0.0850
 -0.7762     0.8238     1.5561    -0.3443     0.6452     0.0404
 -0.7842     2.1451    -0.4480     0.0678     0.0971    -0.2925
 -1.4193    -2.3469     0.3211    -0.6506    -0.0767    -0.6585
 -0.6162     0.1496    -1.2302    -0.4876     0.9920     1.2109
  1.3173    -1.3425    -1.3241     0.3032    -0.8593     1.7676
 -0.1294     0.5533     1.2612    -0.2420    -0.2816     0.3568
  0.0202     1.5900     1.3192    -0.4817     2.0662    -0.0150
 -1.2505    -0.5869    -0.0808    -0.9918    -0.6116     1.9829
  0.3169    -1.8324    -0.5051    -0.2806     0.3156     0.3374
```

```
-1.3864      0.8881     -0.0522      0.6330      0.6603      0.5417
-0.8316      1.5935      0.6289     -1.2398     -1.7222      0.9830
 0.6207      0.5169      2.1800      1.7643     -2.1346     -0.6801
-0.2013     -1.2957     -0.0690     -0.0237      0.0689     -0.1636
 0.2796      0.0546      1.5449      0.1999      0.8678     -0.1346
 0.9558     -0.7846      1.3215      1.3472     -2.2900     -0.2020
-1.1443     -1.0494      0.3222      0.0361     -0.1502      1.0769
-2.0531      2.3305      1.5310      0.8246     -0.2688     -1.6131
-2.0977      1.4027     -0.4212     -1.7027      1.7913      0.7609
 1.3051      0.9426     -1.1588      0.4810      0.6723      1.6471
-0.9816      0.8263     -1.8454      2.4836     -0.2093      0.5148
 0.1204     -0.8115      1.1573      0.4014      0.0122      0.1883
 0.1121      0.4762     -2.1235      0.2152      1.5341     -0.4562
-0.6623      1.0213     -1.1960     -1.8157      0.0773      0.9734
 0.3119      0.6454      1.6422     -0.9117      0.0784     -1.0139
 1.6968      1.0431      0.8837     -0.0490     -0.7793      0.6643
 1.5492     -0.3044      0.5249     -0.4054      0.1666     -0.3709
 1.1324      2.4771     -1.1847      1.1304      0.2653      2.0933
-0.2457      0.9712      2.6558      0.8155      0.8908      1.1466
-0.0088      1.8671     -1.0479      0.0764     -0.4679      0.8574
-0.8241      0.6720     -1.0111      1.4537      0.7584      0.6024
-2.1621     -0.3080      0.6689      0.3741     -0.6417     -0.1753
 1.2677      0.5365      0.1292     -0.1709      0.6277      1.4721
-0.4742      0.8249     -0.4226     -0.5022      0.2483      1.2559
 0.6285     -0.9639     -1.1403      0.5435     -0.7001      0.0717
-2.8804     -0.8551     -1.2937     -0.5052     -0.5674     -0.2139
-1.5603      1.8869     -0.5947      0.7868     -0.2614      0.3096
 0.4371     -0.3918     -1.5008      0.3009     -1.0639      0.8999
 0.3545     -0.9806      0.0159      1.3102     -0.1064     -0.4778
 0.9607      0.6873      0.5402      0.7984      0.7711      0.6837
-1.9131     -0.5050     -1.5473      0.8509      2.7474     -1.6503
 0.0674      2.1577      0.8497     -0.4436     -0.0839     -0.1230
 0.0832     -0.5998      0.8960     -0.4468      0.5436     -0.2654
-1.8068     -0.6945      0.1387      0.0133      0.7529      0.9643
END DATA.
T-TEST PAIRS = V1 V2.
T-TEST PAIRS = V1 V3.
T-TEST PAIRS = V1 V4.
T-TEST PAIRS = V1 V5.
T-TEST PAIRS = V1 V6.
T-TEST PAIRS = V2 V3.
T-TEST PAIRS = V2 V4.
T-TEST PAIRS = V2 V5.
T-TEST PAIRS = V2 V6.
T-TEST PAIRS = V3 V4.
T-TEST PAIRS = V3 V5.
T-TEST PAIRS = V3 V6.
T-TEST PAIRS = V4 V5.
T-TEST PAIRS = V4 V6.
T-TEST PAIRS = V5 V6.
EXECUTE.
```

Example 2: A simulated dataset

```
R
set.seed(43210)
# Start with 100 participant numbers
subno<-paste("SN",1:100,sep="")
# assign a sex to each participant
sex<-sample(c("M","F"),100,TRUE)
# assign an age to each participant in a uniform distribution
age<-sample(16:24,100,TRUE)
# change one age to an impossible value
imp_age<-age[34]
age[34]<--2
# simulate ratings for wine liking, with females preferring wine
like_wine<-rep(0,100)
# fill in the male ratings with a uniform distribution
nmales<-sum(sex == "M")
like_wine[which(sex == "M")]<-
 sample(1:5,nmales,TRUE,prob=c(0.35,0.3,0.2,0.1,0.05))
# for the female ratings, bias the ratings upward
like_wine[which(sex == "F")]<-
 sample(1:5,100-nmales,TRUE,prob=c(0.05,0.1,0.2,0.3,0.35))
# simulate beer rating, biasing the ratings the other way
like_beer<-rep(0,100)
like_beer[which(sex == "M")]<-
 sample(1:5,nmales,TRUE,prob=c(0.05,0.1,0.2,0.3,0.35))
like_beer[which(sex == "F")]<-
 sample(1:5,100-nmales,TRUE,prob=c(0.35,0.3,0.2,0.1,0.05))
# simulate the answers to a question, "Were you drunk last week?"
# giving males a somewhat higher frequency of drunkenness
drunk_lwk<-rep(NA,100)
drunk_lwk[which(sex == "M")]<-
 sample(c("Yes","No"),nmales,TRUE,prob=c(0.6,0.4))
drunk_lwk[which(sex == "F")]<-
 sample(c("Yes","No"),100-nmales,TRUE,prob=c(0.4,0.6))
# combine the separate variables into a rectangular data set
toy_data<-data.frame(subno=subno,sex=sex,age=age,like_wine=like_wine,
 like_beer=like_beer,drunk_lwk=drunk_lwk)
# now save the age of participant SN22 and
# shift the rest of the values one place
changed_age<-toy_data$age[22]
changed_dlw<-toy_data$drunk_lwk[22]
toy_data$age[22]<-toy_data$like_beer[22]
toy_data$like_beer[22]<-toy_data$like_wine[22]
toy_data$like_wine[22]<-toy_data$drunk_lwk[22]
toy_data$drunk_lwk[22]<-NA
# save the data frame and the altered values
# load it again with load("toydata.Rdata")
save(toy_data,imp_age,changed_age,changed_dlw,file="toydata.Rdata")
SPSS
DATA LIST FREE /subno (A5) sex (A1) age (F2.0)
 likewine likebeer (F1.0) drunklwk (A3).
```

```
BEGIN DATA.
SN1 M 19 1 3 Yes SN2 M 16 2 3 No SN3 M 18 5 5 No
SN4 M 19 2 3 Yes SN5 F 23 5 5 No SN6 M 20 1 2 Yes
SN7 M 22 2 2 Yes SN8 F 24 5 1 No SN9 M 21 1 5 Yes
SN10 M 24 2 5 Yes SN11 F 23 5 2 Yes SN12 M 16 2 5 Yes
SN13 M 17 2 5 Yes SN14 F 19 5 4 No SN15 F 23 4 2 No
SN16 M 20 2 3 No SN17 M 23 5 2 No SN18 M 23 1 5 No
SN19 F 21 5 4 No SN20 F 19 3 2 No SN21 F 21 5 1 Yes
SN22 M 19 4 5 Yes SN23 M 17 1 5 Yes SN24 F 18 4 1 Yes
SN25 F 23 4 1 No SN26 M 19 1 3 No SN27 M 20 1 5 No
SN28 M 21 3 3 Yes SN29 M 23 1 3 No SN30 F 21 5 3 Yes
SN31 M 22 1 4 Yes SN32 F 22 5 3 Yes SN33 M 21 3 5 Yes
SN34 F 17 3 2 No SN35 F 19 3 2 No SN36 F 17 5 3 No
SN37 M 20 2 4 No SN38 M 20 1 4 Yes SN39 M 21 1 5 Yes
SN40 M 18 5 1 No SN41 F 19 5 3 No SN42 M 21 3 4 Yes
SN43 M 24 2 5 Yes SN44 M 17 3 5 No SN45 F 19 4 1 No
SN46 M 18 1 4 Yes SN47 M 21 4 5 No SN48 M 16 3 1 Yes
SN49 F 16 5 4 No SN50 M 22 1 4 Yes SN51 F 19 1 1 Yes
SN52 M 23 2 5 Yes SN53 M 20 4 5 Yes SN54 M 17 1 4 Yes
SN55 F 22 3 1 Yes SN56 M 18 3 4 No SN57 M 16 2 5 Yes
SN58 M 16 2 1 No SN59 F 18 2 2 No SN60 M 20 3 5 Yes
SN61 F 20 3 1 No SN62 F 23 2 1 No SN63 M 17 4 3 Yes
SN64 F 18 3 2 No SN65 F 21 4 1 No SN66 F 22 2 3 Yes
SN67 M 16 2 3 Yes SN68 F 23 2 3 No SN69 F 23 3 2 Yes
SN70 F 19 4 2 Yes SN71 M 23 1 5 No SN72 M 21 1 5 Yes
SN73 F 19 4 2 Yes SN74 M 24 3 3 No SN75 M 22 2 1 No
SN76 M 17 3 4 Yes SN77 M 21 4 3 No SN78 M 22 4 5 Yes
SN79 M 17 2 2 Yes SN80 F 19 3 1 Yes SN81 F 19 4 2 No
SN82 M 19 1 5 Yes SN83 F 24 5 1 No SN84 F 21 5 4 No
SN85 M 22 1 5 Yes SN86 F 19 1 3 No SN87 F 18 4 4 No
SN88 M 22 2 5 Yes SN89 M 21 2 5 Yes SN90 M 23 1 4 Yes
SN91 M 17 1 5 Yes SN92 F 24 2 4 No SN93 M 16 2 4 No
SN94 M 20 2 4 No SN95 M 19 1 4 Yes SN96 M 22 2 3 No
 SN97 M 17 3 4 No SN98 M 23 1 3 Yes SN99 M 18 1 4 No
 SN100 M 21 1 4 No
END DATA.
VALUE LABELS /likewine likebeer 1 "Not at all" 2 "A little"
 3 "Somewhat" 4 "Definitely" 5 "Very much".
IF (subno EQ "SN34") age = -2.
IF (subno EQ "SN22") age = likewine.
IF (subno EQ "SN22") likewine = likebeer.
IF (subno EQ "SN22") likebeer = 1.
IF (subno EQ "SN22") drunklwk = "".
SAVE /OUTFILE='toydata.sav'.
```

References

Cohen, J. (1988) *Statistical Power Analysis for the Behavioral Sciences*. Hillsdale, NJ: Lawrence Erlbaum.

Copeland, J., Stevenson, R. J., Gates, P. & Dillon, P. (2007) Young Australians and alcohol: the acceptability of ready-to-drink (RTD) alcoholic beverages among 12–30 year olds. *Addiction*, 102, 1740–1746.

Davey, J., Obst, P. & Sheehan, M. (2000) Developing a profile of alcohol consumption patterns of police officers in a large scale sample of an Australian police service. *European Addiction Research*, 6, 205–212.

Drasgow, F. (1986) Polychoric and polyserial correlations. In: S. Kotz & N. Johnson (eds) *The Encyclopedia of Statistics*, Vol. 7. New York: Wiley, pp. 68–74.

Guinness World Records (2008) *Guiness World Records 2008*. London: Guinness.

Huckle, T., Sweetsur, P., Moyes, S. & Casswell, S. (2008) Ready to drinks are associated with heavier drinking patterns among young females. *Drug and Alcohol Review*, 27, 398–402.

Pinheiro, J. C. & Bates, D. M. (2000) *Mixed Effects Models in S and S-PLUS*. New York: Springer-Verlag.

R Development Core Team (2008) *R: A Language and Environment for Statistical Computing*. Available online: http://www.R-project.org; Vienna: R Foundation for Statistical Computing.

Stevens, S. S. (1946) On the theory of scales of measurement. *Science*, 103, 677–680.

Thode Jr, H. C. (2002) *Testing for Normality*. New York: Marcel Dekker.

Toothaker, L. E. (1993) *Multiple Comparison Procedures*. Newbury Park, CA: Sage.

White, V. & Hayman, J. (2006) *Australian Secondary Students' Use of Alcohol*. Melbourne: Cancer Council Victoria.

Section III
Real World Research Methods

Chapter 12

APPLIED RESEARCH METHODS

David Best and Ed Day

12.1   Introduction

This chapter introduces the reader to research in applied clinical contexts. We base the examples we give and the model we used in a real-life example completed in treatment services in Birmingham – a programme called the Birmingham Treatment Effectiveness Initiative which aimed to introduce a method of delivering structured psycho-social interventions consistently across specialist addiction services in the city. It is a pragmatic model that deals with the context for applied research, which in this case is the staff, clients and services in which we wish to make change, and uses that as part of the process of measurement. We contrast this with more traditional approaches of testing new technologies, such as the randomised controlled trial (RCT).

12.1.1   Why use applied methods?

Given that the RCT is generally held up as the 'gold standard' for evaluating intervention efficacy, the first question we address is why one would ever contemplate using any other method. To illustrate this question, we use an example from research assessing the effectiveness of multi-systemic treatment for delinquent adolescent youth. In this study, the evidence from efficacy studies was much more powerful than from effectiveness studies (see Figure 12.1). Curtis and colleagues (2004) compared the effect size (the difference between the trial condition and the control condition) in RCT-type designs (called 'efficacy studies') with more naturalistic studies (referred to as 'effectiveness' studies) where the intervention is implemented by ordinary clinicians in real-world settings. The findings show that the effect size (or the 'added value' of the intervention) is three times greater in randomised controlled environments than in naturalistic studies. This difference, using the convention of effect sizes defined by Cohen (1988), is such that in trial conditions there is a 'large effect' between multi-systemic treatment and control or no treatment, but that in 'real-world' applications of multi-systemic treatment, this reduces to only a small effect for the new intervention. Why should this be?

Henggeler (2004), commenting on the Curtis paper, suggested that the key mediating factors between trial research and real-world implementation include factors related to individual clinicians working with new treatments, to the organisational context in which the new treatments are trialled and to system factors about services and their effectiveness. He acknowledges that:

> virtually all evidence-based treatments that are currently being transported to community settings place a strong emphasis on programme fidelity ... rigorous evaluations of treatment adherence and program fidelity are absolutely critical to understanding the successes and failures of evidence-based treatments in community practice. (Henggeler, 2004, p. 422)

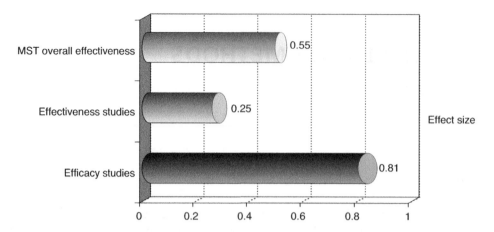

Figure 12.1 Effect sizes of interventions across differing implementation studies reported by Curtis et al. (2004).

This is indicative of an issue that has concerned academics in the addictions field for a number of years. Carroll and Rounsaville (2007) have argued that clinical trial research has yielded a number of 'empirically supported therapies' in the addictions field that are widely available and have a significant evidence base, including motivational interviewing to improve retention in treatment and contingency management as an effective supplement to treatment for stimulant dependence. Yet the authors argue, based on tape-recorded sessions, that such evidenced interventions are rarely used in practice. They argue that this is not simply a question of training or dissemination but involves complex organisational issues and greater understanding of context effects. McLellan (2006) has referred to this as the 'research to treatment gap' and has suggested that the gap should be understood in terms of individual therapist effects (based on training, support and values), the length of the treatment available and the setting it occurs in, and the role of other key components of treatment such as medication, medical and support or wraparound services.

The key conclusion is that what is reported in trials as being effective and what occurs in real-life clinical practice are not one and the same thing, for very good reasons. This chapter reviews a range of approaches to understanding what goes on in clinical addiction settings and how meaningful changes can be brought about.

12.1.2   Overview of the methods to be discussed

We treat the research options available as a process starting from the initiation of the research question, using both needs assessment and qualitative research methods to outline the basic processes involved in developing research questions. In this case, we use the example of how to introduce and implement evidence-based practice in an applied clinical context. The primary method that is described is evaluation research, using a pre-/post-design, and we examine a range of methods for assessing the effectiveness of an intervention, finishing with an overview of qualitative and action methods to determine the effectiveness of the model employed.

Before describing the theoretical model used for the intervention and the evaluation method, we start by considering the ways that we attempted to answer the questions of 'what is currently going on in treatment' and what are the needs for development of the current system.

12.2 Auditing clinical activity in the city

Clinical audit is defined by the UK Department of Health as 'systematically looking at the procedures used for diagnosis, care and treatment, examining how associated resources are used and investigating the effect care has on the outcome and quality of life for the patient' (Department of Health, 1993). In essence, it is a method for reflecting on and reviewing practice in a systematic way and utilising this to improve the quality of service. The key benefits of clinical audit are to:

- Identify and promote good practice
- Provide opportunities for training and development
- Ensure the most efficient use of resources
- Improve communication and working relationships, and the consistency of practice

Audit is not the same as research, as it generally involves the identification of an accepted standard and the measurement of performance against this standard. In contrast, research may have more fluid objectives and is often aimed at the generation of new knowledge (Box 12.1).

However, the key area of interest for us was around what actually took place in those treatment sessions – the so-called black box of treatment. Thus, for the criminal justice agencies participating in the citywide audit described in Box 12.1, we also asked each worker to complete (for every live file on their caseload) a further single-page assessment of what activities they had ever engaged in with their clients and what they had done in the last session. Box 12.2 summarises the findings of this extension of the audit which measured the clinician's perceptions of the activities that occurred in clinical sessions.

Alternative methods that could have been used to assess what occurred in treatment sessions include the use of either audio or videotaping of the workers' sessions with their clients (Miller, 2007). This would have been beneficial to the extent that it would have provided 'objective' data, in that it was not reliant on the workers' accounts (subject as they were to both recall and self-presentational biases). However, this approach would also have had disadvantages. There are ethical questions around the identification of clients and their willingness to have the sessions recorded in this way. There may also be concerns that the act of recording the sessions means that both clients and workers respond to the recording and so it is not indicative of treatment as usual. Finally,

---

Box 12.1   Conducting a citywide audit of addiction service delivery

In a citywide audit in Birmingham, each worker was interviewed about all the clients on their caseload on the day of the interview (Day et al., 2007). The researcher sat down with the worker and completed a data collection pro forma and a current Christo inventory (Christo et al., 2000) for each of their clients. The worker referred to the clinical case notes if there were any questions that they could not answer. This was our attempt to measure what is meant by 'treatment as usual'. In total, data were collected on 2806 clients attending all 15 specialist adult drug services in the city. A majority of the samples (85%, 2391) were receiving a prescription for an opioid replacement therapy, with 1931 (69%) receiving methadone and 470 (17%) buprenorphine. The basic range of non-medical interventions identified as being delivered to clients was that 88.8% received keyworking, 35.9% structured counselling, 39.0% some form of relapse prevention activity, 19.8% support around employment and training, while around 10% were in contact with child and family services and 4.6% with day care provision.

> **Box 12.2   Assessing the content of keyworking sessions**
>
> In total, workers estimated that clients were typically seen for a mean of 44.3 minutes per session, and most were seen on a fortnightly basis or less often. However, when that was broken down – the sessions typically consisted of around four types of activity – the single largest activity was 'case management' (accounting for things like discussion of dosing and supervision arrangements, discussing treatment compliance and drug testing), which typically took around 14 minutes per session. Slightly less time on average (around 12 minutes) was spent on 'signposting' in which the worker discussed with the client's issues around linkage to housing services, employment, probation and other relevant services. Just less than 11 minutes was typically spent on 'other' activities such as paperwork, which meant that in the average treatment session only around 11 minutes was spent on the delivery of evidence-based psycho-social interventions. While this is methodologically limited (it relies on the self-report of workers and does not attempt to account for reporting or memory biases), it shows how audit work can be used to start to answer important questions about the delivery of treatment and what really goes on in sessions. This provided for us the evidence that structured interventions were not being delivered in the city at an optimal level and so provided a significant justification for the subsequent evaluation research process.

and importantly, there is the cost and time involved – not only would there be major resource implications in setting up such a system for 2806 clients, there is also the problem of analysis. How to code and analyse this huge wealth of 'data' is highly problematic and requires considerable expert input. Alternatively, we could have assessed the clients' view (and indeed this is work that we are piloting at present) – not to 'corroborate' the workers' reports but to obtain their perspective on what is going on in sessions. Ultimately, with any complex research design question, there is no perfect solution as each method will have a range of strengths and weaknesses, and, if resources are available, using multiple methods may be the optimal solution. This is known as 'triangulation' (Denzin, 1978) and can be defined as an approach to data analysis that synthesises information from multiple sources. In our case, this second source is needs assessment.

12.3   Needs assessment

Although needs assessments are a well-recognised part of developing treatment services in the addictions field, the adequacy of the science in this area is not good, and relatively little has been published to guide researchers in conducting structured needs assessments. Ford and Luckey (1983) suggested four steps that underpin systematic needs assessment to identify the size of the in-need population:

1. *Determine the geographic size of the area under investigation:* This is basically to ensure that there is a specified geographic area and that each of the candidate sources fall within this boundary – this is generally referred to as the issue of 'co-terminosity'.
2. *Estimate the number of problem users within each population group:* Using existing data sources from epidemiological analysis – which in our example included Home Office assessments of the size of the drug problem (Hay et al., 2008) and local estimates available for alcohol from each Public Health Observatory in the UK.
3. *Estimate the number of users from Step 2 that should be treated within a particular year (defined as the demand population):* This is a complex question that will depend on the data sources available and on the assumptions made – such as whether the number of people requesting

treatment should be weighted according to such factors as mortality, blood-borne viruses, and so on.

4. *Estimate the number of individuals from Step 3 that will require a service from each component of the treatment system:* This part of the analysis will attempt to match what is available in the current system (e.g. number of beds for detox or rehab, number of community treatment slots) against what is known about the characteristics (such as problem severity) of the candidate treatment population.

This approach was extended by Rush (1990) in assessing the need for alcohol treatment in Canada. Using an epidemiological model, Rush (1990) estimated that 15% of problem drinkers in Canada can be considered as the 'target group' for treatment in any given year. While the sources for this estimate were national alcohol-related mortality data, survey data on population drinking levels and population-level consumption data, the model developed was akin to a survival model for treatment, based on individuals making each transition through the process of treatment seeking, assessment, engagement and completion. In this approach, for every 10 000 adult problem drinkers, 1500 (15%) will seek treatment of whom around two-thirds ($n = 1000$, 10%) will make it as far as assessment and just over half to the point of treatment referral. However, the proportions who will seek treatment will vary as a function of local treatment systems, and the methodological challenge will be to work out a mapping process for assessing clients' reasons for seeking treatment and the types of treatment that would be acceptable to them.

In the alcohol treatment system assessed by Rush, just over half of the referrals were to outpatient services, around 30% to day programmes, 10% to short-term inpatient treatment and 5% long-term residential treatment. This approach to needs assessment is highly rigorous and systematic but relies exclusively on the availability and quality of adequate epidemiological data and says nothing about the quality of the treatment service. In developing this kind of approach to needs assessment, the challenge is to combine quantitative measures of existing treatment activity (such as demand and uptake, supplemented by such things as measures of waiting times and early dropout) with more qualitative assessments of perceptions of treatment delivery and need from a range of key stakeholders, such as clients, treatment providers and commissioners, and family members and community representatives.

Best et al. (2007) attempted to develop this model by creating a needs assessment framework that combined qualitative and quantitative methods for assessing the needs of both the in-treatment and out-of-treatment populations of drug users. This involved gathering nationally collated assessments of the size of the problem population and the measures of treatment engagement and retention and combining these with local data sources including expert assessments of effectiveness, treatment gaps and subpopulations whose needs were not being met.

When this method was applied to Birmingham (Loaring & Best, 2007) there was a rationale of:

combining what is known about numbers in treatment with local knowledge to create a locally credible snapshot of activity and gaps, as the foundation for a grounded analysis of treatment needs. Additional local sources of information and expert input provided system mapping around criminal justice clients and locally commissioned research. The second and complementary element of the 'twin track' approach to the needs assessment allowed the process to be driven and informed by a key group of stakeholders. (Loaring & Best, 2007, p. 5)

In other words, the aim was to use a pragmatic model of assessing what was known, developing a method for assessing the quality of what was known and how consistent and compatible information from different data sources was and how this could generate an agenda for new knowledge generation. In the longer term, this new knowledge generation would be primarily quantitative, but in the immediate period of the needs assessment, the aim would be to utilise key informant and 'expert focus group' methods to plug key gaps in local knowledge. Similarly, the method used for missing epidemiological data was to fall back on regional or national data when no local data could be accessed.

A similar approach was adopted by Stimson and colleagues (2006) in evaluating the World Health Organization's rapid assessment and response (RAR) method for assessing injecting drug use and its consequences across ten sites internationally. The aim of the evaluation was to focus on knowledge gain and capacity building, and the authors concluded that the RARs resulted in many new interventions and models being implemented and that is an effective method for linking assessment to the delivery of interventions, and that it was an important public health tool.

However, before going on to describe this work, we quickly overview an alternative approach to this data-driven method, assessing the use of qualitative techniques in the development of research questions.

12.4   Qualitative research approaches

Strauss and Corbin (1998) argue that qualitative research is 'any type of research that produces findings not arrived at by statistical procedures or other means of quantification' (Strauss & Corbin, 1998, p. 10). While this issue is dealt with more generically in the chapter on qualitative methods, it is important to emphasise the role that this approach can play in applied research settings. Qualitative approaches can be used to assess organisations and how they function, social movements and cultural phenomena, and can be used at different stages of the applied research process, as is often used at the start of a programmatic investigation, for example where knowledge about an area is limited (e.g. Stern, 1980).

Thus, it would not be unusual in undertaking a large research project, such as the topic of delivering structured interventions in applied settings, to use qualitative methods at the start and at the end of the research programme. This can be done to generate hypotheses for more structured investigation and also as part of the process of assessing implementation effectiveness. Equally, qualitative methods can be used alongside quantitative methods as a method of assessing the experienced process of the intervention or activity taking place. For instance, the introduction of a new treatment facility may be tested using formalised treatment evaluation processes, but the impact on the local community assessed using more qualitative and perhaps ethnographic methods.

What would be the point of using qualitative methods at the start of the research process? At the outset, when attempting to define the research question, it may be appropriate to use open-ended interviews with a range of stakeholders to allow an initial assessment of what the issues are and what the level of consensus and consistency is across the stakeholder group. Similarly, at the end of the research programme, qualitative methods may be used to assess the impact of the work or, using a reflexive approach, to enable the researchers to consider the impact of the research process on the subject and context (Steier, 1991). It is one of the key differences between qualitative and quantitative methods that the assumption of objectivity and invisibility is not assumed in qualitative methods – in other words, the researcher's own role in the production and interpretation of data is more readily acknowledged. In addiction research, one of the key roles that qualitative research may perform is to give a 'voice' to users – and one of the key politicised objectives of much qualitative research is as an act of empowerment for disenfranchised groups (e.g. Edwards & Potter, 1992).

Thus, for our example about delivery of effective structured interventions, a qualitative approach could involve a combination of interviews with key stakeholders, some observations of both treatment sessions and wider activities within treatment provider organisations. Feeding this back to participants and using the early interpretations as part of a reflexive process would contribute to what is often referred to as 'action' or dynamic research. Action research is a reflective process of progressive problem-solving and takes research from a passive observation of naturally occurring events to an active participant in the process of managed change. In our case example, the process was dynamic but would not be classed as action research as it did not have that participative quality.

12.5 Evaluation research

The basic purpose of evaluation research is to test whether something has worked or not. There are really two separate issues to be addressed – the first is the question of 'implementation fidelity' or whether the method or intervention tested has been implemented as intended and this falls within the area of 'process evaluation', which will attempt to assess how and how well the target intervention has been delivered. The second type of evaluation research is outcome evaluation, which is an assessment of whether the intervention has delivered the desired results. There are a wide range of methods for undertaking this kind of evaluation, but the most straightforward and the one to be explored here is the 'pre-/post-'method. What this involves is assessing the level of functioning or activity prior to the implementation of an intervention, then delivering the intervention and then assessing change in the period following implementation. Please note that this is not a controlled experiment and so does not exclude the possibility that unpredicted or extraneous variables may have influenced the observed change. In other words, this kind of design is susceptible to unpredicted intervening effects. To explain this process, we have cited an example from our own work, using the delivery of a training package around implementing a brief manualised intervention for drug users as the activity to be assessed.

This process is based on a sequenced implementation of training in a novel intervention in which baseline measures are taken of client and staff satisfaction with core aspects of treatment prior to the delivery of a training package. The training is then evaluated in the standard way of assessing receptiveness and impact, but an additional evaluation is then carried out with staff around 3 months later to measure their views on what aspects of the training have actually been implemented. This follow-up is a direct measure of obstacles to training implementation. Finally, the cycle is completed by repeating the initial satisfaction surveys of workers and clients and measuring changes that can be linked to the training implementation (Box 12.3).

This raises the question of why one would use a questionnaire format. The most obvious reason is that it allows large amounts of data to be collected in a consistent manner, reducing the biases that may result from interviewer effects, and offers the possibility of using closed category questions to enable quantification of the results. If existing instruments with established psychometric properties are used (this means there is published information on the reliability and ideally the validity and norms for the scale), then much of the effort and difficulty of generating and testing a new instrument can be avoided. This will also enable the researcher to readily establish electronic databases for the coding and recording of information. If the researchers are unable to find an existing instrument that meets their needs, then guidance should be sought on constructing and testing the measure (see Chapter 7 on survey methods).

There are, however, disadvantages to both using existing questionnaires and using question-naires at all. For established instruments, the disadvantages include lack of sensitivity to the specific

> **Box 12.3　Implementing a model for evaluating the implementation of a new intervention in a clinical setting**
>
> Phase 1: Strategic planning. This involved both the needs assessment and audit activities outlined above. From this we were able to determine that there was a clear need for improvements in the delivery of structured psycho-social interventions in treatment settings in Birmingham and that basic care planning was a key area that needed to be addressed in this process.
>
> Phase 2: Baseline measurement. This involved using structured instruments to measure both workers' assessment of their own situation and that of the agency they worked in and clients' assessments of their motivation, functioning and level of engagement in the treatment process (see below).
>
> Phase 3: Intervention and implementation. For our example study, this involved providing training in a new method of delivering interventions called 'node-link mapping' (Dansereau & Simpson, 2009) and training workers how to apply this in their daily practices. A traditional evaluation of the training was carried out immediately after it had been conducted.
>
> Phase 4: Assessing workers' perceptions of implementation. Three months after the workers had received the training, they were contacted and asked to complete a questionnaire assessing implementation of the measures. This is partially an attempt to address the concerns expressed by Carroll and Rounsaville and by McLellan outlined in the introductory section of the chapter.
>
> Phase 5: Measuring change. A slightly amended version of the worker questionnaire used in Phase 2 and a completely unaltered version of the client questionnaire were distributed a further 4–6 months after implementation to assess the impact that the training and implementation initiative had for clients and workers in the services.

context – particularly if the instruments have been developed in a different setting or country. Amending existing questionnaires must be done with care to avoid reducing the reliability and comparability of the results. More generally, questionnaires can be inflexible, perceived as lacking any personal touch (and researchers may get less of a flavour of the lived experience of respondents) and are subject to a range of research biases including self-presentational effects, boredom effects and acquiescence sets (when respondents agree with all questions or statements).

The model we used was based on the treatment process model developed by Simpson (2004), a key component of which is about the implementation process, based on the idea that treatment delivery occurs in an applied context in which the implementation of training requires organisational commitment and readiness, and can be characterised as involving the following stages:

1. Exposure to training for either individuals or teams.
2. Adoption – the trainees perceive the value of the training and wish to implement it within their daily working practice.
3. Implementation – trainees utilise the techniques or methods in their own practice on a trial or pilot basis.
4. Routine practice – the methods or techniques come to be embedded within the routine activities of the organisation.

Based on a series of developmental studies, Simpson and colleagues have developed a link between organisational functioning and effective implementation of new treatment methods, a process they refer to as 'technology transfer'. The rationale for this approach is outlined in detail in Simpson and Flynn's (2007) paper (see Recommended readings). To implement this model, the team at Texas

---

Box 12.4   Instruments available for testing organisational functioning in addiction treatment services

- Client Evaluation of Self and Treatment (CEST; Joe et al., 2002) measures four aspects of clients' functioning – motivation for treatment, psychological functioning, social functioning and treatment engagement – and has been widely used across the United States.
- Organisational Readiness for Change (ORC; Lehmann et al., 2002) measures four aspects of workers' functioning – motivation for change, resources, staffing factors and organisational climate. This has also been widely used in the United States but has more recently been tested in Italy (Rampazzo et al., 2006).
- Two measures of training evaluation were amended for use in a UK context – the Workshop Evaluation (WEVAL) was distributed to participants immediately after the completion of the training, and the Workshop Assessment Follow-up (WAFU) was distributed to workers around 3 months after the training to assess the extent of implementation of the training process in everyday clinical practice.

Christian University run by Professor Simpson have developed a series of instruments for measuring aspects of the change process (see Box 12.4).

12.5.1   Anonymity and data collection

Another crucial issue that arose in the Treatment Effectiveness study that will affect similar projects is around the identification of participants. While tagged participants are useful for research purposes as it enables a real pre-/post-assessment of change, this will bring potential ethical concerns and linked risks of self-presentation biases on the part of participants who know that they can be identified. If the decision is made to preserve participant confidentiality, the analysis can only assess group level change, and so no matching is possible about the individual effects of participation in the project. It also carries the risk that, in services with a high turnover of clients, those evaluated in the pre-intervention period are markedly different from those assessed in the follow-up and so the comparison is not a valid one. This decision has both ethical and implementation implications, and it is crucial that it is discussed with users and staff organisations as part of the research planning process. It is also possible that different decisions will be taken for the staff and for the clients – based on both research and pragmatic considerations. However, it is crucial to be aware of the possible effects of labelling on both the response set of participants (including successful completion rates for instruments) as part of the pay-off against better quality data that enable stronger analysis to be conducted.

It is also important to be aware in this kind of study of the 'hierarchical' questions the commissioners may want answered. In our study outlined above, one of the key questions was about what the workers' experience of and engagement with the training process would be for the clients on their caseload. In other words, we wanted to be able to test the effects of workers' report on clients' behaviour which necessitated sufficient identifiers on the client and worker forms that we at least knew which clients were on the caseloads of which workers (Box 12.5).

12.5.2   Recruitment and representativeness

Another core question in evaluating treatment effectiveness in applied settings is around the response rates and the implications of non-participation. It is commonly said of the positive results to

Box 12.5   Measuring clients' functioning to test worker engagement with evidence-based intervention training

In the analysis of implementation of training around Treatment Effectiveness, the study measured client ratings of treatment as a function of worker engagement with the training and worker ratings of organisational functioning. Higher client satisfaction was associated with greater worker's perception of both efficacy ($r = 0.07$, $P < 0.05$) and opportunities for growth ($r = 0.07$, $P < 0.05$). There was also a link between client ratings of counsellor rapport and two measures of organisational climate reported by clinical staff on the ORC. Higher client ratings of counsellor rapport were associated with more positive ratings by their workers on measures of cohesion in the team ($r = 0.11$, $P < 0.01$) and communication ($r = 0.09$, $P < 0.05$). The final measure of treatment engagement on the CEST was also linked to how those clients' keyworkers responded on the ORC. Higher client ratings of active participation in the treatment process was linked to more positive worker ratings on cohesion ($r = 0.08$, $P < 0.05$) and communication ($r = 0.07$, $P < 0.05$). Although the actual correlation sizes are small, the scale of the study was sufficient to detect relatively subtle relationships.

satisfaction surveys in the addictions field that the results are meaningless because only those who feel positively about the treatments fill in satisfaction questionnaires and all those who fill in the forms do not say anything bad in case it affects their treatment (e.g. Best et al., 2006). This raises two issues – the first about sampling and the other about 'false-positive' responding, particularly if the work is carried out either by the staff of the service being evaluated or, to a lesser extent, by independent researchers but in a treatment setting. This is another reason for effective planning – and potentially for actively engaging user involvement groups in the preparation and delivery of the evaluation. What is equally important is that, irrespective of the number of responses, a clear strategy is drawn up for not only how many forms are to be returned but also by which subpopulations to ensure adequate coverage for the study. There is no textbook response to this, as this will be partly determined by the nature of the client group, by the question to be answered and by practical factors.

12.5.3   What are the overall implications from this example of evaluation research?

There is some support for the 'technology transfer' method in treatment services in Birmingham, but also for this as a method of assessing implementation. The core lesson from the treatment effectiveness work is that it does not make sense to look only at either clients or even only at workers in assessing the effectiveness of a planned change in service delivery. The crucial lesson for applied research on treatment is that the client–worker relationship is embedded in an organisational and cultural milieu that the research or evaluation team must be aware of (and ideally account for in the project design) for the results to have meaning.

The other core issue in this respect is around the interpretation and the ownership of the results. In applied settings particularly, it is crucial that there is a clear dissemination plan and that the key stakeholders have signed up to this in advance. It is critical that the dissemination process explains what was done, what was found and what the preliminary interpretations for these findings are. It will be essential that the results have credibility and that the stakeholders are sufficiently engaged to believe and to buy into the results. It is here that qualitative methods may be particularly useful as part of the dissemination and implementation process – in other words, in-depth interviews with key stakeholders or focus groups to discuss key findings may not only give richness to the process, they may also increase the chances that the findings can be translated into recommendations that have a real possibility of being implemented within the service. Workers will often complain that researchers come in, cause huge disruption to the clinical process and then disappear with neither the clinical team nor the clients any wiser as to what was found or what these findings actually mean. It is important at the start of the process to be clear about what the process is and what the dissemination methods will be – and that these should be as inclusive as possible.

12.6   The audit cycle

A key component of the information cycle that has significant implications for applied clinical research is around the audit cycle. In many treatment services (including the NHS) there is a governance requirement to engage in a programme of clinical audit in which processes and practices are mapped against established standards – such as the National Treatment Agency's Models of Care (NTA, 2002; updated, 2006). One of the advantages of the method used is that it can be readily evidenced – the care plans and reviews, if that is what is being assessed – will either be in the case files of each client or not and they will either be complete or not. However, this can form the basis for a more sophisticated analysis of quality and also of impact – so the first stage of the applied research process may be to audit one particular aspect of treatment – such as the implementation of care planning. A second stage might be then to evaluate the quality of the care plans, and to use qualitative interviews with clients and workers to assess how important and useful they are. This would provide the foundation for an intervention to improve the process that would itself be the subject of evaluation. The advantage of a care planning cycle is that the routine audit of the target activity would in itself constitute an established and useful measure of effectiveness of change and its durability. In this sense, audit is both the first stage of initiating research agendas but also the basic building block of monitoring and measurement that, if used in a meaningful and cyclical way, can make an important contribution to the planning and delivery of strategic research aims.

12.7   Measuring outcomes in applied settings

Thus, the final question is 'does improving the quality of delivery of structured interventions actually make any difference to treatment outcomes?' In the addictions field, we have a number of recognised outcome monitoring instruments – the Addiction Severity Index (McLellan et al., 1992), the Opiate Treatment Index (Darke et al., 1991) and the Maudsley Addiction Profile (Marsden et al., 1998), as discussed in Chapter 8, each of which measures clients' functioning in a range of core domains that typically will involve substance use, offending, physical and psychological health, risk for disease and blood-borne virus, social functioning and employment. Typically, the aim would be to assess functioning prior to treatment and then at various points during and after treatment, using the same measures to assess the impact of treatment. A number of major treatment outcomes studies have been conducted in the UK (Gossop et al., 2000, 2005) and internationally (Simpson, 2003; Ross et al., 2004) that have typically shown improvements following active treatment engagement. However, these studies typically rely on self-reported data for changes in substance use and offending behaviour and would be classed as observational studies – clients are not assigned to treatment conditions and there is generally no control group to use as a measure of any 'regression to the mean' effect. This can constitute a major challenge when measuring treatment effectiveness, as outcome assessments are costly and time-consuming, and it is often tempting to use 'proxy' measures of outcome such as successful completion of treatment or retention to a particular time threshold to assess the effectiveness of treatment. However, it is critical in assessing the impact of any new intervention that process measures alone are not relied upon and that some measure of outcome is considered in developing an applied research question.

12.8 Overview and conclusions

The methods discussed here should be understood in the context of the daily lives of clients (and staff) whose needs and responsibilities must be respected. As a consequence, there is a need to use methods that are compatible with the context and with the cultures and values of those intended to participate in the project. This means that research will have a wider meaning and will include the use of audit and needs assessment as possible initial foundations for establishing the research question (where qualitative methods would have been a viable alternative), a pre-/post-evaluation method for testing the implementation of a new intervention and process evaluation measures of implementation and training, with an audit cycle used to test and refine the actual implementation in practice. This creates the basis for shifting to an outcome-focused model to complete the answer to the question of 'does it actually work?'

Exercises

1. Your local treatment system consists of a Needle and Syringe Program (NSP), a 7-day residential detox, an Opiate Substitute programme and a treatment service, focused on psycho-social interventions. Choose one of these service elements and design a piece of applied research to evaluate its effectiveness.
2. Design a graphic model of how the effectiveness of one of these services affects others.

References

Best, D., Campbell, A. & O'Grady, A. (2006) *The NTA's First Annual User Satisfaction Survey 2005*. London: National Treatment Agency.

Best, D., Day, E. & Campbell, A. (2007) Developing a method for conducting needs assessments for drug treatment: a systems approach. *Addiction Research and Theory*, 15(3), 263–275.

Carroll, K. & Rounsaville, B. (2007) A vision of the next generation of behavioral therapies research in the addictions. *Addiction*, 102(6), 850–862.

Christo, G., Spurrell, S. & Alcorn, R. (2000) Validation of the christo inventory for substance-misuse services (CISS): a simple outcome evaluation tool. *Drug and Alcohol Dependence*, 59, 189–197.

Cohen, J. (1988) *Statistical Power Analysis for the Behavioral Sciences*, 2nd edn. Hillsdale, NJ: Lawrence Earlbaum Associates.

Curtis, N., Ronan, K. & Borduin, C. (2004) Multisystemic treatment: a meta-analysis of outcome studies. *Journal of Family Psychology*, 18(3), 411–419.

Dansereau, D. F. & Simpson, D. D. (2009) A picture is worth a thousand words: the case for graphic representations. *Professional Psychology: Research and Practice*, 40(1), 104–110.

Darke, S., Ward, J., Hall, W., Heather, N. & Wodak, A. (1991) *The Opiate Treatment Index (Manual) NDARC Technical Report #11*. Sydney, National Drug and Alcohol Research Centre: University of New South Wales.

Day, E., Best, D., Copello, A., Young, H., Khoosal, N. & Modern, N. (2007) Characteristics of drug-using patients and treatment provided in primary and secondary settings. *Journal of Substance Use*, 13(1), 27–35.

Denzin, N. K. (1978) *The Research Act: A Theoretical Introduction to Sociological Methods*. New York: McGraw-Hill.

Department of Health (1993) *Clinical Audit: Meeting and Improving Standards in Health Care*. London: HMSO.

Edwards, D. & Potter, J. (1992) *Discursive Psychology*. London: Sage.

Ford, W. & Luckey, J. (1983) Planning alcoholism services: A technique for projecting specific service needs. *The International Journal of the Addictions*, 18(8), 1073–1084.

Gossop, M., Marsden, J., Stewart, D. & Rolfe, A. (2000) Reductions in acquisitive crime and drug use after treatment of addiction problems: 1-year follow-up outcomes. *Drug and Alcohol Dependence*, 58, 165–172.

Gossop, M., Trakada, K., Stewart, D. & Witton, J. (2005) Reduction in criminal convictions after addiction treatment: 5-year follow-up. *Drug and Alcohol Dependence*, 79, 295–302.

Hay, G., Gannon, M., MacDougall, J., Millar, T., Williams, K., Eastwood, C. & McKeganey, N. (2008) National and regional estimates of the prevalence of opiate use and/or crack cocaine use 2006/2007. Home Office Research Report 9. London: Home Office.

Henggeler, S. (2004) Decreasing effect sizes for effectiveness studies – implications for the transport of evidence-based treatments: comment on Curtis, Ronan, and Borduin (2004). *Journal of Family Psychology*, 18(3), 420–423.

Joe, G. W., Broome, K. M., Rowan-Szal, G. A. & Simpson, D. D. (2002) Measuring patient attributes and engagement in treatment. *Journal of Substance Abuse Treatment*, 22(4), 183–196.

Lehmann, W., Greener, J. & Simpson, DD. (2002) Assessing organizational readiness for change. *Journal of Substance Abuse Treatment*, 22, 197–209.

Loaring, J. & Best, D. (2007) *Needs Assessment for Drug Treatment Services in Birmingham*. Birmingham: Birmingham Drug and Alcohol Action Team.

Marsden, J., Gossop, M., Stewart, D., Best, D., Farrell, M., Lehmann, P., Edwards, C. & Strang, J. (1998) The Maudsley Addiction Profile (MAP): a brief instrument for assessing treatment outcome. *Addiction*, 93(12), 1857–1868.

McLellan, A. T., Kushner, H., Metzger, D., Peters, R., Smith, I., Grissom, G., Pettinati, H. & Argeriou, M. (1992) Addiction Severity Index. *Journal of Substance Abuse Treatment*, 9(3), 199–213.

McLellan, A. T. (2006) What we need is a system: creating a responsive and effective substance abuse treatment system. In: W. Miller & K. Carroll (eds) *Rethinking Substance Abuse: What the Science Shows and What We Should Do About It*. New York: Guildford Press.

Miller, W. (2007) Motivational factors in addictive behaviours. In: W. Miller & K. Carroll (eds) *Rethinking Substance Abuse*. New York: Guildford Press.

National Treatment Agency for Substance Misuse (2002) *Models of Care for Drug Treatment*. London: National Treatment Agency.

Rampazzo, L., De Angeli, M., Serpelloni, G., Simpson, D. D. & Flynn, P. (2006) Italian survey of organizational functioning and readiness for change: a cross-cultural transfer of treatment assessment strategies. *European Addiction Research*, 12(4), 176–181.

Ross, J., Teesson, M., Darke, S., Lynskey, M., Ali, R., Ritter, A. & Cooke, R. (2004) Twelve month outcomes of treatment for heroin dependence: Findings from the Australian Treatment Outcome Study (ATOS). NDARC Technical Report No 196. National Drug and Alcohol Research Centre (NDARC).

Rush, B. (1990) A systems approach to estimating the required capacity of alcohol treatment services. *British Journal of Addiction*, 85(1), 49–59.

Simpson, D. D. (2003) Introduction to 5-year follow-up treatment outcome studies [Editorial]. *Journal of Substance Abuse Treatment*, 25(3), 123–124.

Simpson, D. D. (2004) A conceptual framework for drug treatment process and outcomes. *Journal of Substance Abuse Treatment*, 27(2), 99–121.

Steier, F. (1991) Reflexivity and methodology: an ecological constructionism. In: F. Steier (ed.) *Research and Reflexivity*. London: Sage.

Stern, P. (1980) Grounded theory methodology: its uses and processes. *Image*, 12, 20–23.

Stimson, G., Fitch, C., Des Jarlais, D., Poznyak, V., Perlis, T., Oppenheimer, E. & Rhodes, T. (2006) Rapid assessment and response studies of injection drug use: knowledge gain, capacity building and intervention development in a multisite study. *American Journal of Public Health*, 96(2), 288–295.

Strauss, A. & Corbin, J. (1998) *Basics of Qualitative Research: Techniques and Procedures for Developing Grounded Theory*. Thousand Oaks, CA: Sage.

Recommended readings

Czaja, R. & Blair, J. (1996) *Designing Surveys: A Guide to Decisions and Processes*. Thousand Oaks, CA: Pine Forge Press.

Schuman, H. & Presser, S. (1981) *Questions and Answers in Attitude Surveys: Experiments on Question form, Wording and Context*. Orlando, FL: Harcourt Brace Jovanovich.

Simpson, D. & Flynn, P (2007) Moving innovations into treatment: a stage-based approach to program change. *Journal of Substance Abuse Treatment*, 33(2), 111–120.

Chapter 13

CONDUCTING CLINICAL RESEARCH

Jalie A. Tucker and Cathy A. Simpson

13.1 Conducting clinical research

Clinical research is a comprehensive area of empirical inquiry with the goal of providing high-quality, cost-effective care to persons with physical health, mental health and substance use (MH/SU) disorders. Many people equate clinical research with *randomised controlled clinical trials* (RCTs). However, clinical research is a broader, multidisciplinary enterprise that spans basic laboratory bench science to research that translates basic science findings into clinically meaningful treatments to RCTs to studies of treatment effectiveness in health care settings. Surrounding this ambitious 'bench-to-bedside' research initiative are studies concerned with influences of the broader health care system on patient care and treatment outcomes, the cost of providing quality care and dissemination of therapeutic innovations.

The unifying objective of this broad agenda is to use the best available scientific evidence to guide the provision of *evidence-based practice* (EBP), which seeks to bring health care practices and policies in line with the best scientific knowledge (e.g. Institute of Medicine, IOM, 2001; Jenicek, 2003). Over the past 25 years, the movement has increased the availability of treatment guidelines in health and mental health (e.g. Agency for Health Care Policy and Research, 1993), including those for alcohol and drug use (e.g. U.S. National Institute on Drug Abuse Therapy Manuals for Drug Addiction, 1998–2000a, b; U.S. National Institute on Alcohol Abuse and Alcoholism, NIAAA, 2005) and guidelines for improving organisational systems of care (e.g. U.S. Surgeon General's Report, 1999; IOM, 2001, 2005). For example, to improve quality of care for persons with MH/SU disorders, the IOM (2005) goals include the provision of safe, effective, patient-centred, timely, efficient and equitable care.

As the EBP movement has expanded internationally from its origins in acute medical care and drug therapies to encompass care for chronic health conditions and MH/SU disorders, what constitutes appropriate evidence and how to evaluate its quality remain central issues (Tucker & Roth, 2006). Early conceptions of evidence quality placed experimental research, as epitomised by the RCT, at the top of the 'evidence hierarchy' (e.g. Jenicek, 2003), followed by, in order from high- to low-quality, well-designed clinical trials without randomisation, observational and naturalistic research, and expert opinions, descriptive studies and case reports. Figure 13.1 shows a later elaboration of the hierarchy that placed systematic reviews and meta-analyses of RCTs above individual RCTs and placed laboratory science and research using animal models below studies with humans (Public Health Information and Data Tutorial, 2006).

Recently, a broader, less vertical approach has been advanced that recognises the strengths and limitations of different kinds of research, particularly RCTs, and uses feedback from field applications to guide and shape research questions and methods. Although RCTs have long been the 'gold standard' in clinical research, they have limited utility for investigating some clinical issues, such as how people come to seek care and the effects of environmental context on treatment outcomes.

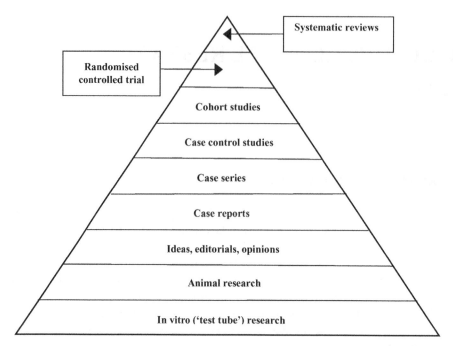

Figure 13.1 The evidence pyramid. Source: Public Health Information and Data Tutorial (2006). *Hierarchy of Evidence*. Retrieved 15 February 2008 from http://phpartners.org/tutorial/04-ebph/2-keyConcepts/4.2.7.html.

Such issues are important because substance use practices and problems are influenced by many factors beyond the treatment context. Different research designs have different strengths and limitations, and it is important for consumers of research, including service providers, to understand and evaluate the quality and usefulness of the different forms of evidence.

This chapter describes the major forms of empirical evidence that contribute to the scientific knowledge base for clinical practice, with emphasis on services for alcohol and drug problems. The chapter is organised around the usual research process, whereby scientific knowledge is developed, evaluated and disseminated from bench to bedside and into the broader community and public health domains. The chapter begins with *translational research*, which is aimed at using basic science findings to guide the development of therapies for patient care. Then, we discuss the strengths and weaknesses of *RCTs* for evaluating treatment efficacy under controlled conditions. *Effectiveness research* is discussed next, which is concerned with how treatments are established as efficacious, using RCTs work in usual care settings with a broader patient mix (see also Chapter 12). Final sections discuss the broader *public health impact* and *effective dissemination of EBPs* to providers and consumers and the special role that practitioner-researchers play in the clinical research process.

13.1.1   Translational research

Translational research seeks to 'translate' findings from basic and pre-clinical laboratory science into clinical studies with applications for patient care. The U.S. Food and Drug Administration (FDA) research process to evaluate new drug therapies epitomises the translational model. When animal research suggests a promising new drug treatment, it is then evaluated for safety with healthy humans before entering a series of therapeutic efficacy studies with the targeted, affected human population.

The developmental progression for new therapies is conceptually similar for pharmacological and behavioural approaches and focuses on translating research findings through increasing levels of scientific rigor, safety evaluation and applicability to the populations of interest (Meadows, 2002).

Pre-clinical research

In the United States, prior to testing a new drug with humans, the FDA requires safety and efficacy demonstrations at multiple pre-clinical research levels. Although treatments for MH/SU problems rarely rely solely on medications, the developmental research necessary to understand the basic behavioural relations of interest often involves animal subjects and is closely regulated by government agencies.

Simulation studies

Pre-clinical research often begins with a conceptual model of how a new drug or treatment might interact with known physical functions or environmental relationships to treat a disorder. This may involve computer simulations of the structure of a new drug or in vitro 'test tube' studies that evaluate drug effects on cellular cultures (CDER Handbook; FDA website http://www.fda.gov/cder/handbook/index.htm). For example, a recent computerised nervous system has simulated neurobehavioural responses to narcotics (Frenger, 2007), and other models have simulated the effects of environmental contingencies such as price increases on smoking (Ahmad & Billimek, 2005).

Animal models

Given promising basic science findings, investigators may begin pre-clinical studies using animals, which are closely regulated to ensure animal safety and minimise discomfort (CDER Handbook; see Chapter 17). In the United States, compliance with federal research guidelines is monitored by the U.S. Department of Agriculture, which certifies animal research laboratories. Institutions may also obtain international certification under the Association for Assessment and Accreditation of Laboratory Animal Care International, the highest level of accreditation for animal research (www.aaalac.org). Pre-clinical research with animals may provide initial information on drug absorption, toxicity, abuse liability and behavioural effects (e.g. sedation). Behavioural science techniques may also be used to model reinforcement contingencies for later translational research on the role of environmental conditions in human substance use (Box 13.1).

13.1.2 Phase 1 and Phase 2 clinical research

Promising pre-clinical research may guide Phase 1 and Phase 2 clinical studies on human substance use, which can focus on pharmacological issues (e.g. drug metabolism), behavioural issues (e.g. abuse liability) or on an interaction of both. Clinical studies with humans that involve drugs or medical devices are FDA regulated in the United States, and pharmacologic and behavioural research follow the same general stages of development and application. Translation merges into application at variable and sometimes overlapping points in this process, but, in general, by the time an innovative treatment is ready for evaluation in a Phase 3 RCT, the translation process is largely completed.

Phase 1 clinical research in pharmacology examines mechanisms of drug action, including dose-related therapeutic and side effects, using a modest number of healthy human volunteers (20–80).

Box 13.1   Context dependence of drug self-administration

An excellent example of pre-clinical translational research is provided by Carroll and colleagues' (reviewed by Carroll, 1994; Campbell & Carroll, 2000) rodent and primate studies on the effects of changes in environmental context on drug self-administration. They found that, in impoverished environments, acquisition of drug self-administration could be delayed by providing a concurrently available non-drug alternative reinforcer (e.g. sweetened water, food). Introduction of such alternatives could also disrupt established drug-taking behaviours.

Carroll et al. (1990) taught primates to self-administer cocaine freebase through a smoking tube. After the behaviour was established, subjects could obtain additional access to cocaine freebase under a progressive ratio procedure that required them to emit increasing numbers of lever presses for each successive dose. Drug self-administration was responsive to changes in 'price', or the responses required per dose. Environmental manipulations that simulated impoverished or low reinforcer density environments (by decreasing subjects' body weight) reliably increased cocaine self-administration, whereas enriched environments that provided non-contingent access to food resulted in the lowest drug self-administration. This research programme provided compelling demonstrations of environmental contingencies that have proved to be relevant to understanding human substance use and its treatment (Campbell & Carroll, 2000).

These studies determine whether further investigation with more participants or with participants who have the target disorder is warranted (CDER Handbook). Phase 1 studies may also translate basic behavioural relationships found with animals to human behaviour; for example under highly controlled conditions, they may seek to model reinforcement contingencies relevant to real-world drug use.

Building on Phase 1 findings, Phase 2 clinical research provides preliminary estimates of the effectiveness, as well as any side effects, of the new approach using larger numbers of participants who have the targeted disease or condition (often 100–200). Successful Phase 1 and Phase 2 studies set the stage for Phase 3 RCTs that examine treatment efficacy in larger samples of affected persons (see Boxes 13.2 and 13.3).

Box 13.2   Phase 1 example: role of unit price and alternative reinforcers on drug self-administration

A series of studies by Bickel and colleagues (e.g. Bickel et al., 1990, 1991) illustrate translational Phase 1 research in addictive behaviours. Nicotine-dependent smokers obtained access to cigarette puffs under conditions that varied the 'unit price' (lever presses required) of the puffs over a range of required responses. As unit price increased, preference, or willingness to work for puffs, decreased in an orderly fashion. Such relationships have been replicated and extended, and generally demonstrate that cigarettes are a 'price-sensitive' commodity, which supports tobacco control policies that involve increased cigarette taxes (e.g. Bickel et al., 1991). Using this general paradigm, Johnson and Bickel (2003) replicated Carroll et al.'s (Carroll et al., 1990; Carroll, 1994) animal laboratory data on the effects of concurrent alternative reinforcers on drug self-administration. Increasing cigarette unit price and making alternative reinforcers (nicotine gum, money) available decreased cigarette consumption.

Box 13.3 Phase 2 example: contingency management (CM) treatment

The work of Higgins and colleagues (e.g. Higgins et al., 1991, 2002) on CM approaches for cocaine dependence illustrates Phase 2 clinical research. CM was developed as an outpatient treatment for cocaine dependence when few other approaches were successful and is based on principles of reinforcement, initially demonstrated under highly controlled laboratory conditions in pre-clinical and Phase 1 studies. CM views real-world drug dependence as a special case of operant (choice) behaviour that is determined by its consequences and by competing environmental alternatives. This Phase 2 approach differs primarily from the Phase 1 work done by Bickel and colleagues in that participants were substance users in real world, largely uncontrolled situations, whereas Bickel and colleagues studied substance users in highly controlled laboratory conditions.

In the initial CM study, new intakes for cocaine dependence treatment were assigned to either CM or usual 12-step counselling (Higgins et al., 1991). CM involved earning points toward retail vouchers for meeting abstinence goals, and points steadily increased for consecutive negative drug screens. In the 12-step control condition, participants received similar payments for drug screens regardless of screen outcomes. Results overwhelmingly supported the CM approach; CM patients were three times more likely to achieve cocaine abstinence and twice as likely to complete the 12-week treatment programme.

13.1.3 Summary

Collectively, the research programmes led by Carroll, Bickel and Higgins illustrate the translational research process for developing treatments for substance use disorders. Basic behavioural science principles were used to conceptualise and treat drug dependence as a 'reinforcement disorder' such that behaviour is 'monopolised' by one kind of reinforcer (Higgins et al., 2002, p. 908).

13.1.4 Phase 3 randomised controlled clinical trials

The RCT to evaluate treatment efficacy is the centrepiece of clinical research. Its cardinal feature is the random assignment of carefully selected patients with a specific disorder to an experimental treatment or a control condition, which may involve usual care, attention or assessment without active treatment, or being put on a waiting list. The RCT addresses whether, under controlled conditions, the treatment causes improvement on outcomes of interest that is independent of other possible causal agents, such as patient characteristics or how patients came to seek services ('self-selection processes'). On the one hand, RCTs have been integral to the US FDA research process to evaluate new drug therapies for humans and are widely used to evaluate other medical and psychosocial treatments (Boutron et al., 2008). On the other hand, RCT methods have limitations and are not the best design for all clinical research questions.

Benefits of the RCT

RCTs seek to maximise the *internal validity* of an evaluation study in order to separate and detect the 'true' effects of a treatment, independent of other possible influences on outcomes. Random assignment to experimental and control groups is thought to 'neutralise' potential confounding variables by distributing their effects evenly across groups. If differences are observed between the treatment and control groups after randomisation and treatment administration, the effect is attributed to the treatment and not to selection processes, participant characteristics or other confounding factors. RCTs may employ additional procedures to help detect treatment-produced effects apart from other sources of variance, such as (a) the use of large samples with 'pure' forms of the targeted condition (e.g. alcohol-dependent persons with no comorbid conditions); (b) 'double-blind' procedures to min-imise placebo and expectancy effects, wherein neither the provider nor the patient knows whether the patient received the active treatment; (c) use of standardised treatment protocols and manuals with 'fidelity checks' on implementation; (d) standardised outcomes assessment using instruments with sound psychometric properties; and (e) wait list or minimal treatment control conditions to assess effects due to the passage of time ('spontaneous' remission).

When used to address an appropriate research question, a well-executed RCT provides stronger evidence of a causal relationship between treatment and outcomes than non-experimental research. Thus, non-experimental designs were placed at lower levels of the evidence hierarchy, both because of their non-experimental status and because they were thought to have a greater risk of selection bi-ases. However, in many health care areas, well-conducted, non-randomised cohort and case-control studies have found 'effect sizes' or treatment benefits comparable to RCTs (Concato et al., 2000; Shadish et al., 2000). The findings from the two designs converged across a wide range of treatments and conditions supporting increased confidence about causal inferences and generalisability. When differences were observed, effect sizes tended to be lower, not higher, in the quasi-experimental stud-ies (Shadish et al., 2000). Thus, the concern that observational studies without random assignment will overestimate treatment effects through selection bias appears to be overstated as long as sound research methods are used.

Limitations of the RCT

RCTs use research volunteers who will accept random assignment to a promising new treatment or a control condition. However, treatments are never prescribed randomly in real-world environments and are typically selected and sought by patients with input from providers, family and other social network members. These factors are eliminated through random assignment and cannot be studied using RCTs.

A second limitation is that RCTs often use carefully selected patients who lack complicating comorbid conditions that may contribute to poor outcomes (Humphreys et al., 2005). These ho-mogenous samples may yield results that suggest stronger treatment effects than would be observed in usual practice settings with heterogeneous 'case mix' samples. Exclusion of patients with risky comorbidities from RCTs may increase the risk of unanticipated adverse outcomes when the treat-ment is marketed commercially and prescribed to patients with such comorbidities (Horn et al., 2005).

A third artificiality of the RCT comes from treatment 'fidelity' procedures used to standardise research experiences across participants. This approach works well when the focus is on an acute surgical or pharmacological intervention that may be improved by fine adjustments in technique or dosing. However, when the treatments and disorders are distributed through time and outcomes are context-dependent, as they often are for MH/SU disorders, strict treatment standardisation can result in insensitivity to the dynamic nature of the controlling variables of behaviour change (Tucker & Roth, 2006).

A final concern about RCTs is that the use of random assignment may convey a false sense that there is a reduced need for the guidance of theory in research. Even if the treatment itself is well grounded in theory, serious missteps can occur in the treatment validation and dissemination process if the mechanisms of therapeutic action are not known (Box 13.4).

Box 13.4 RCT example: Project MATCH

The best-known RCT in the alcohol treatment literature is Project MATCH (e.g. Project MATCH Research Group, 1997), which investigated patient characteristics identified at treatment intake (e.g. readiness to change, dependence) as a basis for matching patients to treatments that presumably had different mechanisms of therapeutic action. As summarised in Table 13.1, Project MATCH was a large multi-site study in which participants with alcohol problems ($N = 1726$) were randomly assigned to one of three psychosocial treatments (12-step facilitation, cognitive–behavioural or motivational enhancement therapy). No control group was included. Although conceptually defensible, this proved a serious design limitation when outcomes over the 3-year follow-up showed very few matching effects. Rather, similar improvements were found in all three treatment conditions, but without a control group, the role of treatment in producing the improvements remained ambiguous.

Table 13.1 Design features and major findings of Project MATCH (Matching Alcoholism Treatment to Client Heterogeneity)

Research goal: evaluate the 'matching hypothesis' using RCT methodology	Do problem drinkers with different characteristics respond better to one of three psychosocial treatments that have different putative mechanisms of therapeutic action?
Sample	A total of 1726 patients at nine treatment facilities in the United States (75% male, 15% ethnic/racial minorities) drawn from parallel outpatient treatment or inpatient aftercare arms
Three-group design	Random assignment to 12-step facilitation, cognitive–behavioural or motivational enhancement therapy; no control group; intensive baseline and follow-up assessments every 90 days after treatment completion and again 3 years post-treatment
Matching variables assessed at baseline	Severity of alcohol involvement, cognitive impairment, conceptual level, gender, meaning seeking, motivation, psychiatric severity, social support for drinking versus abstinence, sociopathy, alcoholic typology
Results	All treatments led to similar improvements in drinking outcomes; little evidence for patient–treatment matching effects; exception: a treatment moderation effect at 3 years showed that participants with social networks highly supportive of drinking had better outcomes following 12-step facilitation than the other two interventions
Conclusions	Professional psychosocial treatment is beneficial, but the type is relatively unimportant
Cost	US$27 million over 8 years (US$15 643 for each of 1726 enrolled patients)

Sources: Project MATCH Research Group (1997), Marlatt (1999).

The study generally suggested that professional psychosocial treatments yield benefits, but failed to reveal a basis for patient-treatment matching. Marlatt (1999) and others have suggested that the use of random assignment took away patient choice, making the RCT a poor choice for studying differential treatment selection processes that may be vital to enhancing outcomes. These aspects of Project MATCH point to why RCTs should be complemented with other research strategies that are better suited to studying treatment choice and benefits in real-world settings.

Table 13.2 Efficacy versus effectiveness studies of treatment effects

	Efficacy studies	Effectiveness studies
Purpose	Detect the 'true effects' of treatment by reducing extraneous variance	Assess treatment effectiveness in usual care settings
Typical characteristics	• Homogeneous samples • Random assignment, blinded • Manualisation, standardised treatment, fidelity checks	• Heterogeneous samples • Circumstances leading to and surrounding care studied • Compliance measured, not forced
Better suited for studying	• Technical interventions with acute effects (e.g. surgery and pharmacotherapy) • Interventions with effects that are fairly independent of context • Interventions amenable to fine adjustments to improve outcomes	• Psychosocial problems and interventions distributed through time (e.g. functional recovery after injury) • Problems and interventions that are influenced by context • Care studied as a process, not just as an outcome
Validity and inference	Higher internal validity but lower generalisation potential and capacity to inform science-to-practice linkages	Lower internal validity but higher generalisation potential and capacity to inform science-to-practice linkages

Source: Adapted from Tucker (2008, p. 25).

13.1.5 Phase 4: Evaluating treatment effectiveness in usual care settings

Once Phase 3 RCTs establish a new treatment as efficacious, research next assesses whether the therapeutic benefits generalise to less controlled, usual care practice settings and whether unanticipated adverse effects are detectable using larger samples of usual care patients (100–1000). Phase 4 studies use larger, more diverse samples and dosages to better examine the generalisability and sustainability of *treatment effectiveness*.

Table 13.2 summarises key differences between efficacy and effectiveness studies. While both may use similar methodologies, effectiveness studies typically include a broader mix of patients with comorbid disorders who often are excluded from samples used in efficacy research. This broader mix may entail greater risk to internal validity, but effectiveness studies tend to have greater external validity through use of samples that are more representative of treatment-seeking patients (Humphreys et al., 2005; Seligman, 1995).

Trade-offs between experimental control and real-world conditions are of minor concern when the treatment under study does not depend on patient motivation, compliance, active behaviour change, or the environmental circumstances surrounding treatment delivery. But the more these dimensions matter in outcomes, as they often do in addictive behaviour change, the less well-suited RCTs are for investigating the linkages among therapeutic and extra-therapeutic variables. This is the case because the random assignment in RCTs treats persons' attributes and contextual factors as potential confounding variables that need to be neutralised. However, these factors are important to treatment-seeking and outcomes in their own right (Tucker & King, 1999; Miller & Rollnick, 2002). For example, less than 25% of persons with alcohol problems seek help, and treatment seekers tend to have more serious problems for which abstinence is an appropriate goal. In contrast, natural recovery without treatment is the dominant pathway to remission in the larger population of persons with alcohol problems, and moderation drinking is a relatively more common outcome (Sobell et al., 1996) (Box 13.5).

Box 13.5 Treatment effectiveness example: Project TrEAT

As shown in Table 13.3, Fleming et al. (2002) investigated the effectiveness of screening and brief interventions (SBIs) for alcohol problems in primary care clinics. Over 17 500 patients were screened using questions that have since been recommended for use in non-specialty medical care (NIAAA, 2005). Patients who screened positive were randomly assigned to an experimental BI or a usual care control condition. In the BI condition, physicians gave patients feedback and made recommendations about reducing or quitting drinking, discussed drinking goals and a behaviour change plan, and arranged follow-up appointments or specialty referrals as needed. Nurses made brief follow-up phone calls.

Table 13.3 Design features and major findings of Project TrEAT (Trial for Early Alcohol Treatment)

Research goal	Does brief physician advice delivered to patients in primary care who screen positive for alcohol problems improve drinking-related outcomes and reduce health services utilisation over a 4-year follow-up interval? What is the benefit–cost ratio for the intervention?
Sample	17 695 patients screened in 17 community-based primary care clinics in Wisconsin were screened for possible drinking problems (>14 drinks/week for men, >11 drinks/week for women); 772 of 2450 who screened positive were enrolled.
Three-group design	Random assignment to experimental brief intervention (BI) or usual care control condition; follow-up assessments over next 4 years (83% found at 4 years)
Intervention procedures	Two 15-minute physician sessions held 1 month apart using a scripted workbook with homework, followed by two 5-minute nurse reinforcement follow-up phone calls; behaviourally oriented BI included clear statement about need to stop/cut down on drinking, norms for safer drinking, personalised goals, self-monitoring, specialist referral as needed.
Results	Compared to usual care, BI resulted in significant reductions in alcohol use and binge drinking at 6 months; reductions maintained over 4 years; similar benefits for men and women; BI associated with fewer hospital days, emergency department visits, motor vehicle events and crime.
Benefit–cost analysis	Very favourable benefit–cost ratio; for about 70K US dollars, a health care organisation can screen and treat about 10K adults (costs = 50% for screening, 40% for intervention, 10% for staff training)
Conclusions	Brief screening and physician advice in primary care yield sustained reductions in alcohol use, health services utilisation, motor vehicle events, crime and monetary costs

Source: Fleming et al. (2002).

Compared to usual care, BI resulted in significant reductions in alcohol use and binge drinking at 6 months, which were maintained over the 4-year follow-up. In addition, BI was associated with fewer hospital days, emergency department visits, and motor vehicle events and crime. BI also had a highly favourable cost–benefit ratio, with net medical benefits of $546 and net societal benefits (taking into account positive effects on non-medical outcomes) of $7780 per patient. This landmark effectiveness study showed that alcohol screenings could be widely implemented in primary care and that brief physician advice had sustained benefits on drinking, other areas of functioning and associated costs.

13.1.6 Beyond Phase 4: Economic, public health and treatment dissemination research

There are a number of broader issues that affect whether a new treatment finds a market niche and makes its way into clinical practice. These include treatment costs relative to benefits, whether the treatment is adopted by providers or preferred by health care consumers, and the impact on population-level public health.

Treatment systems, costs and utilisation patterns

Health care has been shown to function as a 'normal good' subject to the laws of supply and demand when the distorting effects of insurance or other third-party payers are taken into account (Morrisey, 2007). For example, including a behavioural health benefit that covers substance-related services in health plans reduces the use of costly medical services (Fiedler & Wight, 1989), and providing addiction treatment reduces costs related to substance use and to other variables not directly tied to use (e.g. crime) (McCollister & French, 2003). Evidence of such *cost-offset effects* has helped expand coverage of services for MH/SU disorders, including *parity* legislation in the United States that seeks to bring MH/SU service coverage in line with historically more generously reimbursed medical services.

Public health approaches

Public health research and practice are concerned with the population of persons with health and MH/SU problems or who are at risk for problems. Public health interventions are typically community based and aimed at those who do not seek clinical care, often before problems become serious, and who could benefit from less intensive and less costly interventions that emphasise screening and prevention (e.g. SBIs). For instance, most persons with alcohol and drug problems do not seek help, and this untreated majority contributes the bulk of harm and cost at the population level (Humphreys & Tucker, 2002). Although public health interventions have modest effects on individuals, the overall impact on population health can be greater than the impact of clinical care received by a small minority. Such interventions can also serve as gateways to clinical care.

Disseminating evidence-based practices

Another important research area focuses on how to disseminate treatments established as efficacious in RCTs into usual practice settings. Efficacious but underutilised treatments are available for many behavioural health problems, including alcohol and drug problems. The dissemination process usually takes 8–9 years for new pharmacological treatments regulated by the FDA to complete the development process and enter into clinical use. For behavioural interventions, it typically takes about twice as long (Addictions Technology Transfer Center, ATTC, 2008). This lag has been attributed to theoretical differences between researchers and practitioners, lack of education and training in the provider workforce, structural and financial barriers, and policies that impede change (Squires et al., 2008).

Nevertheless, many resources are available to professionals to learn about evidence-based interventions for alcohol and drug problems. For example, SAMHSA maintains the '*Guide to Evidence-Based Practices (EBP) on the Web*' site, which provides an overview of EBPs to increase implementation. The guide is searchable by age (youth or adult) and area of practice/population (e.g. corrections,

---

Box 13.6 Disseminating EBP: the New England Regional ATTC

As an example of EBP dissemination, the New England Regional ATTC recently facilitated the dissemination of a manualised CM approach to 54 substance abuse clinics in the northeastern United States (Squires et al., 2008). The technology transfer process involved provision of information on the utility of EBPs, expert multi-component staff training in CM, bidirectional communication to facilitate organisational problem-solving for the change process, and agency feedback to ATTC regarding their satisfaction with the dissemination process. Among agencies that completed the training, staff and management satisfaction was high, and the availability of an easy-to-follow 'menu of practice options' was overwhelmingly endorsed as most helpful in promoting adoption (Squires et al., 2008).

---

dually diagnosed and methamphetamine issues), and it contains links to websites that provide free information about EBPs (SAMHSA, 2008).

Through its Center for Substance Abuse Treatment (CSAT, 2008), SAMHSA also funds the ATTC Network, a national, multidisciplinary resource for addiction professionals aimed at increasing public and professional awareness of EBPs, strengthening addiction treatment workforce skills, and assisting with organisational changes necessary for community-based agencies to adopt and use EBPs (ATTC, 2008) (Box 13.6).

13.2 Discussion and conclusions: The role of the practitioner-researcher

Different kinds of research work in concert to inform clinical practice. The different types of studies are diverse conceptually and methodologically. Each type of research has a proper place in the development, evaluation and dissemination of evidence that informs practice. However, if methods are misapplied or poorly suited to the research questions at hand, or if a single methodology like the RCT is forced on the array of clinically relevant research, the knowledge base that guides clinical practice is compromised. For this reason, clinical research is shifting away from a sharply hierarchical view of evidence that values the RCT over all other approaches to a broader horizontal view referred to as '*evidentiary pluralism*' (Tucker & Roth, 2006), a more balanced and diverse evidence base for practice that selects methodologies in service of research content questions, and not the other way around. Each research approach discussed in this chapter has something important to contribute, but none are universally applicable to all clinically relevant research questions.

Effectively evaluating the evidence places a significant burden on the research consumer. Researchers and service providers alike need to gain a working knowledge of the strengths and limitations of different research approaches and the empirical questions they can best address, including which forms of evidence inform different aspects of clinical care. Professionals who deliver health services and are also involved in clinical research occupy a special position at the interface of science and practice that is essential to effective EBP. By virtue of their experience in delivering services, they are a primary source for detecting trends in patients' needs, preferences and demand for services, identifying delivery challenges posed by financial and organisational systems, and generating new patient-oriented research questions. Practitioner-researchers also serve as critical conduits for the dissemination of innovations into real-world practice, for example by participating in clinical research networks that involve their service organisation or by modelling the early adoption of new EBPs.

A challenge for practitioner-researchers is the implementation of sound research protocols in practice settings without compromising clinical care. For example, at the level of individual patients, it is routine to establish firm boundaries between informed consent for treatment and informed consent for research participation and to maintain separate confidentiality protections between the two endeavours. Information disclosed in one venue should not affect the other, except under high-risk circumstances disclosed as part of the consent process (e.g. legally required disclosure of child or elder abuse or sexually transmitted disease reporting).

At another level, practitioner-researchers can help develop RCT protocols that strive to maintain *clinical equipoise*, which requires that (a) there is evidence-based disagreement or uncertainty about best practices and (b) no participant is 'randomized to an intervention known to be inferior to one of the treatments under investigation or the established, scientifically-validated standards of care' (Miller & Brody, 2007, p. 153). This is a complex determination, often best made by research-informed clinicians, and one that has come to favour RCTs that compare a 'usual treatment' with a new experimental treatment. Wait list, minimal or no-treatment control groups have fallen out of favour because they do not readily maintain clinical equipoise. Equipoise is also difficult to achieve when there is no usual treatment against which to compare a new treatment. This occurs in addiction treatment when a new drug problem develops in a heretofore unaffected region or population subgroup about which little is known, such as methamphetamine use in the United States.

These complex situations can be addressed through the unique clinical and research knowledge of practitioner-researchers. Because the evidence guiding practice is ever changing, practitioners and researchers must stay abreast of key developments over the span of their careers. Although challenging, growing web-based resources to promote cutting-edge EBP technology transfer and continued government subsidisation of EBP development and dissemination make continuing professional development possible for the motivated practitioner-researcher, if coupled with self-study across the spectrum of evidence.

Acknowledgements

Preparation of this chapter was supported in part by grant R01 AA08972 from the U.S. National Institute on Alcohol Abuse and Alcoholism and grant R21 DA R21-DA021524 from the U.S. National Institute on Drug Abuse.

Exercises

Exercise 1: Using the CONSORT statement

Many scientific journals require treatment-related research to be reported in line with the '*Consolidated Standards of Reporting Trials*' (CONSORT; Moher et al., 2001). The CONSORT statement includes a checklist in which randomisation and other typical RCT features figure prominently. The original version was recently elaborated to better accommodate features common to behavioural treatments, as shown in Table 13.4 (Boutron et al., 2008). To increase understanding of RCT methodologies, we recommend that readers review the seminal publication on Project MATCH (1997) and then complete the 2008 CONSORT checklist for non-pharmacological trials shown in Table 13.4. How does Project MATCH measure up?

Table 13.4 Extending the CONSORT statement to trials of non-pharmacological treatment[a]

Section	Item	Standard CONSORT description	Extension for non-pharmacologic trials
Title and abstract	1	How participants were allocated to interventions (e.g. 'random allocation', 'randomised' or 'randomly assigned')	In the abstract, description of the experimental treatment, comparator, care providers, centres and blinding status
Introduction Background	2	Scientific background and explanation of rationale	
Methods Participants	3	Eligibility criteria for participants and the settings and locations where the data were collected	When applicable, eligibility criteria for centres and those performing the interventions
Interventions	4	Precise details of the interventions intended for each group and how and when they were actually administered	Precise details of both the experimental treatment and comparator
	4A		Description of the different components of the interventions and, when applicable, descriptions of the procedure for tailoring the interventions to individual participants
	4B		Details of how the interventions were standardised
	4C		Details of how adherence of care providers with the protocol was assessed or enhanced
Objectives	5	Specific objectives and hypotheses	
Outcomes	6	Clearly defined primary and secondary outcome measures and, when applicable, any methods used to enhance the quality of measurements (e.g. multiple observations and training of assessors)	
Sample size	7	How sample size was determined and, when applicable, explanation of any interim analyses and stopping rules	When applicable, details of whether and how the clustering by care providers or centres was addressed

(Continued)

Table 13.4 (*Continued*)

Section	Item	Standard CONSORT description	Extension for non-pharmacologic trials
Randomisation-sequence generation	8	Method used to generate the random allocation sequence, including details of any restriction (e.g. blocking and stratification)	When applicable, how care providers were allocated to each trial group
Allocation concealment	9	Method used to implement the random allocation sequence (e.g. numbered containers or central telephone), clarifying whether the sequence was concealed until interventions were assigned	
Implementation	10	Who generated the allocation sequence, who enrolled participants and who assigned participants to their groups	
Blinding (masking)	11A	Whether or not participants, those administering the interventions, and those assessing the outcomes were blinded to group assignment	Whether or not those administering co-interventions were blinded to group assignment
	11B[b]		If blinded, method of blinding and description of the similarity of interventions[b]
Statistical methods	12	Statistical methods used to compare groups for primary outcome(s); methods for additional analyses, such as subgroup analyses and adjusted analyses	When applicable, details of whether and how the clustering by care providers or centres was addressed
Results Participant flow	13	Flow of participants through each stage (a diagram is strongly recommended) – specifically, for each group, report the numbers of participants randomly assigned, receiving intended treatment, completing the study protocol, and analysed for the primary outcome; describe protocol deviations from study as planned, together with reasons	The number of care providers or centres performing the intervention in each group and the number of patients treated by each care provider or in each centre

Table 13.4 (*Continued*)

Section	Item	Standard CONSORT description	Extension for non-pharmacologic trials
Implementation of intervention	New item		Details of the experimental treatment and comparator as they were implemented
Recruitment	14	Dates defining the periods of recruitment and follow-up	
Baseline data	15	Baseline demographic and clinical characteristics of each group	When applicable, a description of care providers (case volume, qualification, expertise, etc.) and centres (volume) in each group
Numbers analysed	16	Number of participants (denominator) in each group included in each analysis and whether analysis was by 'intention-to-treat'; state the results in absolute numbers when feasible (e.g. 10/20, not 50%)	
Outcomes and estimation	17	For each primary and secondary outcome, a summary of results for each group and the estimated effect size and its precision (e.g. 95% confidence interval)	
Ancillary analyses	18	Address multiplicity by reporting any other analyses performed, including subgroup analyses and adjusted analyses, indicating those prespecified and those exploratory	
Adverse events	19	All important adverse events or side effects in each intervention group	
Discussion Interpretation	20	Interpretation of the results, taking into account study hypotheses, sources of potential bias or imprecision, and the dangers associated with multiplicity of analyses and outcomes	In addition, take into account the choice of the comparator, lack of or partial blinding, and unequal expertise of care providers or centres in each group

(*Continued*)

Table 13.4 (*Continued*)

Section	Item	Standard CONSORT description	Extension for non-pharmacologic trials
Generalisability	21	Generalisability (external validity) of the trial findings	Generalisability (external validity) of the trial findings according to the intervention, comparators, patients, and care providers and centres involved in the trial
Overall evidence	22	General interpretation of the results in the context of current evidence	

ᵃAdditions or modifications to the CONSORT checklist. CONSORT ☐ Consolidated Standards of Reporting Trials.
ᵇThis item anticipates a planned revision in the next version of the standard CONSORT checklist.
Table reproduced from Boutron et al. (2008).

Exercise 2: Real-world relevance of Project TrEAT

Project TrEAT was an RCT and used random assignment and careful measurement that are the hallmarks of efficacy research. Nevertheless, the study has many other elements that resulted in findings that have relevance to real-world treatment effectiveness. Review the distinctions in Table 13.2 between efficacy and effectiveness studies, which should be viewed as complementary, not opposing, categories. Which Project TrEAT features are more relevant to addressing treatment effectiveness in usual practice environments? How well did the design balance internal and external validity? How do the Project TrEAT findings compare to Project MATCH in providing evidence for practice?

References and other readings

Abrams, D. B. & Emmons, K. M. (1997) Health behaviour and health education: the past, present, and future. In: K. Glanz, B. K. Rimer & F. M. Lewis (eds) *Health Behaviour and Health Education: Theory, Research, and Practice*. San Francisco: Jossey-Bass, pp. 453–478.

Addictions Technology Transfer Center (ATTC) Network (2008) Available online: http://www.attcnetwork.org (accessed 1 July 2008).

Agency for Health Care Policy and Research (1993) *Clinical Practice Guideline Development* (AHCPR Publication No. 93-0023). Rockville, MD: U.S. Department of Health and Human Services.

Ahmad, S. & Billimek, J. (2005) Estimating the health impact of tobacco harm reduction policies: a simulation approach. *Risk Analysis*, 25, 801–812.

Bickel, W. K., DeGrandpre, R. J., Higgins, S. T. & Hughes, J. R. (1990) Behavioral economics of drug self-administration. I. Functional equivalence of response requirement and drug dose. *Life Sciences*, 47, 1501–1510.

Bickel, W. K., DeGrandpre, R. J., Hughes, J. R. & Higgins, S. T. (1991) Behavioral economics of drug self-administration. II. A unit-price analysis of cigarette smoking. *Journal of the Experimental Analysis of Behaviour*, 55, 145–154.

Boutron, I., Moher, D., Altman, D. G., Schulz, K. F. & Ravaud, P. (2008) Extending the CONSORT statement to randomized trials of nonpharmacologic treatment: explanation and elaboration. *Annals of Internal Medicine*, 148, 295–309.

Brownson, R. C., Baker, E. A., Leet, T. L. & Gillespie, K. N. (2003) *Evidence-Based Public Health*. New York: Oxford University Press.

Budney, A. J., Higgins, S. T., Mercer, D. E. & Carpenter, G. (1998) *Manual 2: A Community Reinforcement Approach: Treating Cocaine Addiction* (NIDA Therapy Manuals for Drug Abuse). National Institute on Drug Abuse NIH Publication No. 98-4309. Available online: http://www.drugabuse.gov/TXManuals/CRA/CRA1.html.

Campbell, U. C. & Carroll, M. E. (2000) Acquisition of drug self-administration: environmental and pharmacological interventions. *Experimental and Clinical Psychopharmacology*, 8, 312–325.

Carroll, M. E. (1994) Pharmacological and behavioural treatment of cocaine addiction: animal models. *NIDA Research Monograph*, 145, 113–130.

Carroll, M. E., Krattiger, K. L., Gieske, D. & Sadoff, D. A. (1990) Cocaine-base smoking in rhesus monkeys: Reinforcing and physiological effects. *Psychopharmacology*, 102, 443–450.

CDER (n.d.) *The CDER Handbook*. Available online: http://www.fda.gov/cder/handbook/index.htm (accessed 5 July 2008).

Centers for Substance Abuse Treatment (CSAT) (2008) *CSAT Inventory of Effective Substance Abuse Treatment Practices*. Available online: http://csat.samhsa.gov/treatment.aspx (accessed 1 July 2008).

Collins, C., Harshbarger, C., Sawyer, R. & Hamdallah, M. (2006) The diffusion of effective behavioral interventions project: development, implementation, and lessons learned. *AIDS Education and Prevention*, 18(Suppl. A), 5–20.

Concato, J., Shah, N. & Horwitz, R. I. (2000) Randomized, controlled trials, observational studies, and the hierarchy of research designs. *New England Journal of Medicine*, 342, 1887–1892.

Donatelle, R. J., Prows, S. L., Champeau, D. & Hudson, D. (2000) Randomized controlled trial using social support and financial incentives for high risk pregnant smokers. *Tobacco Control*, 9(Suppl. III), iii67–iii69.

Dworkin, S. L., Pinto, R. M., Hunter, J., Rapkin, B. & Remien, R. H. (2008) Keeping the spirit of community partnerships alive in the scale up of HIV/AIDS prevention: critical reflections on the roll out of DEBI (Diffusion of Effective Behavioral Interventions). *American Journal of Community Psychology*, 42(1–2), 51–59.

Fiedler, J. L. & Wight, J. B. (1989) *The Medical Offset Effect and Public Health Policy*. New York: Praeger.

Fleming, M. F., Mundt, M. P., French, M. T., Manwell, L. B., Stauffacher, E. A. & Barry, K. L. (2002) Brief physician advice for problem drinkers: long-term efficacy and benefit-cost analysis. *Alcoholism: Clinical and Experimental Research*, 26, 36–43.

Frenger, P. (2007) Human narcotic use emulator. *Biomedical Sciences Instrumentation*, 43, 278–283.

Ghitza, E., Epstein, D. & Preston, K. (2008) Contingency management reduces injection drug HIV risk behaviors in heroin and cocaine using outpatients. *Addictive Behaviors*, 33, 593–604.

Higgins, S. T., Alessi, S. M. & Dantona, R. L. (2002) Voucher-based incentives: a substance abuse treatment innovation. *Addictive Behaviors*, 27, 887–910.

Higgins, S. T., Delaney, D. D., Budney, A. J., Bickel, W. K., Hughes, J. R., Foerg, F. & Fenwick, J. W. (1991) A behavioural approach to achieving cocaine abstinence. *American Journal of Psychiatry*, 148, 1218–1224.

Higgins, S. T. & Petry, N. M. (1999) Contingency management: incentives for sobriety. *Alcohol Research and Health*, 23, 122–127.

Horn, S. D., DeJong, G., Ryser, D. K., Veazie, P. J. & Teraoka, J. (2005) Another look at observational studies in rehabilitation research: going beyond the Holy Grail of the randomized controlled trial. *Archives of Physical Medicine and Rehabilitation*, 86(Suppl. 2), S8–S15.

Humphreys, K. & Tucker, J. A. (2002) Toward more responsive and effective intervention systems for alcohol-related problems. *Addiction*, 97, 126–132.

Humphreys, K., Weingardt, K. R., Horst, D., Joshi, A. A. & Finney, J. A. (2005) Prevalence and predictors of research participant eligibility criteria in alcohol treatment outcome studies. *Addiction*, 100, 1249–1257.

Institute of Medicine (2001) *Crossing the Quality Chasm: A New Health System for the 21st Century*. Washington, DC: National Academies Press.

Institute of Medicine (2005) *Improving the Quality of Health Care for Mental Health and Substance Use Conditions*. Washington, DC: National Academies Press.

Jenicek, M. (2003) *Foundations of Evidence-Based Medicine*. New York: Parthenon.

Johnson, M. W. & Bickel, W. K. (2003) The behavioural economics of cigarette smoking: the concurrent presence of a substitute and an independent reinforcer. *Behavioural Pharmacology*, 14, 137–144.

Leichsenring, F. (2004) Randomized controlled versus naturalistic studies: a new research agenda. *Bulletin of the Menninger Clinic*, 68, 137–151.

Marlatt, G. A. (1999) From hindsight to foresight: a commentary on Project MATCH. In: J. A. Tucker, D. M. Donovan & G. A. Marlatt (eds) *Changing Addictive Behaviour: Bridging Clinical and Public Health Perspectives*. New York: Guilford, pp. 45–66.

McCollister, K. E. & French, M. T. (2003) The relative contribution of outcome domains in the total economic benefit of addiction interventions: a review of first findings. *Addiction*, 98, 1647–1659.

Meadows, M. (2002) The FDA's drug review process: ensuring drugs are safe and effective. *FDA Consumer*, 36(FDA Publication No. 02-3242).

Miller, F. G. & Brody, H. (2007) Clinical equipoise and the incoherence of research ethics. *Journal of Medical Philosophy*, 32, 151–165.

Miller, W. R. & Rollnick, S. (2002) *Motivational Interviewing: Preparing People for Change*, 2nd edn. New York: Guilford.

Miller, W. R. & Wilbourne, P. L. (2002) Mesa Grande: a methodological analysis of clinical trials of treatments for alcohol use disorders. *Addiction*, 97, 265–277.

Moher, D., Schulz, K. F. & Altman, D. (2001) The CONSORT statement: revised recommendations for improving the quality of reports of parallel-group randomized trials. *JAMA: Journal of the American Medical Association*, 285, 1987–1991.

Moos, R. H., Finney, J. W. & Cronkite, R. (1990) *Alcoholism Treatment: Context, Process, and Outcome*. London: Oxford University Press.

Morrisey, M. A. (2007) *Health Insurance*. Chicago, IL: Health Administration Press.

National Institute on Alcohol Abuse and Alcoholism (NIAAA) (2005) *Helping Patients Who Drink Too Much: A Clinician's Guide*. Rockville, MD: NIAAA/National Institutes of Health/U.S. Department of Health and Human Services. Available online: http://pubs.niaaa.nih.gov/publications/Practitioner/Clinicians Guide2005/clinicians_guide.htm.

National Institute on Alcohol Abuse and Alcoholism (1994–1998) *Project MATCH Series Treatment, Assessment, and Implementation Manuals*. Rockville, MD: NIAAA/National Institutes of Health/U.S. Department of Health and Human Services. Available online: http://pubs.niaaa.nih.gov/publications/match.htm.

National Institute on Drug Abuse (NIDA) (1998–2000a) *The NIDA Clinical Toolbox: Science-Based Materials for Drug Abuse Treatment Providers*. Rockville, MD: NIDA/ National Institutes of Health/U.S. Department of Health and Human Services. Available online: www.nida.nih.gov/TB/Clinical/ClinicalToolbox.html.

National Institute on Drug Abuse (1998–2000b) *Therapy Manuals for Drug Addiction*, Vol. 1–3. Rockville, MD: NIDA/ National Institutes of Health/U.S. Department of Health and Human Services.

Petry, N. M. (2005) Methadone plus contingency management or performance feedback reduces cocaine and opiate use in persons with drug addiction. *American Journal of Psychiatry*, 162, 340–349.

Petry, N. M., Martin, B., Cooney, J. L. & Kranzler, H. R. (2000) Give the prizes, and they will come: contingency management treatment of alcohol dependence. *Journal of Consulting and Clinical Psychology*, 68, 250–257.

Preston, K. L., Silverman, K., Umbricht, A., DeJesus, A., Montoya, I. D. & Schuster, C. R. (1999) Improvement in naltrexone treatment compliance with contingency management. *Drug and Alcohol Dependence*, 54, 127–135.

Project MATCH Research Group (1997) Matching alcoholism treatment to client heterogeneity: Project MATCH posttreatment drinking outcomes. *Journal of Studies on Alcohol*, 58, 7–29.

Public Health Information and Data Tutorial (2006) *Hierarchy of Evidence*. Available online: http://phpartners.org/tutorial/04-ebph/2-keyConcepts/4.2.7.html (accessed 15 February 2008).

Roll, J. M. (2007) Contingency management: an evidence-based component of methamphetamine use disorder treatments. *Addiction*, 102(Suppl. 1), 114–120.

Seligman, M. (1995) The effectiveness of psychotherapy. *American Psychologist*, 50(12), 965–974.

Shadish, W. R., Navarro, A. M., Matt, G. E. & Phillips, G. (2000) The effects of psychological therapies under clinically representative conditions: a meta-analysis. *Psychological Bulletin*, 126, 512–529.

Sobell, L. C., Cunningham, J. A. & Sobell, M. B. (1996) Recovery from alcohol problems with and without treatment: prevalence in two population surveys. *American Journal of Public Health*, 86, 966–972.

Spring, B., Pagoto, S., Kaufmann, P. G., Whitlock, E. P., Glasgow, R. E., Smith, T. W., Trudeau, K. H. & Davison, K. W. (2005) Invitation to a dialogue between researchers and clinicians about evidence-based behavioral medicine. *Annals of Behavioral Medicine*, 30, 125–137.

Squires, D. D., Gumbley, S. J. & Sorti, S. A. (2008) Training substance abuse treatment organizations to adopt evidence-based practices: The Addiction Technology Transfer Center of New England Science to Service Laboratory. *Journal of Substance Abuse Treatment*, 34, 293–301.

Substance Abuse and Mental Health Services Administration (2008) *SAMHSA: A Pocket Guide to Evidence-Based Practices (EBP) on the Web*. Available online: http://www.samsah.gov/ebpwebguide/index.asp (accessed 4 July 2008).

Tucker, J. A. (1999) Changing addictive behaviour: historical and contemporary perspectives. In: J. A. Tucker, D. M. Donovan & G. A. Marlatt (eds) *Changing Addictive Behaviour: Bridging Clinical and Public Health Perspectives*. New York: Guilford, pp. 3–44.

Tucker, J. A. (2001) Resolving problems associated with alcohol and drug misuse: understanding relations between addictive behaviour change and the use of services. *Substance Use and Misuse*, 36, 1501–1518.

Tucker, J. A. & King, M. P. (1999) Resolving alcohol and drug problems: influences on addictive behaviour change and help-seeking processes. In: J. A. Tucker, D. M. Donovan & G. A. Marlatt (eds) *Changing Addictive Behaviour: Bridging Clinical and Public Health Perspectives*. New York: Guilford, pp. 97–126.

Tucker, J. A. & Reed, G. M. (2008) Evidentiary pluralism as a strategy for research and evidence-based practice in rehabilitation psychology. *Rehabilitation Psychology*, 53, 279–293

Tucker, J. A. & Roth, D. L. (2006) Extending the evidence hierarchy to enhance evidence-based practice for substance use disorders. *Addiction*, 101, 918–932.

U.S. Surgeon General (1999) *Mental Health: A Report of the Surgeon General*. Rockville, MD: Substance Abuse and Mental Health Services Administration, National Institutes of Health.

Victoria, C. G., Habicht, J.-P. & Bryce, J. (2004) Evidence-based public health: moving beyond randomized trials. *American Journal of Public Health*, 94, 400–405.

Westen, D., Novotny, C. M. & Thompson-Brenner, H. (2004) Empirical status of empirically supported psychotherapies: assumptions, findings, and reporting in controlled clinical trials. *Psychological Bulletin*, 130, 631–663.

Recommended readings

Addictions Technology Transfer Center (ATTC) Network (2008) Available online: http://www.attcnetwork.org

Association for Assessment and Accreditation of Laboratory Animal Care (AAALAC) (2008) Available online: http://www.aaalac.org

Boutron, I., Moher, D., Altman, D. G., Schulz, K. F. & Ravaud, P. (2008) Extending the CONSORT statement to randomized trials of nonpharmacologic treatment: explanation and elaboration. *Annals of Internal Medicine*, 148, 295–309.

Budney, A. J., Higgins, S. T., Mercer, D. E. & Carpenter, G. (1998). *Manual 2: A Community Reinforcement Approach: Treating Cocaine Addiction*. NIDA Therapy

Centers for Substance Abuse Treatment (CSAT) (2008) *CSAT Inventory of Effective Substance Abuse Treatment Practices*. Available online: http://csat.samhsa.gov/treatment.aspx

Fleming, M. F., Mundt, M. P., French, M. T., Manwell, L. B., Stauffacher, E. A. & Barry, K. L. (2002) Brief physician advice for problem drinkers: long-term efficacy and benefit-cost analysis. *Alcoholism: Clinical and Experimental Research*, 26, 36–43.

Manuals for Drug Abuse. National Institute on Drug Abuse NIH Publication Number 98-4309. Available online: http://www.drugabuse.gov/TXManuals/CRA/CRA1.html

Project MATCH Research Group (1997) Matching alcoholism treatment to client heterogeneity: Project MATCH posttreatment drinking outcomes. *Journal of Studies on Alcohol*, 58, 7–29.

Recommended websites

http://www.ncrr.nih.gov/clinical_research_resources/
National Center for Research Resources website maintained by the U.S. National Institutes of Health, Department of Health and Human Services
http://www.nimh.nih.gov/health/trials/index.shtml
Clinical trials information maintained by the U.S. National Institute on Mental Illness, National Institutes of Health, Department of Health and Human Services
http://www.clinicaltrials.gov/
Registry of ongoing clinical trials in the United States and around the world; includes a link for a glossary of terms
http://www.dcri.duke.edu/
Website for the Duke University Clinical Research Institute, the world's largest academic clinical research organisation
http://www.drugabuse.gov/TB/Clinical/ClinicalToolbox.html
Link for the U.S. National Institute on Drug Abuse 'Clinical Toolbox' that provides science-based materials for treatment providers
http://pubs.niaaa.nih.gov/publications/Practitioner/CliniciansGuide2005/clinicians_guide.htm
Link for the U.S. National Institute on Alcohol Abuse and Alcoholism 2005 guide 'How to Help Patients Who Drink Too Much: A Clinical Approach'
http://www.fda.gov/cder/handbook/index.htm
Link to the 'The CDER Handbook', which describes the stages and rationale of the FDA research process
http://www.attcnetwork.org
Link to technology transfer information in the Addictions Technology Transfer Center (ATTC) Network and regional technology transfer assistance centres

Section IV
Biological Methods

Chapter 14

PSYCHOPHARMACOLOGY

Jason White and Nick Lintzeris

14.1 Introduction

Psychopharmacology broadly describes the study of drugs that affect the brain. It includes both those used for treatment of medical conditions (e.g. analgesics for pain) and mental health disorders (e.g. antipsychotics, antidepressants) as well as drugs used non-medically. In this chapter we are concerned only with the second group (drugs used non-medically), as well as those used in the treatment of addiction. Only studies in humans are considered here and we focus on laboratory-based studies; clinical and survey methods are discussed in other chapters in this volume.

The chapter is divided into four sections. The first provides an overview of both the aims of psychopharmacology research and the various measures used in this research (i.e. behavioural and physiological measures, drug concentrations and measures of neurotransmitter function). The second focus is on measurement of the changes in subjective experience and objective effects produced by drugs, including a consideration of adverse drug effects, such as cognitive and psychomotor and physiological impairment. The final two sections describe two areas of study central to addiction: drug self-administration and drug withdrawal and craving.

14.2 Psychopharmacology: drugs, behaviour, physiology and the brain

14.2.1 Aims of psychopharmacology

There are a number of reasons to carry out psychopharmacology research as part of the study of drug addiction and its treatment. One reason is to understand or predict the degree to which a drug is going to be used non-medically and the likelihood of this use resulting in addiction. Collectively, this research has been known under the term 'abuse liability testing'. For new drugs that have a central nervous system action suggesting significant abuse liability, this is an essential part of the research that precedes approval by regulatory authorities. However, it is also important in understanding relative abuse liability of existing drugs and the factors that affect the likelihood of abuse, as well as the links between brain mechanisms and abuse liability.

A second major focus of psychopharmacology research consists of determining and describing the adverse effects of drugs. Most such research focuses on the effects that occur following single drug administration, although there are also increasing numbers of studies in users that focus on long-term changes associated with neurotoxic drug effects. The adverse effects can range from life-threatening changes (e.g. respiratory depression following administration of an opioid) to less dramatic, but more common physical (e.g. nausea and skin rashes) ailments or impairment of cognitive and psychomotor functions. Many studies of the latter type have been motivated by concerns related to motor vehicle driving (Ogden & Moskowitz, 2004), but the implications are much broader. Impairment in a range of functions affects the person's likelihood of carrying out paid work or study, being able to care

---

Box 14.1   Pharmacokinetics and pharmacodynamics

Pharmacokinetics is the study of how drug concentrations change in the body. It includes absorption of the drug, its distribution through the body, as well as metabolism and other ways in which drugs are eliminated.

Pharmacodynamics is the study of drug action: what actions does the drug have in the body and what effects are produced as a consequence?

---

for children and function socially. Drugs may interfere with a range of such day-to-day activities, and the degree can be predicted from laboratory studies of performance.

The third focus is to understand mechanisms in the broad sense. How do particular effects of drugs come about? What brain systems are involved? Two such areas are outlined below: relating observed changes produced by drugs to the change in concentration of the drug following administration and relating changes in drug effects to neurotransmitter changes. Another mechanism involves interactions between drugs. Much non-medical use of drugs involves the administration of multiple drugs. Based on an understanding of the pharmacology of the drugs, both pharmacokinetics and pharmacodynamics (see Box 14.1), we can predict certain interactions that may result in an effect of different magnitude than would be expected or the emergence of a novel effect from the drug combination. Such interactions may be unintended consequences of drug use or may be intended by the user to produce specific outcomes. The study of such interactions is an essential part of psychopharmacology, even though one that has received limited attention to date.

14.2.2   Linking outcomes to drug concentration and neurotransmitter changes

Behavioural, physiological and subjective outcome measures can be related to changes in drug concentrations. Such relations can help establish a causal mechanism of change. The information is also of importance in determining which people are likely to experience particular effects after administering a drug. While the ideal measure is the concentration of drug in the central nervous system, this is currently unobtainable. Other biological media have to be used as proxies for what is happening in the brain (see also Chapter 10).

There are various types of biological samples that can be assayed to determine drug concentration, but some have little relevance to psychopharmacology research because they reflect long-term changes. Hair and sweat samples may be analysed for longer-term changes in drug concentration that may be useful clinically, but are of limited interest when studying more immediate drug effects (Pragst & Balikova, 2006). Urine drug concentrations also fail to reflect immediate changes. For psychopharmacology research, blood is of the most value, with some potential for saliva to be used (Cone & Huestis, 2007).

Assays for blood (usually in the form of plasma) to quantify drug concentration are based on chromatographic methods. Drug molecules travel at different rates through chemical media depending on the chemical properties of the drug. Each drug has a specific time/distance of travel through a chemical medium that enables identification of the drug. The concentration in a sample can then be calculated based on the results from known concentrations in the same system. Commonly used methods include TLC (thin layer chromatography), HPLC (high-performance liquid chromatography), GC/MS (gas chromatography/mass spectrometry) and LC/MS (liquid chromatography/mass spectrometry).

Box 14.2   Polarity

Polarity refers to the degree of a charge in the drug molecule. A polar molecule is more positive at one end and more negative at the other. A non-polar molecule will not have any difference in charge.

While blood plasma is the best medium to use in determining drug concentration in the body, it should be recognised that the drugs of interest in psychopharmacology research have their major site of action in the brain. The various functions of the blood–brain barrier mean that *concentrations in the blood may not accurately reflect brain concentrations*. The blood–brain barrier limits access of drugs to the brain based on their chemical properties. Thus, morphine, a very polar molecule (see Box 14.2), does not readily cross the blood–brain barrier, whereas diacetylmorphine (heroin) is much less polar and is more readily able to cross. Drug molecules are prevented from acting on neural tissue also by the action of transporters that move drug molecules from brain tissue into blood. The activity of these transporters is largely genetically determined, leading to significant variation between individuals. The permeability of the blood–brain barrier (see Box 14.3) is also subject to change, with the actions of drugs themselves being one means by which permeability may be increased. All these factors can lead to significant to inter- and intra-individual variability in the brain–plasma drug concentration ratio. As a consequence, plasma concentrations need to be interpreted with some degree of caution. This also means that for some drugs there is a good correlation between plasma concentration and effect (e.g. methadone), whereas for others the relation is poor (e.g. tetrahydrocannabinol).

Even given these limitations, correlations of plasma drug concentration and effect can be valuable. Understanding how concentration influences a drug effect gives the ability to predict outcomes based on known changes in concentration. Differences in drug concentration may also be a major driver of variability. Determining concentration then allows control of this factor, increasing the power of experimental studies in psychopharmacology. Finally, knowledge of concentration–effect relations can help in the translation of laboratory-based findings into application in the clinical environment (e.g. dose requirements of a medication).

Understanding the mechanisms underlying drug effects is greatly facilitated if we can link these changes to levels of neurotransmitter activity. Traditionally, this has been largely carried out through animal models with human research limited to less invasive methods. Brain imagining technology is advancing rapidly, and while neurotransmitter action cannot be measured directly, it can be inferred through changes in activities of specific brain regions and receptor occupancy (see Chapter 15).

This leaves only indirect methods for assessing neurotransmitter function in humans. One approach is to measure the neurotransmitter and/or its metabolites in blood. If there is greater brain

Box 14.3   The blood–brain barrier

The walls of blood vessels in the brain are composed of closely spaced cells that make it difficult for potentially toxic substances to enter the brain. This is known as the blood–brain barrier. In addition, there are transporters that serve to remove potentially toxic molecules from the brain. The effectiveness of the blood–brain barrier varies according to conditions in the body and can be diminished by some illnesses and drugs.

> **Box 14.4   Dopamine and serotonin**
>
> Dopamine and serotonin are two of the key neurotransmitters (chemical messengers that allow communication between neurons) in the brain. Dopamine is found in distinct pathways that play a role in movement (degeneration causes Parkinson's disease), mental state (dopamine dysfunction is the main cause of psychosis) and drug addiction. Serotonin is more widely distributed in the brain. It has a role in mood (antidepressants generally produce their effects by modifying serotonin function), sleep and cognitive function.

activity in dopamine or serotonin systems (see Box 14.4), for example, we would expect to find higher concentrations of the metabolites, 5-HIAA (5-hydroxyindoleacetic acid) for serotonin and DOPAC (3,4-dihyroxyphenylacetic acid) and HVA (homovanillic acid) for dopamine. There are obvious limitations in the assumption that blood and brain concentrations of these metabolites are closely related and that concentrations in the blood will reflect overall activity in the brain, rather than in specific regions. Nevertheless, the concentrations in blood provide reasonable markers of brain activity.

When long-term changes in the brain neurotransmitter function are of interest, drugs themselves can be used as probes. For example, the response to amphetamine administration may be used as a measure of dopamine functioning in an individual and the response to a compound called 5-HTP to measure serotonin function. However, these methods cannot be used to assess neurotransmitter function following drug administration.

14.3   Measuring drug effects

Psychotropic drugs exert effects which a person experiences or feels after their administration (subjective effects), and effects which may be apparent to an onlooker (objective effects). Drugs may exert beneficial effects to the individual, and/or may produce negative consequences or adverse effects, either due to immediate drug effects (e.g. intoxication), through long-term use, or following cessation of long-term use (rebound or withdrawal phenomena).

Acute drug effects may be readily examined under controlled laboratory conditions following the administration of a drug, often at different doses in order to obtain a dose–response relationship, and by measurement of various subjective and objective parameters before and after drug administration. Such research is often conducted in 'healthy volunteers' (Phase I research) or in individuals with the target condition, such as examining the effects of a new medication in a target group of chronic methamphetamine users (Phase II research). See also Chapter 13 for a full description of the different phases of clinical research.

Assessment of the effects of long-term drug use is often more difficult. It is generally unethical to get healthy volunteers to take psychoactive drugs for extended periods for the purposes of research. Consequently, such studies require examination of drug effects in individuals who have themselves been taking the drugs chronically. However, individuals taking long-term medication (e.g. methadone and antidepressants) or chronic non-medical substance users often have a range of other medical or mental health conditions, and a history of other (poly)substance use which confounds the interpretation of findings. Comparisons to healthy 'controls' are frequently made when examining the effects of chronic non-medical use (e.g. cannabis use) or the effects of long-term medication (e.g. years of benzodiazepine or methadone use), although difficulties in appropriately matching groups is a potentially major confounder (Meyer, 2001).

Randomised prospective trials comparing active drug to a control (e.g. placebo) or comparing different doses of a drug are ideally required to examine long-term drug effects (e.g. adverse events), although such studies are unfortunately rarely conducted in psychopharmacology. Prospective randomised controlled trial designs allow for the detection of high-incidence adverse events, but not of rare-adverse events, which require case study and post-marketing surveillance (Phase IV) studies.

The following provides an overview of the techniques used to assess subjective, cognitive performance and physiological drug effects. Our better understanding of the links between these overlapping domains, and developments in behavioural, neurotransmitter and imaging, electrophysiological and genetic research has led to greater interest in combined approaches to psychopharmacological assessment (Curran & Mintzer, 2006).

14.3.1   Subjective drug effects

Measurement of subjective effects of a drug typically involves asking an individual how he/she feels before a drug is administered, and then to repeat the question(s) at regular intervals after its administration. However, asking individuals to describe drug effects in their 'own words' can produce results that are difficult to collate, interpret and compare between individuals. Consequently, more structured questioning is routinely employed. *Symptom checklists* ask whether an individual is experiencing a particular symptom or adverse event (e.g. headache and dry mouth) at a particular point in time, with either 'yes/no' responses or grades of response (e.g. absent, mild, moderate and severe). *Adjective checklists* can be used for individuals to describe their current mental state by means of predetermined adjectives. Examples include the Profile of Mood States (McNair et al., 2003) and the Addiction Research Centre Inventory (Haertzen et al., 1963) (see Box 14.5). A further refinement involves the use of *semantic differentials* – in which individuals are asked to choose between contrasting terms (e.g. 'sleepy' or 'wide-awake'; 'sad' or 'cheerful'). Visual analogue scales (Aitken, 1969) are a version of a semantic differential, in which the individual is asked to rate (using a mark on a 100-mm line) between two extremes denoted at either end of the line). They are commonly used in research as they are quick to administer, generally reliable and easy to analyse quantitatively. Whilst standardisation of questionnaires simplifies quantitative comparisons between individuals and groups, it nevertheless limits the individual's description of subjective effects and/or obscure individual variations, such that most studies will also include some open-ended description of subjective effects.

Objective measures of drug effects

Drugs can affect behaviour that requires some level of performance, which can be assessed using various performance tests. These can be broadly classified into tests that measure overlapping domains of general performance, perception, aspects of thought and intelligence, characteristics of memory and characteristics of motor function. Tests of general performance record the degree of

---

Box 14.5   Addiction Research Center Inventory (ARCI) questions (Haertzen et al., 1963)

True/false	I am full of energy
True/false	I feel more clear headed than dreamy
True/false	My speech is slurred
True/false	People might say that I am a little dull today
True/false	My head feels heavy
True/false	It seems harder than usual to move around

Box 14.6   Cancellation of 4s task

Instructions. 'When I say "Go", I want you to cross out all the 4s as quickly as you can. Work along each line from left to right'. Then say 'Go' and start stopwatch.

```
98932787243566768344238423768341497873218786178914 3
33783121323342487977423879027207902890408091986490 7
84497784262346324879089079823789742432179823083434 2
52709215179007432767583281908038826310901427870929 9
67242218244978092786920894932789275676233424347828 2
29238743210908932122341989092190532210921307634213 0
42397643252398908789863483083890723176521307321093 7
32162319023241289135679801534275687901264987218374 5
```

---

alertness, concentration or exertion, and include simple arithmetic, cancellation (e.g. Cancellation of 4s – see Box 14.6) and coding tasks (e.g. Digit Symbol Substitution Test). Assessing processes of perception examines speed, extent and quality of perception, often as an assessment of wakefulness or tiredness, commonly using tachistoscopic trials and visual flicker tests (see Lezak, 2004).

The acute effects of drug use upon various aspects of learning and memory are commonly assessed using digit span, word list, paired associate and logical memory tests. These approaches are commonly used for drugs known to affect memory (e.g. sedative hypnotics and stimulants). Through appropriate timing of drug administration and memory assessment, the different components of memory – intake (registration), processing (encoding), storage and retention, and retrieval – can be examined.

Motor performance is subject to many cognitive, emotional and physical systems. Many methods of testing motor performance come from driving and work place settings, such as measurement of reaction times, tapping and aiming tests. These tests often suffer from pronounced practice effects through repeated testing. More sophisticated and complex tests are available through computerised simulators (e.g. driving simulators) that can differentiate aspects of psychomotor function and impairment.

14.3.2   Physiological assessment

Many drugs affect physiological function, and these are sometimes examined in research as a way of measuring the strength of drug effect (e.g. pupil size as a measure of level of opiate activity), or in assessing adverse drug effects. Examples of measures of physiological drug effects include:

Cardiorespiratory measures (e.g. heart rate, blood pressure and electrocardiograph readings) and measures of respiration (e.g. respiratory rate, peripheral oxygen and carbon dioxide levels) are employed where there are particular concerns regarding overdose toxicity (e.g. opioids and sedatives) or cardiac conduction abnormalities (e.g. stimulants, synthetic opioids, and antipsychotic medications implicated in QT prolongation).

Neurophysiological testing increasingly uses neuroimaging techniques to identify structural or functional changes in brain activity, and has largely superseded earlier approaches such as electroencephalograms (EEGs). However, EEG studies continue to be of use clinically (e.g. assessment of alcohol or benzodiazepine withdrawal seizures), and in related areas such as polysomnograph sleep studies, in which EEGs are linked to other parameters of cardiorespiratory function, eye and muscle activity. Polysomnographs are particularly relevant in assessing the effects of sedative-hypnotic, stimulant and opioid medications implicated in sleep disorders.

Hepatic function is commonly assessed using **blood liver function tests,** as many individuals with substance use problems have underlying hepatic disease (due to alcohol or viral pathogens), and it is important to exclude that medications used to treat addictive disorders do not cause further hepatic injury.

It has long been recognised that non-medical use of various substances (most notably heroin and alcohol) is associated with various endocrine changes (e.g. sex hormones and bone metabolism) and immune changes (e.g. impaired T-cell function in long-term heroin users). However, as many endocrine and immune changes arise from long-term substance use in individuals with complex medical and polysubstance histories, it is difficult to examine in humans, and most work continues in animal models.

14.4 Human drug self-administration

14.4.1 Methods

Drug self-administration is the way in which drug use is directly studied under controlled laboratory conditions. Prior to the development of this approach, drug use could only be studied in naturalistic settings that did not permit the variation in conditions that the laboratory allows. Such naturalistic research could only address a limited number of questions; significant advance has required the development of self-administration methods that have borrowed extensively from the animal self-administration studies that began in the 1960s.

The experimental paradigm for animal and human self-administration research is based on operant conditioning methods. The drug is provided as a reinforcer that is contingent on a prescribed behaviour. In the experimental situation this is commonly a simple behaviour such as key pressing. The schedule determines the relation between the behaviour and the delivery of the drug reinforcer. For example, 200 button-presses may be required before a person receives a dose of heroin. In human research, the route of administration is typically the one employed by users of the drug: oral for alcohol, smoke inhalation for cannabis, intravenous infusions for opioids, and so forth.

More complex experimental arrangements offer subjects a choice, for example, between two different doses of a drug, or between a drug and money. This allows the experimenter to determine the relative reinforcing strength of a particular drug dose. Schedules may also be arranged to determine the maximum amount of work the person will do to obtain the reinforcers. This allows comparison between the reinforcing strength of different doses of a drug, different routes of administration and different drugs. To date, this approach has been much less extensively used in humans compared to animal research.

Human self-administration research is limited by factors such as the difficulty in gaining ethical approval, recruiting appropriate subjects, controlling their drug use and providing an environment in which self-administration can be studied. Most of the laboratories that have a strong record of research in this area use residential laboratory environments for their studies. Typically, the subjects are drug users who have extensive drug use experience, but who are not necessarily physically dependent. They reside in a facility for the duration of a study and engage in experimental sessions periodically over that time. This allows a large body of data to be gained for each subject under conditions in which the person's pattern of drug use is entirely controlled. Other alternative types of participants are naïve subjects and drug users in a less controlled environment. The former group is at risk of experiencing adverse effects because of the lack of tolerance, and there are ethical issues regarding the risk of addiction. The latter approach provides real-life validity, but with the potential for considerable variability due to lack of control of prior and current drug use.

Box 14.7   Sedative self-administration (Hursh et al., 2005)

In one of these early studies, subjects with a history of sedative abuse who were living on a research ward for a period of weeks had the opportunity to self-administer a sedative drug. Each subject had an exercise cycle and was able to earn a token for each 2 minutes of riding. If not used for drug purchase, tokens could be exchanged for other on-ward privileges. The number of tokens per dose varied from one to ten. When the cost was 1 token per dose subjects consumed all or nearly all the available doses, but as the cost increased the number of doses purchased decreased, in some cases to zero. This and other similar studies have shown that even among people with a history of abuse and dependence, drug use is not an inflexible pattern. It is strongly influenced by external factors such as the cost or amount of effort required to obtain the drug.

14.4.2   Outcomes

The self-administration model has been shown to transfer readily to the human laboratory. Drug users will self-administer the drugs that are subject to 'abuse' in the natural environment. Importantly, this self-administration has been shown to be sensitive to environmental contingencies. One of the factors that has been studied extensively is the cost of the drug. In an experimental situation this is usually operationalised in terms of the amount of work required to obtain a dose of the drug. Typically, it is found that as the work requirement per unit dose is increased, the overall frequency of drug intake decreases. In economic terms, drugs show some degree of price elasticity. This occurs even in people regarded as dependent on the drug and the finding contrasts with popular views that regard dependent users as insensitive to such external cost factors. These early findings from the 1970s have been extended over the years to a much more sophisticated study of the behavioural economics of drug self-administration (Hursh et al., 2005) (see Box 14.7).

Self-administration studies have also played a key role in the development of new pharmacotherapies for drug addiction. Two important questions can be addressed by this experimental approach:

1.   Is the pharmacotherapy effective in suppressing self-administration of the drug?
2.   What is the likelihood that the medication itself will be associated with dependence and abuse?

An important example of the first type of study is the research that demonstrated that opioid users who were maintained on buprenorphine largely ceased heroin self-administration, even when it was readily accessible in a laboratory environment (Mello & Mendelson, 1980) (see Box 14.8). This outcome led directly to clinical trials of buprenorphine as an opioid maintenance medication. Many other drugs have been tested in a similar manner. For example, the GABA-B agonist baclofen has been shown to reduce cocaine self-administration in cocaine-dependent volunteers.

Box 14.8   Examining effect on self-administration (Mello & Mendelson, 1980)

In 1980, Mello and Mendelson published the results of a study which was critical to the eventual development of buprenorphine as a medication for the treatment of opioid dependence. Up to that time buprenorphine had only been used for the treatment of pain. In the study, heroin-dependent subjects lived in a research ward for a number of days during which they could work to earn money or heroin. Those subjects administered buprenorphine rarely chose heroin, whereas those given placebo chose heroin over money on nearly every occasion. This demonstrated the ability of buprenorphine to block heroin self-administration in opioid-dependent people.

Tests of the second type evaluating the abuse liability of novel therapeutic agents for addiction treatment are essential in assessing the costs and benefits of a new medication. For example, buprenorphine alone and the buprenorphine + naloxone combination are both self-administered with equivalent reinforcing efficacy, and in non-dependent users buprenorphine has reinforcing effects equal to those of methadone.

14.5   Drug withdrawal and craving

14.5.1   Withdrawal syndromes

Drug withdrawal syndromes typically comprise a mixture of behavioural and subjective symptoms; many also include physiological signs. Withdrawal is often broken into acute and protracted phases. The acute phase is the major focus of withdrawal research. It begins soon after cessation of drug use and typically continues for a number of days. The exact time of onset and the duration are determined by the pharmacokinetics of the drug used, such that shorter acting drugs are associated with a more rapid onset and shorter duration of withdrawal, but higher peak withdrawal intensity. The protracted phase of withdrawal may last some months; the symptoms are typically of subclinical intensity and, therefore, considerably harder to measure. To date, there has been relatively little study of protracted withdrawal for any drug class.

Withdrawal scales are widely used clinically and in research. For some drugs these are well established and have been used for some years. They include the CIWA-Ar for alcohol withdrawal (see Box 14.9) (Sullivan et al., 1989) and the CIWA-B for benzodiazepine withdrawal (Busto et al., 1989). Various opioid withdrawal scales are commonly used, such as the Objective and Subjective Opioid Withdrawal Scales, and the Clinical Opioid Withdrawal Scale (Wesson & Ling, 2003). For other drugs, there is less information available. A cocaine withdrawal scale (Kampman et al., 1998) has been described, and recently an amphetamine withdrawal scale has also been developed and validated (McGregor et al., 2008).

Withdrawal syndromes differ significantly across drug classes, but can largely be predicted based on drug effects. Withdrawal is understood to result from the adaptations that occur following long-term drug administration (Koob & Le Moal, 2001). The manifestation of these adaptations in the absence of the drug effect constitutes the withdrawal syndrome. Thus, withdrawal symptoms are largely opposite in direction to the direct effects of the drug.

There are two major approaches to studying withdrawal. One is to study spontaneous withdrawal by preventing physically dependent users from gaining access to the drug. The development of signs and symptoms can then be studied over a period of days. Given the nature of many withdrawal syndromes, this can only be conducted in a clinical environment. The second approach is

---

Box 14.9   The Clinical Institute Withdrawal Assessment of Alcohol Scale, Revised

The CIWA-Ar is the short name for the Clinical Institute Withdrawal Assessment of Alcohol Scale, Revised. It was first published in 1989 and is now the most widely used alcohol withdrawal scale. It has ten items: (1) nausea and vomiting, (2) tremor, (3) paroxysmal sweats, (4) anxiety, (5) agitation, (6) tactile disturbances, (7) auditory disturbances, (8) visual disturbances, (9) headache, fullness in head, (10) orientation and clouding of sensorium. The first nine of these are scored 0–7 and the tenth 0–4. Higher scores indicate more severe withdrawal and greater need for medication. The scale is not copyrighted: it is readily available on the web and can be reproduced freely. A training programme is available at www.ciwa-ar.com.

administration of an antagonist to precipitate withdrawal. This has a number of advantages, including exact timing of withdrawal and control over severity through the dose of the antagonist. It can also be used to study withdrawal-like changes in non-dependent volunteers following drug administration. However, a major limitation is that for many drugs there is no competitive antagonist available for this purpose. When examining the effects of medications for alleviating withdrawal, study designs using control groups (e.g. randomised controlled trials) are required given the considerable inter-individual variability in withdrawal severity seen in clinical studies.

14.5.2   Craving measures

Approaches to the measurement of craving have been the subject of considerable debate. The simple approach adopted in many studies has been to use a visual analogue scale (VAS) with the subject indicating the degree of craving on the scale at various times or following various experimental manipulations. For example, craving may be measured in response to presentation of drug-related stimuli. Prior to, during and following stimulus administration, the subjects can be asked to indicate their level of craving on the VAS. More sophisticated methods have been developed to allow craving measures in the natural environment. For example, there are electronic alternatives to the usual paper and pencil methods of craving assessment. Data are recorded in real time in the subject's usual environment and can be timed by the use of electronic reminders.

While the VAS is still widely used, researchers with a specific interest in craving have moved beyond this simple approach. This has largely been driven by recognition that craving is not a unitary phenomenon. Craving can accompany withdrawal and be thought of as one aspect of the syndrome, but it also occurs in other situations. Craving may be elevated by administration of the drug the subject normally uses or a drug with similar action. These findings suggest a 'positive' aspect of craving; that is, it is prompted by drug effect and not just by the absence of such effects during withdrawal.

In addition, there is no agreed-on definition of what constitutes the phenomenon of craving. Many consider that it comprises solely the intrusive thoughts of drug use that occur following presentation of drug-related stimuli or in drug-associated environments. However, there are also other components of craving, and scales have been developed to measure these various aspects. For example, Ooteman et al. (2006) developed a 24-item questionnaire to measure alcohol craving. This included four components: emotional urge, physical sensations, temptation to drink and uncontrolled thoughts. The complexity of this scale reflects the difficulty in characterising craving as unitary phenomenon.

Unfortunately, the attempts to develop more complex craving scales have been hampered by the lack of consistency in research. There has been a tendency for different researchers to develop their own craving scales, making comparisons across different studies extremely difficult. Thus, while craving remains a central concept to the understanding of addiction, its measurement is still at a relatively early stage of development.

14.6   Summary

Psychopharmacology encompasses a range of research methodologies that investigate the effects of drugs that affect the brain. It allows us to better understand important factors such as the impact of dose and route of administration, the underlying mechanisms by which drugs act, how drugs may interact with each other, and enables us to better understand individual variations in these parameters based on genetic, psychological and physiological conditions. Psychopharmacology plays a critical role in the development of safer pharmaceutical products used in other areas of medicine (but that may be subject to misuse), and in the development of medications for the treatment of substance use disorders. These approaches are an important aspect of understanding how and why drug use occurs, alongside epidemiological, sociological and clinical research approaches

---

Excercises

Recent media reports suggest that there is a new drug being used in dance clubs called 'Zed' – reports suggest that it causes users to feel elated, to have increased stamina and sexual arousal, but has also been linked to 'blackouts', agitation and seizures. Reports suggest that it comes from veterinary supplies. You have been able to identify the drug as 'methoprixam', which is also licensed for humans as a local anaesthetic.

Describe studies that would examine the psychopharmacological effects of this medication, its abuse liability, and effects when combined with alcohol.

References

Busto, U. E., Sykora, K. & Sellers, E. M. (1989) A clinical scale to assess benzodiazepine withdrawal. *Journal of Clinical Psychopharmacology*, 9(6), 412–416.

Cone, E. J. & Huestis, M. A. (2007) Interpretation of oral fluid tests for drugs of abuse. *Annals of the New York Academy of Science*, 1098, 51–103.

Curran, V. & Mintzer, M. (2006) Psychopharmacology of memory. *Psychopharmacology*, 188, 393–396.

Haertzen, C. A., Hill, H. E. & Belleville, R. E. (1963) Development of the Addiction Research Center Inventory (ARCI): selection of items that are sensitive to the effects of various drugs. *Psychopharmacology*, 4, 155–166.

Hursh, S. R., Galuska, C. M., Winger, G. & Woods, J. H. (2005) The economics of drug abuse: a quantitative assessment of drug demand. *Molecular Intervention*, 5(1), 20–28.

Kampman, K. M., Volpicelli, J. R., McGinnis, D. E., Alterman, A. I., Weinrieb, R. M., D'Angelo, L. & Epperson L. E. (1998) Reliability and validity of the Cocaine Selective Severity Assessment. *Addictive Behaviors*, 23(4), 449–461.

Koob, G. F. & Le Moal, M. (2001) Drug addiction, dysregulation of reward, and allostasis. *Neuropsychopharmacology*, 24(2), 97–129.

Lezak, M. D. (2004) *Neuropsychological Assessment*. New York: Oxford University Press.

McGregor, C., Srisurapanont, M., Mitchell, A., Longo, M. C., Cahill, S. & White, J. M. (2008) Psychometric evaluation of the Amphetamine Cessation Symptom Assessment. *Journal of Substance Abuse Treatment*, 34, 443–449.

McNair, D. M., Heuchert, J. P. & Shilony, E. (2003) *Profile of Mood States: Bibliography 1964–2002*. New York: North Tonawanda: Multi Health Systems, Inc.

Mello, N. K. & Mendelson, J. H. (1980) Buprenorphine suppresses heroin use by heroin addicts. *Science*, 207(4431), 657–659.

Meyer, F. P. (2001) Psycho- and immunopharmacological factors relevant to selection of volunteers in clinical studies. *International Journal of Clinical Pharmacology and Therapeutics*, 39(7), 300–310.

Ogden, E. J. & Moskowitz, H. (2004) Effects of alcohol and other drugs on driver performance. *Traffic Injury Prevention*, 5(3), 185–198.

Ooteman, W., Koeter, M. W., Vserheul, R., Schippers, G. M. & Van Den Brink, W. (2006) Measuring craving: an attempt to connect subjective craving with cue reactivity. *Alcoholism, Clinical and Experimental Research*, 30(1), 57–69.

Pragst, F. & Balikova, M. A. (2006) State of the art in hair analysis for detection of drug and alcohol abuse. *Clinica Chimica Acta*, 370(1–2), 17–49.

Sullivan, J. T., Sykora, K., Schneiderman, J., Naranjo, C. A. & Sellers, E. M. (1989) Assessment of alcohol withdrawal: the revised clinical institute withdrawal assessment for alcohol scale (CIWA-Ar). *British Journal of Addiction*, 84(11), 1353–1357.

Wesson, D. R. & Ling, W. (2003) The Clinical Opiate Withdrawal Scale (COWS). *Journal of Psychoactive Drugs*, 35(2), 253–259.

Recommended readings

Curran, V. & Mintzer, M. (2006) Psychopharmacology of memory. *Psychopharmacology*, 188, 393–396.

Lezak, M. D. (2004) *Neuropsychological Assessment*. New York: Oxford University Press.

Chapter 15

IMAGING

Alastair Reid and David Nutt

15.1 Introduction

The aim of this chapter is to give the reader a practical understanding of neuroimaging techniques and to show the reader why these techniques might be useful in addiction research. A brief summary of the contribution of neuroimaging to addiction research is given, plus a list of recommended readings to complement this.

Addiction can be thought of, from both a psychological and pharmacological viewpoint, as occurring primarily in the brain, and is in a sense *psychopharmacology gone awry*. It makes sense that we would want to investigate what goes on in the brains of addicts and also to learn more about what effects substances of abuse have on the brain. Neuroimaging methods allow us to carry out these sorts of investigations *in vivo*, and give us the opportunity to explore a very rich set of hypotheses, some of which are derived from animal experiments and some from other branches of neuroscience and psychiatry.

15.2 Introduction to neuroimaging

There are two main divisions in neuroimaging techniques – *structural* and *functional*.

One of the great advantages of functional neuroimaging is that cognitive tasks can be performed by subjects while they are in the scanner. We can then measure task performance and relate this to brain activity in terms of neuronal activity (fMRI) or receptor binding or neurotransmitter release (PET & SPET). This can be done in both addicted and control groups. Pharmacological modulation of either task performance or brain activity or both can also be applied to explore the psychopharmacology of addiction.

Although the neuroimaging approach is very powerful and has many advantages, there are also some drawbacks. For example, there is the 'dirty brain' problem – most addicts have abused or continue to abuse multiple substances, which means there are multiple confounders and problems in examining the effects of a particular substance on the brain. Careful selection of subjects and good study design can mitigate against this. Also, although neuroimaging studies can give us much correlational information they say much less about causality unless longitudinal studies are undertaken, and these, because they are difficult and expensive, are rare.

15.3 Imaging techniques

15.3.1 Positron emission tomography (PET) and single positron emission computed tomography (SPET)

The basis of positron emission tomography (PET) is that a radioisotope based on ^{11}C or ^{18}F is attached to a compound with known pharmacological properties (the ligand) to create a *tracer*. The tracer is then injected into the bloodstream of a subject and the radioactive isotope decays to give off positron particles. A positron particle will combine with a nearby negatively charged electron and in the process both particles are annihilated and two photons are emitted 180° apart. A ring of crystal detectors can detect coincident photons that are 180° apart, and the point from which they emanate can be calculated. A three-dimensional image of the radiation concentrations within the brain is then created. This image has only moderate anatomical resolution, so an anatomical template is superimposed to obtain results with good anatomical specificity. Usually, a T1-weighted structural magnetic resonance imaging (MRI) of the same subject is co-registered with the PET image, and then anatomical templates can be applied on the basis of the MRI.

Single positron emission computed tomography (SPECT or SPET) imaging is very similar to PET. Technecium-99 (^{99m}Tc) is often used to create a tracer that measures regional brain metabolism. [^{123}I]IZBM is another commonly used tracer that binds to dopamine D_2 and D_3 receptors. As these compounds undergo radioactive decay a single photon is released from each atom and this is detected in a similar way to that in PET; however, with only a single particle emitted, detecting the origin of the radioactive decay is harder, so precision is lower. SPECT has advantages over PET in terms of lower cost and lower technology requirements and the fact that the tracers have longer half-lives, though subjects are usually exposed to higher levels of radiation. SPECT scans can be of use in measuring receptor density, location of receptor binding and regional cerebral blood flow.

The pros and cons of these different neuroimaging techniques are summarised in Table 15.1.

15.3.2 Measuring endogenous neurotransmitter release

Early PET studies in addiction used radioactively labelled water ($H_2{}^{15}O$) to measure regional cerebral blood flow (rCBF) as a way of localising brain activity. However, with the advent of more pharmacologically specific tracers it is now possible to measure endogenous neurotransmitter release effectively using PET techniques. In particular, [^{11}C]raclopride has been very useful in addiction research to further understanding of the role of dopamine in addiction. Figure 15.1 illustrates the way in which [^{11}C]raclopride binding gives a measure of in vivo endogenous dopamine release. The amount of dopamine bound at the D_2 receptor is proportional to the amount of endogenous dopamine released. The amount of [^{11}C]raclopride that can bind to the D_2 receptor is inversely proportional to the amount of endogenous dopamine that is bound at the receptor, and also the amount of endogenous dopamine released. The binding potential (BP) is a measure which reflects both receptor availability and ligand affinity at that receptor (Laruelle et al., 2002). Using a reference region, where the receptor density is negligible – the cerebellum in this case – the BP can be calculated without the need for taking arterial blood samples. The BP is a useful measure to compare dopamine release in different brain regions. Figure 15.2 illustrates what happens to dopamine release when a stimulant drug is taken and how this causes [^{11}C]raclopride binding to decrease. A summary of tracers that have been used in addiction research is shown in Table 15.2.

Usage

By looking at where the radioactivity is localised in the brain, we can examine and define the regional distribution of receptors, or the level of binding to those receptors under different conditions to examine differences between healthy volunteers and a subject population. Other comparisons can include subjects at rest versus performing a cognitive or mental task, or subjects receiving placebo versus active drug or medication.

Table 15.1 Pros and cons of commonly used neuroimaging techniques

Type of scan	Pros	Cons
PET	The only way to do true 'psychopharmacological' studies where we can examine/modulate effects in both pharmacology and psychology in the living individual Reasonable spatial resolution (voxel size 2 mm^3)	Use of radiation is risky Large infrastructure needed: cyclotron, physicists, chemists, mathematicians (image analysis and modelling), clinicians Development of ligands is required Expensive Studies require venous, and often also arterial, cannulation – so quite invasive for the subjects
SPECT	Cheaper and easier to make SPECT tracers compared with PET	Higher levels of radiation exposure required compared with PET Lower resolution of image (voxel size >5 mm^3)
MRI	Relatively cheap and safe Non-invasive Less infrastructure needed compared to PET Good spatial resolution – voxel sizes 2 mm^3	The scanning environment is claustrophobic and noisy – patients and volunteers sometimes find it too anxiogenic Contraindicated in individuals with metal implants and pacemakers No temporal dimension
fMRI	Good combination of high anatomical localisation of activity and reasonable temporal resolution	As per structural MRI and the following: • Study design can be complex – needs to be carefully set up and careful consideration given to the cognitive tasks used • Interpretation of results can be difficult • The linkage between the BOLD signal and underlying neurophysiological events is not fully understood

15.3.3 Structural magnetic resonance imaging (MRI)

MRI works on the basis that nuclear spins have magnetic properties, and these become aligned (flipped) when placed in a magnetic field. When a radio signal is passed through the magnetic field, this causes the spins to flip back to their original state. When applying this to the brain, the amount of energy from the radio signal required to revert the spins is proportional to the density of the brain matter through which it is passing. This means that the different substrates of the brain, for example white matter, grey matter or CSF, can be clearly distinguished and a high-definition image can be obtained. The intensity of the radio signal has to be limited to prevent soft tissue damage, so

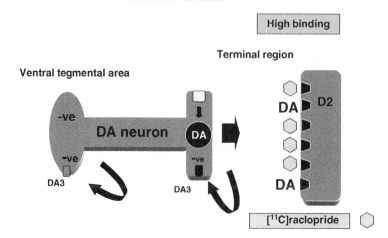

Figure 15.1 [^{11}C]raclopride binding under normal conditions.

to increase image resolution the magnetic field strength must be increased. 1.5-T and 3-T scanners are in common use, and some facilities are now using 5-7 T machines. T1-weighted images show fat as bright and water as dark and are good for viewing white matter and grey matter parts of the brain. T2-weighted images are the opposite.

Usage

Structural MRI can be used in case-control studies to investigate potential structural differences in the brains of certain populations. Such studies have usually taken a region of interest (ROI) approach, for example examining the size of predefined regions of interest such as the hippocampus. A recent

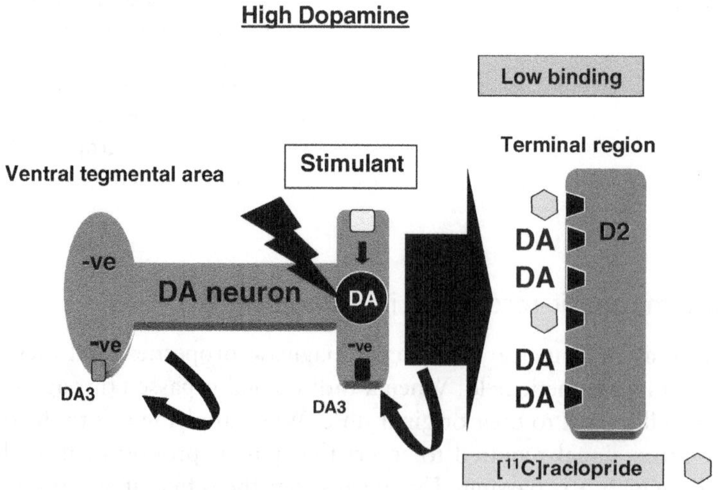

Figure 15.2 [^{11}C]raclopride binding when a stimulant drug is taken.

Table 15.2 PET and SPET tracers used in addiction research

Receptor/target	PET (^{11}C)	SPET (^{123}I)
GABA-benzodiazepine	Flumazenil	Iomazenil
Dopamine (D$_1$-like)	SCH 23390	
Dopamine (D$_2$-like)	Raclopride	IBZM
	FLB	Epidepride
Dopamine transporter	Cocaine	FP-CIT
Dopamine/5HT transporter		Beta-CIT
5HT1A	WAY 100635	
5HT2A	Altanserin	5-1-R91150
Opioid (mu, kappa, delta)	Diprenorphine	
Opioid (mu)	Carfentanyl	
Acetyl choline (M1)		QNB

popular semi-automated method of comparing groups of structural MRIs is to use voxel-based morphometry. This is a voxel-by-voxel method (see below), which can detect structural differences in brain regions in an a priori rather than hypothesis-led way. There is some controversy in the use of voxel-based morphometry, hinging around the fact that in order for the images to be averaged they all need to be mapped into a common image space; however, this mapping will distort the structural information contained in the image. There is also the issue of correction for multiple comparisons.

Structural MRI images are also used for co-registration in PET studies to help more accurately map anatomical templates onto the PET image. They can also be used to ensure there are no anatomical anomalies in the brains of subjects who have undergone other scans.

15.3.4 Functional MRI (fMRI)

Functional MRI (fMRI) works along similar lines to MRI but exploits a magnetic property of blood to provide a measure of localised cerebral activity. There is a difference in the magnetic properties of oxygenated compared with deoxygenated blood. This difference can be detected using an MRI paradigm and is known as the BOLD (blood oxygen level dependent) signal. The strength of this signal at a particular location indicates the relative level of deoxygenated blood at that location. It is assumed that neuronal activity requires oxygenated blood, which then becomes deoxygenated, although the precise nature of this coupling is not known. The BOLD signal therefore reflects cerebral activity at that location. During the same scan a structural MRI is obtained and this is used to help generate a highly anatomically defined image of cerebral activity. fMRI has reasonably good temporal (1–4 seconds) and spatial resolution (3–6 mm^3), but it can be difficult to interpret scans if there is conflict between physiological rhythms and the BOLD signal, and the study design needs to be sensitive to the interscan interval.

Usage

Studies aiming to examine brain activity while performing a cognitive task.

15.3.5   Arterial spin labelling, diffusion tensor imaging and pharmaco-MRI

These are recently developed neuroimaging modalities and are all based on MRI.

Arterial spin labelling studies use other spin properties of the atomic nucleus to provide a high-resolution and non-invasive image of arterial blood supply in the brain. Diffusion tensor imaging relies on differences in the diffusion gradient of white matter tracts to give high-resolution images of these tracts in vivo. Pharmaco-MRI is essentially the use of pharmacological agents to modulate brain activity and/or cognitive performance in an fMRI study.

15.3.6   Neuroimaging and addiction research

Functional neuroimaging has been widely applied to map craving and cognitive processes in addiction, and shows involvement of prefrontal cortex and some allocortical structures, such as amygdala, that are variably correlated with self-reported levels of craving. Breiter et al.'s (1997) pharmaco-fMRI study identified limbic, orbitofrontal and striatal regions as being involved in the neural response to cocaine. These regions are major components in the 'reward circuitry' of the brain, and correspondingly, this study identified different subregions of this circuit to be correlated with the sensations of *high* versus *craving*. A more recent study used the same approach and identified similar regions activated during craving (nucleus accumbens, orbitofrontal cortex (OfCx) and anterior cingulate (ACC); Risinger et al., 2005). Other studies have also investigated the neural correlates of craving using cue-exposure techniques and have produced similarly overlapping but not identical results (Grant et al., 1996; Childress et al., 1999; Wexler et al., 2001; Kilts et al., 2004). These regional variations may reflect the complex interplay between environmental, psychological and biological factors that intersect in phenomena such as drug craving. One potent modifying factor that should be taken into account is that of *anticipation* or *expectation*. Volkow et al. (2003) discovered that the reported experience of high in cocaine addicts receiving methylphenidate was 50% higher when they were expecting the methylphenidate compared with when they were not. In addition, Wilson et al. (2000) point out that cue exposure activates dorsolateral prefrontal cortex and OfCx in non-treatment-seeking addicts, but not in addicts in treatment. Thus, craving in addicts may have a different neural substrate depending on whether they are in treatment or not. This type of study highlights the complex interplay between the pharmacologically induced neuroplasticity that underlies addiction and the sociological circumstances regulating drug-seeking behaviour.

Several studies have looked at neuropsychological aspects of heroin addiction. For instance, exposing heroin addicts to personalised heroin-related auditory stimuli (cues) increased rCBF in the ACC and OfCx (Daglish et al., 2001), with increases in ACC independent of craving. This suggests the ACC may be responding more specifically to the cue, while OfCx may be involved in the experience of craving. Of interest is the observation that the ACC activation increased rather than decreased with duration of abstinence, suggesting enduring changes in the brain following addiction to heroin. A similar finding with cocaine craving was described by Wexler et al. (2001). A series of studies (Ersche et al., 2005a, b, 2006) have investigated performance on cognitive tasks in opiate and amphetamine users. They found that current opioid and amphetamine users were impaired on a set of executive and memory tasks, and that this impairment persisted in subjects who had been abstinent for over a year. These studies suggest that there are long-term changes in cognitive processing and possible corticofugal glutamate transmission, in particular on working memory and decision-making tasks, in the brains of heroin and amphetamine users, and that these changes persist into abstinence.

Jovanovski et al. (2005) have provided a synthesis of studies looking at the neuropsychological changes in cocaine addiction. They found the largest effect size was for measures of attention, then for visual memory and working memory tasks, and then for tests of verbal fluency. These results agree with the general finding of altered activation in ACC and OfCx. For healthy individuals, OfCx is involved in impulse control and ACC is implicated in attentional processes. In trying to establish a theory of the cognitive neuropsychology of addiction, which takes into account these findings, it has been suggested that increased activity in OfCx may reflect hypersensitivity to reward (Bolla et al., 2003), whereas reduced activity in ACC may reflect hyposensitivity to losses (Garavan & Stout, 2005) (Boxes 15.1 and 15.2).

15.4 Image analysis

The analysis of data generated by imaging studies is very complex and requires several levels of mathematical processing before we can obtain a useful measure of significant change.

These levels can be thought of in three distinct categories:

1. **Image generation.** Conversion of the raw signal from the scanner into a basic image.
2. **Image processing.** This involves refining the basic image. Movement correction algorithms, for example frame-by-frame realignment, can be applied here. Images will be 'tidied up' and transformed, or warped, into a common three-dimensional coordinate space so that direct comparisons can be made between specific points in different brains. Coordinate systems based on an average of multiple brains are much preferable to the Talairach system, which was based on the brain from a 60-year-old woman with a smaller than average cranium. The Montreal Neurological Institute (MNI) have produced a template based on the averaging of 152 normal brains (the MNI152 template), and it has been suggested to make this system the standard (Devlin & Poldrack, 2007). It is also at this stage of the processing sequence that activity data can be parcellated according to ROI.
3. **Statistical analysis.** At this level the images will have been processed to the point where direct comparisons can be made between images, or groups of images, using forms of standard statistical test such as T-test, ANOVA or ANCOVA. If the study incorporated a cognitive task, or there are other measures that the experimenter wants to examine in relation to the brain images, then these can be added to statistical models at this stage.

ROI *versus voxel-by-voxel*

In order to detect areas of difference between two sets of neuroimaging data there are two basic approaches. The ROI approach is hypothesis led and requires the use of hand-labelled regions. Hand-labelling is very laborious and prone to bias as each labeller is likely to define a region slightly differently. More than one labeller should be used when creating ROIs, and inter-rater reliability scores should be calculated. This approach may miss regions of significant difference. One new approach to the extraction of regions of interest is that, rather than hand-drawing a template, a *probabilistic atlas* (Hammers et al., 2003) is used. This atlas has been generated from the regional analysis of many brains and gives a probability value for a particular area in the brain belonging to a particular neuroanatomical region. This atlas can be mapped onto any image to be studied in a semi-automated way.

Box 15.1   fMRI study example (Breiter et al., 1997)

Breiter et al. used fMRI to examine the activity in the neural circuitry associated with addiction and reward during cocaine use, and to link this activity to the subjective effects of the drug. They chose fMRI as the imaging technique as this provided them with greater structural resolution than PET or SPET, which was important as they planned to examine activity in specific anatomical structures, some of which are small and hard to demarcate, for example nucleus accumbens and amygdala.

Procedure: The study is a double-blind randomised trial using 17 cocaine-dependent individuals. Subjects were screened to exclude anxiety and depression and other comorbid medical and neurological disorders. Subjects were assessed for cocaine dependence using the Mini-Structured Clinical Interview for DSMIV (SCID) and the Addiction Severity Index. Subjects were selected to be heavy long-term cocaine users (mean years of use 7.8). Subjects were not currently seeking, or in treatment for cocaine addiction. They had to have one positive urine test for cocaine prior to the experiment and to be abstinent from cocaine and alcohol for at least 18 hours prior to the start of the experiment. The study obtained the following measures: fMRI BOLD signal; cognitive measure of 'rush', 'high', 'low', 'craving'; physiological measures; plasma cocaine levels. Each scan period consisted of five separate scans, lasting in total 90 minutes. Subjects received a cocaine infusion 5 minutes into an 18-minute long BOLD scan. The BOLD scan was preceded and followed by flow-sensitive alternating inversion recovery and visual stimulation BOLD scans, which were required to give a measure of global signal in order to separate global effects from the signal of interest.

Results:

1. An increase in heart rate and BP in response to cocaine, which returned to baseline within 2 hours.
2. Peak 'rush' and 'high' sensations at 3 minutes post-infusion. Peak 'low' was at 11 minutes post-infusion and peak 'craving' was at 12 minutes post-infusion.
3. Brain regions with signal change during cocaine infusion:
   (a) Increased signal: nucleus accumbens/subcallosal cortex, thalamus, hippocampus, insula, cingulate gyrus and parahippocampal gyrus.
   (b) Decreased signal: amygdala, temporal pole and medial frontal cortex.
4. Correlations between signal change in brain region and behavioural states: The behavioural state of 'Rush' had early transient maxima, whereas 'craving' had later maxima.

Points of interest:

1. Only seven matched sets of usable scan and infusion data were collected from 17 volunteers who underwent scanning with infusion, due to uncorrectable subject movement. This highlights the problem of subject movement and the need for good **movement correction** techniques during image analysis.
2. Subject **blinding** only lasted a few minutes past the start of the infusion.
3. **Test–re-test data** provide valuable information about the stability of the scanning methodology and help to identify the presence of potential confounders, for example signal change due to the novelty of the scanning environment.
4. The Talairach brain coordinate system (Talairach & Tournoux, 1988) was used – alternatives such as the **MNI152 template** would be preferable (see below).
5. Efforts were made to separate BOLD fMRI signal due to cocaine, from signal changes due to a global effect of cocaine on cerebral vasculature, since cocaine is a potent vasoconstrictor. Correction for global signal change is particularly important in any imaging study where blood flow may be influenced by the study paradigm.

Box 15.2   PET study example (Brody et al., 2004)

The study of Brody et al. (2004) illustrates the use of ligand PET in addiction research to investigate the release of dopamine in the ventral striatum during smoking. They used [^{11}C]raclopride to show an increase in dopamine release in one group of subjects who smoked a cigarette versus a control group who did not.

Procedure: This study used 20 smokers ($\geq$15 cigarettes per day). Subjects were screened using the Structured Clinical Interview for DSM-IV and certain exclusion criteria were applied. The main measure of interest was the [^{11}C]raclopride BP. Other measures included the Urge to Smoke Scale, the state questions from the Spielberger State–Trait Anxiety Inventory, and the Hamilton Depression Rating Scale, exhaled carbon monoxide, and a rough measure of recent smoking intensity. Subjects were required to smoke as usual in the morning of the PET session and to smoke a cigarette immediately before the PET scan session. [11C]raclopride was given as a slow bolus over 1 minute followed by a continuous infusion for 90 minutes. After 50 minutes the subjects were taken out of the scanner and had a 10-minute break, with the infusion still running. Ten of the subjects had a cigarette during this break and ten did not. Subjects were then re-positioned in the scanner and scanning was continued for another 30 minutes. Subjects also underwent a structural MRI scan to ensure correct cerebral neuroanatomy and for use in localising the regions of interest on the PET images.

Image analysis: The PET scans consist of a series of 5-minute frames. The frames of interest were the two immediately preceding smoking the cigarette and the two frames immediately following the cigarette break. ROIs were drawn onto PET images that had been summed for the frames of interest. ROIs were bilateral ventral caudate/nucleus accumbens and ventral putamen. Dorsal caudate and dorsal putamen were also defined for use as control regions. The BP for each ROI was calculated and then BPs for the smoking group and the control group were put to statistical comparison.

Results:

(1)   The smoking group had a significantly reduced craving scores between pre- and post-break;
(2)   A multivariate repeated-measures MANCOVA test for the two main regions of interest – bilateral ventral caudate/nucleus accumbens and ventral putamen both pre-break and post-break (four variables and two repeated measures) – showed an overall between-group difference in change in [^{11}C]raclopride BP between the smokers and non-smokers.
(3)   Left ventral caudate/nucleus accumbens and left ventral putamen showed a significant **reduction** in the BP of smokers, suggesting increased dopamine release.
(4)   There was a significant correlation with reduction in the Urge to Smoke Scale score, suggesting that dopamine release is associated with a decrease in craving.

Points of interest:

(1)   A crossover design (i.e. each subject has a smoking and non-smoking scan) would have increased the power of the study and may have lessened the impact on the results of individual variation in dopamine release.
(2)   Significant movement artefact is likely to be generated when the subject is moved in and out of the scanner. Even when good motion correction algorithms are available, the most important factor in reducing movement artefact is to avoid the subject moving in the first place.
(3)   The ROI approach has limitations (see below).
(4)   A study by the same group (Brody et al., 2006) showed a smaller effect size, which was restricted to people with a specific genetic variation. See also Brody et al. (2009).

With the advent of increased computing power and the development of suitable statistical algorithms, a voxel-by-voxel whole-brain approach is also possible. This entails comparing every voxel in one brain with a similarly positioned voxel in every other brain. This approach is less dependent on initial assumptions and can be semi-automated to give good consistency, although will lack power to find small differences due to the problem of multiple comparisons.

The voxel-by-voxel approach may be seen as hypothesis generating, whereas ROI is hypothesis testing. It would not be good statistical practice to use both approaches on the same dataset.

In order to carry out image processing, many imaging laboratories have developed their own software. However, there are several suites of software available for free download. The foremost of these are the Statistical Parametric Mapping tools (http://www.fil.ion.ucl.ac.uk/spm/). The image data are assumed to be parametric and are 'groomed' further using techniques from Gaussian Random Field theory to ensure it is suitable for parametric testing. Massively, univariate statistical tests are then applied with various corrections for multiple testing. There is a non-parametric version of Statistical Parametric Mapping for datasets that are not parametric. Other centres have followed a non-parametric approach, for example the BAMM software (http://www.idoimaging.com) developed at Cambridge University. Other useful tools include: FreeSurfer Libraries (http://www.fmrib.ox.ac.uk/fsl/), MarsBar (http://marsbar.sourceforge.net/), WfU Pickatlas (http://fmri.wfubmc.edu/cms/software) and the Automated Anatomical Labelling (http://www.cyceron.fr/freeware/). Processing pipelines which automatically take the image data from one step in the sequence and input it into the next step can improve the efficiency and reliability of image analysis, and are being developed.

15.5   Some considerations when setting up an imaging study

Imaging methodology: Is there a suitable radioligand available? Suitability of functional tasks – how good is the task at measuring what you want it to? Can it be performed in the scanner? Will the scanning environment interfere with performance on the task?

Image analysis: Do you have enough statistical power? Tasks should be piloted, as should scanning, to get an idea of effect size (which will be necessary for the power calculation).

Subject availability and recruitment: Do you have access to a large enough pool of subjects? Will they be able to tolerate the scanning environment? Will they be able to perform the tasks you would like them to?

References

Bolla, K. I., Eldreth, D. A., London, E. D., Kiehl, K. A., Mouratidis, M., Contoreggi, C., Matochik, J. A., Kurian, V., Cadet, J. L., Kimes, A. S., Funderburk, F. R. & Ernst, M. (2003) Orbitofrontal cortex dysfunction in abstinent cocaine abusers performing a decision-making task. *Neuroimage*, 19, 1085–1094.

Breiter, H. C., Gollub, R. L., Weisskoff, R. M., Kennedy, D. N., Makris, N., Berke, J. D., Goodman, J. M., Kantor, H. L., Gastfriend, D. R., Riorden, J. P., Mathew, R. T., Rosen, B. R. & Hyman, S. E. (1997) Acute effects of cocaine on human brain activity and emotion. *Neuron*, 19(3), 591–611.

Brody, A. L., Mandelkern, M. A., Olmstead, R. E., Allen-Martinez, Z., Scheibal, D., Abrams, A. L., Costello, M. R., Farahi, J., Saxena, S., Monterosso, J. & London, E. D. (2009) Ventral striatal dopamine release in response to smoking a regular vs a denicotinized cigarette. *Neuropsychopharmacology*, 34(2), 282–289.

Brody, A. L., Mandelkern, M. A., Olmstead, R. E., Scheibal, D., Hahn, E., Shiraga, S., Zamora-Paja, E., Farahi, J., Saxena, S., London, E. D. & McCracken, J. T. (2006) Gene variants of brain dopamine pathways and smoking-induced dopamine release in the ventral caudate/nucleus accumbens. *Archives of General Psychiatry*, 63(7), 808–816.

Brody, A. L., Olmstead, R. E., London, E. D., Farahi, J., Meyer, J. H., Grossman, P., Lee, G. S., Huang, J., Hahn, E. L. & Mandelkern, M. A. (2004) Smoking-induced ventral striatum dopamine release. *American Journal of Psychiatry*, 161(7), 1211–1218.

Childress, A. R., Mozley, P. D., McElgin, W., Fitzgerald, J., Reivich, M. & O'Brien, C. P. (1999) Limbic activation during cue-induced cocaine craving. *American Journal of Psychiatry*, 156, 11–18.

Daglish, M. R. C., Weinstein, A., Malizia, A. L., Wilson, S., Melichar, J. K., Britten, S., Brewer, C., Lingford-Hughes, A., Myles, J. S., Grasby, P. & Nutt, D. J. (2001) Changes in regional cerebral blood flow elicited by craving memories in abstinent opiate-dependent subjects. *American Journal of Psychiatry*, 158(10), 1680–1686.

Daglish, M. R. C., Williams, T. M., Wilson, S. J., Taylor, L. G., Eap, C. B., Augsburger, M., Giroud, C., Brooks, D. J., Myles, J. S., Grasby, P., Lingford-Hughes, A. R. & Nutt, D. J. (2008) Brain dopamine response in human opioid addiction. *British Journal of Psychiatry*, 193, 65–72.

Devlin, J. T. & Poldrack, R. A. (2007) In praise of tedious anatomy. *Neuroimage*, 37(4), 1033–1058.

Ersche, K. D., Clark, L., London, M., Robbins, T. W. & Sahakian, B. J. (2006) Profile of executive and memory function associated with amphetamine and opiate dependence. *Neuropsychopharmacology*, 31(5), 1036–1047.

Ersche, K. D., Fletcher, P. C., Lewis, S. J. G., Clark, L., Stocks-Gee, G., London, M., Deakin, J. B., Robbins, T. W. & Sahakian, B. J. (2005a) Abnormal frontal activations related to decision-making in current and former amphetamine and opiate dependent individuals. *Psychopharmacology*, 180, 612–623.

Ersche, K. D., Roiser, J. P., Clark, L., London, M., Robbins, T. W. & Sahakian, B. J. (2005b) Punishment induces risky decision-making in methadone-maintained opiate users but not heroin users or healthy volunteers. *Neuropsychopharmacology*, 30(11), 2115–2124.

Garavan, H. & Stout, J. C. (2005) Neurocognitive insights into substance abuse. *Trends in Cognitive Science*, 9(4), 195–201.

Gazdzinski, S., Durazzo, T. C. & Meyerhoff, D. J. (2005) Temporal dynamics and determinants of whole brain tissue volume changes during recovery from alcohol dependence. *Drug and Alcohol Dependence*, 78, 263–273.

Grant, S., London, E. D., Newlin, D. B., Villemaqne, V. L., Liu, X., Contoreggi, C., Phillips, R. L., Kimes, A. S. & Margolin. (1996) Activation of memory circuits during cue-elicited cocaine craving. *Proceedings of the National Academy of Sciences USA*, 93(21), 12040–12045.

Hammers, A., Allom, R., Koepp, M. J., Free, S. L., Myers, R., Lemieux, L., Mitchell, T. N., Brooks, D. J. & Duncan, J. S. (2003) Three-dimensional maximum probability atlas of the human brain, with particular reference to the temporal lobe. *Human Brain Mapping*, 19(4), 224–247.

Jovanovski, D., Erb, S. & Zakzanis, K. K. (2005) Neurocognitive deficits in cocaine users: a quantitative review of the evidence. *Journal of Clinical and Experimental Neuropsychology*, 27, 189–204.

Kilts, C. D., Gross, R. E., Ely, T. D. & Drexler, K. P. (2004) The neural correlates of cue-induced craving in cocaine-dependent women. *American Journal of Psychiatry*, 161, 233–241.

Laruelle, M., Slifstein, M. & Huang, Y. (2002) Positron emission tomography: imaging and quantification of neurotransporter availability. *Methods*, 27(3), 287–299.

Lingford-Hughes, A. R., Hume, S. P., Feeney, A., Hirani, E., Osman, S., Cunningham, V. J., Pike, V. W., Brooks, D. J. & Nutt, D. J. (2002) Imaging the GABA-benzodiazepine receptor subtype containing the alpha5 subunit in vivo with [11C]Ro15-4513 positron emission tomography. *Journal of Cerebral Blood Flow and Metabolism*, 22(7), 878–879.

Nader, M. A. & Czoty, P. W. (2005) PET imaging of dopamine D2 receptors in monkey models of cocaine abuse: genetic predisposition versus environmental modulation. *American Journal of Psychiatry*, 162, 1473–1482.

Risinger, R. C., Salmeron, B. J., Ross, T. J., Amen, S. L., Sanfilipo, M., Hoffmann, R. G., Bloom, A. S., Garavan, H. & Stein, E. A. (2005) Neural correlates of high and craving during cocaine self-administration using BOLD fMRI. *Neuroimage*, 26, 1097–1108.

Talairach, J. & Tournoux, P. (1988) *Co-planar Stereotaxic Atlas of the Human Brain: 3-Dimensional Proportional System – an Approach to Cerebral Imaging*. New York: Thieme Medical Publishers.

Volkow, N. D., Fowler, J. S., Wang, G. J., Baler, R. & Telang, F. (2009) Imaging dopamine's role in drug abuse and addiction. *Neuropharmacology*, 56(Suppl 1), 3–8.

Volkow, N. D., Wang, G.-J., Ma, Y., Fowler, J. S., Zhu, W., Maynard, L., Telang, F., Vaska, P., Ding, Y. S., Wong, C. & Swanson, J. M. (2003) Expectation enhances the regional brain metabolic and the reinforcing effects of stimulants in cocaine abusers. *The Journal of Neuroscience*, 23(36), 11461–11468.

Wexler, B. E., Gottschalk, C. H., Fulbright, R. K., Prohovnik, I., Lacadie, C. M., Rounsaville, B. J. & Gore, J. C. (2001) Functional magnetic resonance imaging of cocaine craving. *American Journal of Psychiatry*, 158, 86–95.

Williams, T. M., Daglish, M. R. C., Lingford-Hughes, A., Taylor, L. G., Hammers, A., Brooks, D. J., Grasby, P., Myles, J. S. & Nutt, D. J. (2007) Brain opioid receptor binding in early abstinence from opioid dependence. *British Journal of Psychiatry*, 191, 63–69.

Wilson, W., Matthew, R., Turkington, T., Hawk, T., Coleman, R. E. & Provenzale, J. (2000) Brain morphological changes and early marijuana use: a magnetic resonance and positron emission tomography study. *Journal of Addiction Disorders*, 19(1), 1–22.

Recommended readings

Daglish, M. R. C., Williams, T. M., Wilson, S. J., Taylor, L. G., Eap, C. B., Augsburger, M., Giroud, C., Brooks, D. J., Myles, J. S., Grasby, P., Lingford-Hughes, A. R. & Nutt, D. J. (2008) Brain dopamine response in human opioid addiction. *British Journal of Psychiatry*, 193, 65–72.
– *Recent PET imaging study provides new insight into the role of the opioid system in addiction.*

Ersche, K. D., Fletcher, P. C., Lewis, S. J. G., Clark, L., Stocks-Gee, G., London, M., Deakin, J. B., Robbins, T. W. & Sahakian, B. J. (2005a) Abnormal frontal activations related to decision-making in current and former amphetamine and opiate dependent individuals. *Psychopharmacology*, 180, 612–623.
– *Use PET imaging to examine the function of brain regions which mediate a risk-based decision-making task in drug-using individuals and controls.*

Gazdzinski, S., Durazzo, T. C. & Meyerhoff, D. J. (2005) Temporal dynamics and determinants of whole brain tissue volume changes during recovery from alcohol dependence. *Drug and Alcohol Dependence*, 78, 263–273.
– *A longitudinal MRI study showing recovery of brain volume after alcohol dependence.*

Lingford-Hughes, A. R., Hume, S. P., Feeney, A., Hirani, E., Osman, S., Cunningham, V. J., Pike, V. W., Brooks, D. J. & Nutt, D. J. (2002) Imaging the GABA-benzodiazepine receptor subtype containing the alpha5 subunit in vivo with [11C]Ro15-4513 positron emission tomography. *Journal of Cerebral Blood Flow and Metabolism*, 22(7), 878–879.
– *Show that PET imaging techniques can be used to study α-5 GABA-benzodiazepine receptors, which may have a role in the neurobiology of alcohol addiction.*

Nader, M. A. & Czoty, P. W. (2005) PET imaging of dopamine D2 receptors in monkey models of cocaine abuse: genetic predisposition versus environmental modulation. *American Journal of Psychiatry*, 162, 1473–1482.
– *Examine the effect of social environment on dopamine function, referring primarily to work in monkeys.*

Risinger, R. C., Salmeron, B. J., Ross, T. J., Amen, S. L., Sanfilipo, M., Hoffmann, R. G., Bloom, A. S., Garavan, H. & Stein, E. A. (2005) Neural correlates of high and craving during cocaine self-administration using BOLD fMRI. *NeuroImage*, 26, 1097–1108.
– *This fMRI study updates the Breiter et al. (1997) study but uses a self-administration paradigm to create a more naturalistic setting.*

Volkow, N. D., Fowler, J. S., Wang, G. J., Baler, R. & Telang, F. (2009) Imaging dopamine's role in drug abuse and addiction. *Neuropharmacology*, 56(Suppl 1), 3–8.
– *Excellent review of the literature on imaging and the role of dopamine in addiction written by a pioneer of the field.*
Williams, T. M., Daglish, M. R. C., Lingford-Hughes, A., Taylor, L. G., Hammers, A., Brooks, D. J., Grasby, P., Myles, J. S. & Nutt, D. J. (2007) Brain opioid receptor binding in early abstinence from opioid dependence. *British Journal of Psychiatry*, 191, 63–69.
– *Recent PET imaging study provides new insight into the role of the opioid system in addiction.*

Chapter 16

GENES, GENETICS, GENOMICS AND EPIGENETICS

David Ball and Irene Guerrini

16.1 Introduction

This chapter provides the information to enable a working understanding of the research methods currently used in this rapidly developing field. Firstly, it examines the genetically informative animal approaches used to model addiction. Secondly, it describes the human methods employed to quantify the contribution of genes and environment to complex behaviours, such as addiction, including family, twin and adoption studies under the heading 'Quantitative genetics'. Thirdly, having established the importance of the genetic contribution, it addresses the molecular genetic methodologies currently employed for gene hunting that attempt to map the genes involved. Read in parallel with the current literature, this should enable the reader to appreciate the current position of this field, evaluate ongoing reports and perhaps integrate genetic research into planned or ongoing projects.

The aetiology of addiction is complex, with many different factors determining initial substance use and why some progress to dependence. These include the availability and acceptability of the substance or behaviour, comorbidity, self-medication of symptoms such as depression or anxiety, personality traits and genes. Whilst this chapter focuses on the latter, the contribution of genes must be seen within the environmental context in which they operate in order to appreciate the complex gene–environment interactions that occur during the development of addictive behaviours.

In 1866, the priest Mendel, published his eponymous laws of heredity but sadly died unaware of the profound influence that his work would have on subsequent biological research (Mendel, 1866) (Figure 16.1) (Box 16.1).

The biochemical basis of these laws began to be unravelled when DNA (deoxyribonucleic acid) was determined to be the hereditary material as reported in 1944 by Avery and colleagues (Avery et al., 1944). Indeed, the iconic double-helix structure of DNA, a thing of both beauty and function, was eventually described by Watson and Crick, aided by the work of Wilkins and Franklin (Watson, 1968). The molecule they described consisted of two strands of DNA running in opposite directions, which have a strong sugar–phosphate backbone, to which the four bases that make up the genetic code are attached. These strands in turn are held together weakly by hydrogen bonds between the bases on the opposite strands (Figures 16.2 and 16.3) (Box 16.2).

This structure provides an excellent mechanism for the DNA to be copied, transcribed and translated with a high fidelity. Thus, separating the strands, by breaking these weak hydrogen bonds, each single strand can operate as a template for further copies that can be passed on to other cells. The four bases are adenine (A), cytosine (C), guanine (G) and thymine (T). As such A forms two hydrogen bonds with T, and G forms three with C; the two bases, bonding across the helix, are called base pairs and they form the 'steps of the double-helix ladder'. The sequence of these bases provides the information that, amongst other things, is translated into specific amino acids that form the basic building blocks of proteins; the latter perform important structural

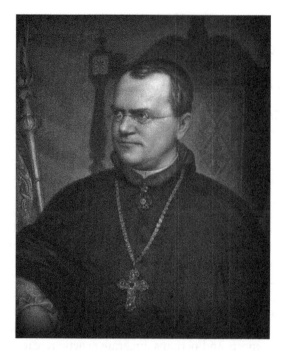

Figure 16.1 Mendel. (Reproduced with permission.)

Box 16.1   Gregor Johann Mendel (1822–1884)

Gregor Mendel, an Augustian monk, has been called the 'father of modern genetics'. He explored the variation that occurred in pea plants in a systematic way through experiments conducted in the monastery garden of Brno. Using pure breeding parental plants, he counted the characteristics, for example whether the seeds were wrinkled or smooth, of the plants he produced from them; counting was one of his innovative strengths and he counted a great many pea plants.

Of several characteristics observed, he noted that some were dominant to others that were re-cessive, without intermediates produced by blending of these characteristics. For example, crossing a wrinkled seed pea with a smooth seed pea resulted in all smooth seeded peas. However, when this generation was crossed within itself, three-fourths were smooth and one-fourth were the wrinkled type. Thus, the smooth characteristic was dominant to the recessive wrinkled type. When comparing plants which had more than one characteristic, Mendel also noted that the inheritance of each characteristic he studied occurred independently of each other.

From his observations, Mendel deduced that two 'elements' combine in the offspring cells and his conclusions are enshrined in what are now termed the Mendelian laws of segregation and independent assortment. The first of these describes the presence of hereditary elements that determine characteristics such that when the parent produces offspring they pass on one of the two elements. The second law describes how these elements are passed on independently of each other during this process, something we now know to be inaccurate for those genes that are on the same chromosome. This deviation is exploited in the molecular genetic techniques of linkage and association.

Why Mendel's work was largely ignored until it was rediscovered in 1900 is not clear. Certainly, working outside the mainstream scientific arena and publishing in an obscure journal are likely to have been detrimental to any citation index at that time.

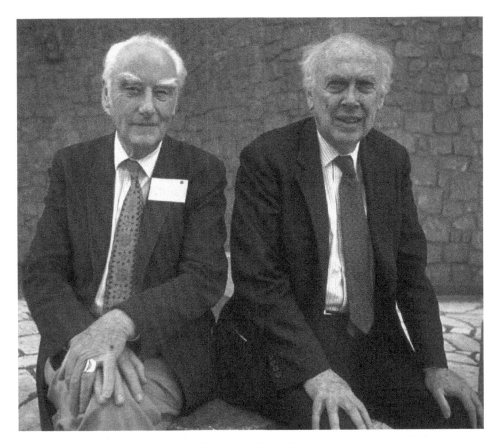

Figure 16.2 Watson and Crick. (Reproduced with permission.)

and functional roles in cells. Subsequently, methods for DNA sequencing were described by Sanger, and whilst pondering about sequencing during a late night drive, Kary Mullis conceived the idea of polymerase chain reaction, which remains a ubiquitous tool for amplifying specific fragments of DNA (Sanger & Coulson, 1975; Newton et al., 1997) (Figure 16.4).

In 2001, The International Human Genome Mapping Consortium and Celera Genomics published the working draft sequence of the human genome (McPherson et al., 2001; Venter et al., 2001). Indeed, the advances in the field of molecular genetics have been fast paced, profound and truly exciting.

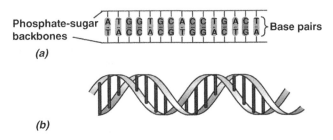

Figure 16.3 DNA double helix. (Reproduced with permission.)

Box 16.2   The double helix

The American James Watson (born 1928) began working with Francis Crick (1916–2004) after he came to Cambridge, joining the Medical Research Council unit at Cavendish Laboratory in 1951. Watson attended a colloquium at King's College London, at which both Maurice Wilkins (1916–2004) and Rosalind Franklin (1920–1958) presented their DNA research findings. Shortly after this, Watson and Crick produced their first model of DNA in late 1951. This was a triple-helical model with the bases on the outside and the phosphates inside. When Wilkins and Franklin were asked for their opinion, they quickly discounted this model. However, data from Franklin provided the dimensions for their second iconic model, the double helix, reported in 1953. Watson, Crick and Wilkins were jointly awarded, one-third each, the Nobel Prize for Medicine in 1962 'for their discoveries concerning the molecular structure of nucleic acids and its significance for information transfer in living material'; Franklin sadly having died in 1958 could not be included.

Science is undertaken by real people and the tense relationships between some of these research giants makes for fascinating reading. Furthermore, the circumstances surrounding Watson's viewing of Franklin's beautiful photograph 51, that was instrumental in motivating him to pursue the helical structure of DNA, will remain wonderfully controversial. Watson's own account of this period is graphically described in his book, *The Double Helix: A Personal Account of the Discovery of the Structure of DNA* (Watson, 1968). Alternatively Victor McElheny has written an excellent portrayal of Watson entitled 'Watson and DNA: Making a Scientific Revolution' (McElheny, 2003).

16.2   Animal studies[1]

It is very well established that animal models are particularly useful in dissecting complex, multifactorial traits. Among the main advantages of animal models is the fact that animals can be easily bred and kept in a controlled environment; furthermore, it is possible to 'simplify' a complex behaviour into its single components, using selective breeding techniques.

Historically, selective breeding of rodents has been used to produce genetic models of complex traits. Breeding pairs of rats/mice are chosen to create lines of animals with a specific phenotype or observed characteristic, such as alcohol preference, sensitivity to the hypnotic effects of ethanol, alcohol withdrawal seizures and alcohol tolerance. More recently, other approaches have been developed including inbred strains, RI strains and knockout mice (Tabakoff & Hoffman, 2000).

An inbred strain is a population of genetically identical animals that have been created by mating brothers to sisters for at least 20 generations. Researchers look for variations in behaviour between different inbred strains reared in identical environments, as evidence of genetic components of behaviour (Tabakoff & Hoffman, 2000). They also look for variations in behaviour within inbred strains. Since members of an in-bred strain are genetically alike, observed differences in behaviour are classically attributed to environmental factors.

Recombinant inbred (RI) strains are derived from standard inbred strains where each individual is homozygous at all genetic loci. The two progenitor strains are then interbred to generate a genetically identical population (F1). The following step is to breed the F1 population in order to have a genetically heterogeneous population F2 where some areas of the parental chromosomes have been recombined. Using the brother–sister mating of F2, it is possible to obtain individuals, genetically identical for one or the other parental alleles at each locus. This approach yields a unique pattern of recombination of the parental chromosomes in each RI strain.

The RI methodology is a very useful tool to analyse polygenic traits in which every single gene has a small influence on the genetic susceptibility of the trait. Furthermore, multiple genes influence the

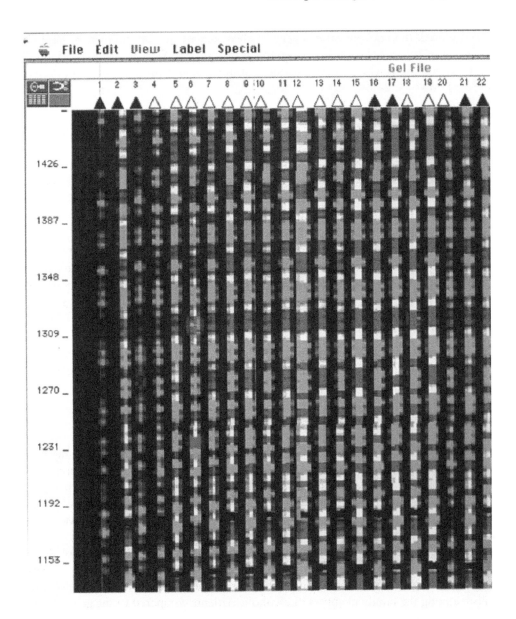

Figure 16.4 DNA sequencing gel. (Courtesy of Linzy Hill.)

expression of the traits, and the vast majority of phenotypes/traits behave quantitatively; in other words, they vary over a continuous range of values (quantitative traits). To identify the genetic loci (quantitative trait loci) associated to those, the allelic variation is correlated with the phenotypic variability in the RI strains (Tabakoff et al., 2003).

Other strategies for evaluating a gene's contribution to complex traits include the production of transgenic and knockout animals. These strategies are particularly important to understand the role of candidate genes, i.e. those believed to contribute to the development of the trait/disease.

In order to produce a transgenic mouse, a foreign gene is integrated into the mouse's own genome. Transgenic animals express the inserted gene, and the influence of the gene on the development of the trait can be explored. In knockout mice, a gene has been inactivated or modified. Several knockout mice have been used in alcohol studies, for example dopamine and serotonin (e.g. D2-5 and 5HT1b) receptor knockouts, in which sensitivity to alcohol and alcohol drinking behaviours have been analysed (Tabakoff et al., 2000).

16.3 Quantitative genetics

Many common, complex diseases or traits are believed to have a genetic susceptibility, but unlike disorders with a Mendelian inheritance, they cannot be understood using single gene models (Dick et al., 2006). Quantitative genetics is a useful tool to explore if a common disorder aggregates in families and to evaluate the contribution of genetic and environmental factors in its development.

The hunt for genetic susceptibility to complex diseases starts with family studies, that is studies investigating the clustering of a disorder in families. The second step is to discriminate, via twin and adoption studies, the impact of environmental and genetic factors on the susceptibility.

In the following paragraphs the methodologies of family, twin and adoption studies are described.

16.3.1 Family studies

The family study approach is based on the principle that if a disease or a trait has a genetic component, the trait is present among family members more frequently than in the general population. In fact, in the case of familial aggregation, the proportion of cases having a relative with the same disease is higher than in controls.

Several methodologies have been used to explore the familial aggregation of a disease or trait in families. Abbreviated family history involves obtaining information from the probands themselves about the presence/absence of a trait/disease in their first- or second-degree relatives; the proportion of probands with a disease/trait-carrying relative is compared with controls. Alternatively, each family member is interviewed with the aim of building an accurate family tree (pedigree). This contains each member's affection status, and includes first-degree (parents, siblings, and children) and second-degree relatives (aunts, uncles, grandchildren, grandparents, and nephews or nieces), as well as more distant family members (Farrer & Cupples, 1998).

Numerous family studies have been carried out in probands affected by alcohol dependence. In fact, it has long been observed that alcohol disorders cluster in families, and the systematic investigation of biologically related individuals has consistently documented the higher prevalence of alcoholism among the family members of alcoholic patients compared to the general population (Hesselbrock, 1995; Kalsi et al., 2008). Offsprings of alcoholics are approximately five times more likely to develop alcohol-related problems than the children of non-alcoholics (Kalsi et al., 2008).

Family studies are particularly important for linkage analysis (see Section 16.4, 'Molecular genetics'). The familiar recurrence risk or risk ratio is an index of the strength of the genetic effect, and it is defined as the ratio of the risk to relatives compared to the population risk (λR). For instance, in a complex disorder like alcohol dependence the risk ratio has been calculated to be between three and nine. A risk ratio higher than two is indicative of a significant genetic component in the aetiopathogenesis of the disease/trait (Farrer & Cupples, 1998)

Another approach to estimate the genetic component of quantitative traits is the heritability (h^2). Heritability indicates the proportion of the phenotypic variance due to genes versus the environment. The greater the h^2 value, the more significant the genetic component; for example if h^2 is 0.60, this means that 60% of the phenotypic variance of the trait is due to the genetic component.

16.3.2 Segregation analysis

Segregation analysis evaluates large contributions of genes to the expression of the phenotype. The method analyses the pedigree structure in order to ascertain whether the mode of transmission of a disorder is congruent with a particular Mendelian modality.

An early example was reported by Kroon in 1924 with the description of a single pedigree with 22 cases of 'dipsomania' (Hesselbrock, 1995). In this study, the author suggested a 'sex-limited' form of inheritance, in which dipsomania displays dominant inheritance in males, but recessive inheritance in females (Hesselbrock, 1995). More recent findings favour a mixed model of transmission with a possible dominant major gene effect and a multi-factorial (polygenic) background.

Moreover, the validity of segregation analyses is dubious in the study of genetic effects in complex diseases such as addiction. Such statistical procedures depend on large numbers of variables and assume that a population under study is homogeneous in terms of the mode of transmission of the disorder. Such assumptions are not warranted in the case of addiction.

16.3.3 Twin and adoption studies

Even traits or disorders that are familial in nature are not necessarily influenced or transmitted by genetic factors alone, but twin and adoption studies help elucidate the importance of those factors in the transmission of psychiatric disorders including addiction (Agrawal & Lynskey, 2008).

Twin studies are based on the fact that identical, or monozygotic (MZ), twins are genetically identical while non-identical, or dizygotic (DZ), twins on average have half of their DNA in common. A basic assumption in these studies is that since pairs are raised alongside each other, the environment where they are raised has a similar influence on each member of the pair. If both the twins have the trait under study, they are said to be concordant. Genetic influence is indicated when the concordance rate, or correlation coefficient, for MZ twins exceeds that for DZ twins. The higher the concordance rate for MZs compared to DZs, the greater the genetic component. If the disease/trait had Mendelian transmission, the concordance rate would be 100% in MZ twins. As an example, the concordance rate for alcohol dependence in MZ twins is reported around 70%, while in DZ twins it is around 30% (Hesselbrock, 1995).

An elegant method to tell genetic from environmental influences studies adopted child separated near birth from the affected parent. In fact, if a trait/disease has a genetic component, the risk of developing the same trait/disease is higher in biological relatives than in adopted relatives.

There are four basic separation study methodologies: (1) adoptive family method – the prevalence of the trait/disorder under study is compared in both the biological and adoptive relatives of affected adoptees and controls; (2) adoptee study method – compares the prevalence of trait/disorder under study among the adopted-away children of an affected parent either to the adoptee of controls or to the general population; (3) adoptive parents' method – begins with affected probands and compares the prevalence of trait/disorder under study in their biological and adoptive parents; (4) the cross-fostering method – identifies two groups of adoptees (e.g. children of an alcoholic parent raised by a non-alcoholic adoptive parent and children of a non-alcoholic biological parent raised by an alcoholic parent) in which the prevalence of the trait/disorder under study is compared between the groups (Hesselbrock, 1995; Agrawal & Lynskey, 2008).

Adoption study approaches are particularly useful if the trait or disease under study has a large environmental component as in many neuropsychiatric disorders including alcoholism. The most widely cited series of studies of adopted-away children of an alcoholic biological parent were the Copenhagen Adoption Registry and the Swedish adoption study (Agrawal & Lynskey, 2008). One

---

Box 16.3 The Swedish adoption study

A large cohort of adopted men born in Stockholm, Sweden, were studied jointly by Bohman and Cloninger in the early eighties. The 852 children had been separated from their biological parents at an early age and adopted by non-relatives. Information on alcohol abuse, criminality, and physical and mental complaints was routinely collected in Sweden as part of health and social policy, and data were made available for the purpose of the adoption study.

Information about the genetic background of adoptees was measured using the available data about their biological parents. Conversely, information about their rearing environment was measured by data about their adoptive parents and familial environment. Cloninger developed a new methodology to analyse the impact of environmental and genetic backgrounds, combined or separately, called a 'cross-fostering' analysis.

The main outcome of the study was the description of two forms of alcoholism with different clinical features and modes of inheritance. Type 1 alcoholism is characterised by an adult onset, rapid progression of dependence, no association with criminal behaviour, and family history negative for alcoholism, whereas type 2 alcoholism has an early onset (below the age of 25 years), frequently associated with social and forensic complications, affecting mainly males, highly heritable in men.

In 1996, the original study was replicated by the same group producing confirmatory evidence in support of type 1 and type 2 alcoholism as two distinct clinical subtypes.

---

of the most significant findings in the Swedish adoption study was the evidence produced for two subtypes of alcoholism: type 1 or 'milieu limited', has a later age of onset, being only mildly genetic in origin; type 2, being strongly genetic and associated with criminality in the adoptee and their biological father (Box 16.3).

16.4 Molecular genetics

16.4.1 DNA extraction

In humans, the DNA, stored in the cell nucleus, is packaged into 46 chromosomes (23 pairs), one of each pair being inherited from one parent, including the two sex chromosomes (females being XX and males XY) (Figure 16.5).

The hereditary material, DNA, can therefore be readily extracted from body cells that contain a nucleus, with adequate quantities being obtained from a 10-mL venous blood sample, collected into an EDTA (ethylenediaminetetraacetic acid) tube that is commonly used for routine blood investigations (e.g. full blood count). Less, and poorer quality, DNA can be obtained from cheek cells, obtained from rubbing several cotton buds (Q-Tips) around the inside of the mouth. However, using the latter method, in the form of a kit, means that DNA can be obtained at a distance and even by post.

16.4.2 DNA markers

Markers are sites within the DNA that vary and are identifiable. As such they represent changes in the base sequence of the DNA. For example, one group of markers called the single nucleotide polymorphisms (SNPs) have a change in a single base at a particular location. Other markers consist of differences in length, for example varying numbers of DNA repeat sequences, insertions and

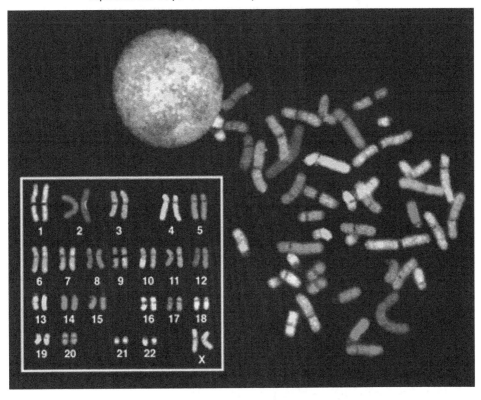

During cell division the chromosomes condense and can be
separated into 23 pairs that make up the human DNA complement

Figure 16.5 Chromosomes in nucleus. (Reproduced with permission of John Wiley & Sons, Inc.)

deletions. The different variants within a gene are called alleles and the particular combinations that
the individual possesses, for most sites one inherited from each parent, are termed the genotype.

16.4.3 Endophenotypes

In genetic studies, a phenotype, or observed characteristic, is selected for study that is the result
of genes and environmental interaction. This could be addiction per se but is usually substance,
or behaviour-specific and may even be quite well defined such as alcohol-related liver disease in
alcohol-dependent individuals. As the addictions are complex behaviours, they may be better studied
by exploring the genetic contribution to individual components of behaviour or endophenotypes.
This latter term has been defined by Gottesman and Gould as 'measurable components unseen by the
unaided eye along the pathway between disease and distal genotype' (Gottesman & Gould, 2003). In
essence, this attempts to get closer to the genes and thereby enhance the chance of identifying genetic
influence. Examples of endophenotypes include measuring an individual's responses to alcohol doses
such as body sway or standing steadiness, electrophysiological measures and personality traits such
as impulsive sensation seeking. These may be substance specific, for example responses to alcohol
dose, or may span several addictive behaviours, for example the personality trait of sensation seeking.

16.4.4   Quantitative trait loci

Some conditions are caused by a single defect in a gene, for example Huntington's disease, a condition characterised by late-onset dementia, choreiform (dance-like) involuntary movements and psychiatric symptoms. In this case, the condition is caused by three DNA bases being repeated in the gene more than 37 times, and this produces an abnormal protein that causes the premature loss of neurons in specific brain areas. However, addictive behaviours are likely to be caused by multiple genes that interact with environmental factors, during a process of development. Thus, quantitative genetics and molecular genetics have combined to identify genes that contribute to these complex behaviours in an interchangeable and additive way, thereby increasing the risk of developing these conditions. Such a gene acting in concert with other genes is called a quantitative trait locus. The techniques employed then to seek out the quantitative trait loci that underpin addiction must therefore be sensitive to the relatively small effects that are envisaged for individual genes. Traditionally, two main approaches have been adopted, namely, linkage analysis and association.

16.4.5   Linkage analysis

When two sites, also known as loci, are close to each other on a chromosome, they do not obey Mendel's law of independent assortment, as they are often inherited together rather than this occurring randomly. This coinheritance, due to closeness or proximity, is termed linkage, and linkage analysis attempts to identify coinheritance between a behaviour or disorder and a marker, that is a locus of DNA that varies between individuals and therefore can be identified and tracked. Stated simply, the linkage approach attempts to identify coinheritance, within a family, between a variant of a marker and the disorder or behaviour. To this end, DNA samples are collected from family members of pedigrees that contain several affected individuals; although some methods employ 'fragments' of families, for example, sibling pairs (Figure 16.6).

The finding of significant linkage, between a marker and addiction, implies that there is a gene, somewhere in the vicinity of the linked marker, that has a role in the development of the condition. As such linkage can identify new genes that are involved in conditions for which there has been no previous reason to suspect any contribution. For example, Figure 16.4 shows a condition such as Huntington's disease in which the disease is inherited along with the particular marker variant c. Huntington's disease was successfully mapped to chromosome 4 using this approach. However, as indicated above, addictive behaviours are not like a single gene disorder, and therefore advanced

Linkage analysis looks for a coinheritance between a particular marker variant and the condition. In this pedigree, males are designated as squares and females as circles. Those affected are coloured in blue and the marker variants are shown alongside the individuals. In this family marker, there are four variants at this particular marker and variant c is inherited along with the disease from the first affected male downwards.

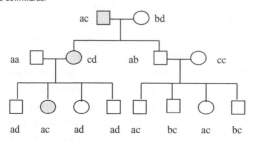

Figure 16.6 Linkage analysis. (Reproduced with permission.)

> **Box 16.4   Collaborative Studies on Genetics of Alcoholism**
>
> While exhaustive reviews of linkage studies in the addictions world would immediately need updating, the Collaborative Studies on Genetics of Alcoholism is perhaps the best example. Collecting multiply affected pedigrees since 1989, the study has now amassed more than 3000 individual from more than 300 families. These subjects have been carefully studied and, in addition to comprehensive clinical assessments, have undergone neuropsychological, electrophysiological and biochemical testing. Early findings from this study provided evidence for linkage to alcohol dependence on chromosomes 1 and 7, with modest evidence for chromosome 2 and a protective locus on chromosome 4 in the region of the cluster of alcohol-metabolising genes that code for alcohol dehydrogenase (Reich et al., 1998).

statistics are employed to detect any subtle coinheritance. A linkage scan of all the human chromosomes can be undertaken using a mere 300 markers and therefore this approach is systematic, but this advantage has to be balanced against the limited sensitivity to detect genes of relatively small effect and those masked by complex gene–environment interactions (Box 16.4).

16.4.6   Association

The second strategy adopted to identify genes, predisposing to addiction, is that of allelic association. The different genetic variants at a particular DNA site, or locus, are called alleles, and allelic association refers to the association between one of these and the phenotype, in this case usually an addiction. Such studies rely on a genetic change occurring many generations ago that confers an increased, or decreased, susceptibility to addiction. This change originally occurs on the background of a specific pattern of alleles up and down the same chromosome. Over the subsequent generations, that unique pattern of genetic variations is lost through DNA recombination that occurs during the process of meiosis, which generates both eggs and sperms. This particularly affects those alleles further away from the predisposing allele, whilst those closer are less likely to become dissociated. As a result those alleles, which are close to the vulnerability causing genetic variation, will be inherited as a block and therefore these may occur at a different frequency in those with the addiction when compared with those not affected (Figure 16.7).

Practically speaking, allelic association studies are performed by obtaining samples from those affected by an addiction, such as alcohol dependence, and comparing them with non-affected individuals. In essence, these are unrelated individuals, although the approach is based on individuals being related many generations previously. Thus, in contrast to linkage studies, it is relatively easy to collect a bank of DNA samples from alcohol-dependent individuals, for example by recruiting those attending treatment services. This ease of collection means that it is very tempting to piggyback such research onto clinical services or other research projects and not invest sufficiently in characterising the samples, for example by direct assessment and documentation of the clinical features. In addition, appropriately matched control panels are, if anything, more difficult to obtain. For example, for a DNA sample of smokers, would the best controls be those who have never smoked; sometimes such controls are called 'supernormals', or those who smoke but do not progress to dependence, for example 'chippers' who do not smoke at a frequency characteristic of nicotine dependence? Should control subjects for an alcohol dependence study be matched for alcohol exposure prior to the progression to dependence? All too often, researchers have settled for unscreened population samples that were poorly matched to their sample and contained unidentified, affected individuals and those

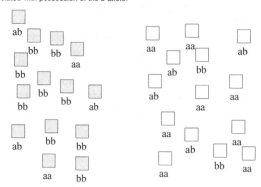

Samples of DNA are collected from affected individuals, depicted in blue, and controls. The distributions of marker variants are compared across the two samples and positive association detected if there is a significant difference. In this case, the affected individuals have a greater frequency of the b allele and therefore the condition is associated with possession of the b allele.

Figure 16.7 Allelic association.

prior to presentation. Indeed, some early studies even recruited controls from among their work colleagues, which as a result would be very poor controls for their addiction counterparts. Fortunately, some research bodies are now very wisely investing in well-characterised, community-based samples that they are willing to make available more generally.

Having obtained a sufficiently large sample of subjects and controls, the distribution of genetic variants is examined in both and compared. Often the variants examined are in candidate genes chosen because their function suggests a potential role in addiction. Often multiple alleles, in an individual gene, are studied and these are often combined with other genes to analyse systematically a particular brain pathway; for example, the dopamine system includes genes for enzymes involved in synthesis and metabolism along with dopamine transporters and receptors. A simple chi-square test can be used to test for significant allele frequency differences that indicate an association between the addiction phenotype and the allele. A positive association indicates that the allele studied itself, or another close by, increases the vulnerability to addiction.

It is now possible, using DNA chips, also known as arrays, to undertake a systematic association study covering the whole genome. Essentially, an array consists of short fragments of DNA that are spotted at very high density onto a glass or plastic surface. These identify different alleles by their ability to match and pair up with the DNA extracted from an individual. By using this technique, a million markers can be examined in one reaction. This can be made even more efficient and cost-effective by methods that create DNA pools from affected individuals and compare the allele profiles with those from control pools (Figure 16.8).

Unfortunately, association studies are hampered by their high false-positive rate, although this may be diminished by careful sample selection and characterisation, especially when applied to the control population. Paul Buckland has attempted to model this inherent difficulty and has provided an estimate of the probability that a reported association with, in this case, alcohol dependence has occurred by chance (Buckland, 2001). The parameters of the model he proposed suggests that there are 20 genes that genuinely contribute to the risk of alcohol dependence, that there are 80 000 genes in the human genome (we now know that this is an overestimate as the subsequent sequencing of the entire human DNA suggests around 25 000) and that you can test each gene's involvement using a single marker (several are generally required). This implies that 'we would expect to find a true-positive result in 1 in every 4000 experiments or 0.025% of the time' and 'any result with P-value of 0.05 has a 99.5% likelihood of having occurred by chance'. Even correcting for the gene

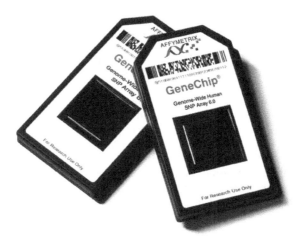

Figure 16.8 Affymetrix® GeneChip® Genome-Wide Human SNP Array 6.0. (Courtesy of Affymetrix with permission.)

number, we would only expect to find a true-positive result in 1 in every 1250 experiments or 0.08% of the time and any result with P-value of 0.05 has a 98.4% likelihood of having occurred by chance.

Typically, association studies are not systematic but examine the role of candidate genes in addiction. However, using DNA microarrays it is now feasible to undertake a systematic whole genome approach. Association studies are more sensitive than linkage studies and can potentially identify the relatively small genetic contributions that are anticipated to contribute to addictive behaviour. However, a major limitation is their high false-positive rate. There follows an example of the most robust finding in the field of addictions and indeed in psychiatric genetics. Other genes that have been implicated by association studies are the 'usual suspects' including those in the dopamine, GABA, cannabinoid, opiate and serotonin neurotransmitter systems as well as those involved in alcohol metabolism (Figure 16.9) (Box 16.5).

16.4.7 Epigenetics

Genetic effects may not just be manifestations of changes at the DNA level but rather may reflect differences in the way that the DNA is expressed through reversible changes in the configuration of DNA. The British embryologist, Conrad Hal Waddington, coined the term 'epigenetics' in 1942

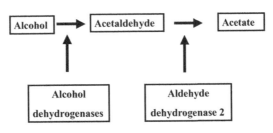

The main route for alcohol metabolism involves oxidation by alcohol dehydrogenases to form acetaldehyde followed by further oxidation by aldehyde dehydrogenase 2 to form acetate.

Figure 16.9 Metabolism of alcohol.

Box 16.5   The example of aldehyde dehydrogenase 2 (ALDH2)

A genetic variant in the ALDH2 gene confers protection against alcohol dependence. Following rapid absorption of alcohol, in the small intestine, the major pathway for alcohol metabolism takes place in the liver, via alcohol dehydrogenase, not one but a family of enzymes, to acetaldehyde, followed by further metabolism to acetate by ALDH2.

Back in the 1970s, Wolff, in a study of oriental ethnic groups (Japanese, Taiwanese and Koreans), recognised the high rate of facial flushing within this population and raised the possibility that this may be related to the risk of developing alcoholism (Wolff, 1972). This 'oriental flush reaction' was subsequently demonstrated to be due to an inactive variant of ADLH2 that results in the accumulation of acetaldehyde, an unpleasant and toxic compound, which is also the cause of the adverse disulfiram reaction that this drug produces by 'suicidal' inhibition of ALDH2. Indeed, possession of this inactive variant not surprisingly reduces the risk of developing alcohol dependence. Subsequently, the molecular genetic underpinning of this inactive variant has been clarified and it is due to a single base change in the gene from a G to an A (Yin & Agarwal, 2001; Higuchi et al., 2004). This lone base change in the ALDH2 gene changes the amino acid in the protein at that point from a glutamate to a lysine, and this disrupts the activity of the enzyme. Most individuals with the low-activity variant also possess a normal activity variant, as they have two copies of the gene, one from each parent. However, there was great excitement in the field some years ago when an individual bearing two copies of the inactive variant managed to attract a diagnosis of alcohol dependence, even though under DSM-III-R criteria (Chen et al., 1999). In summary, a single base change, a typo as it were, in the ALDH2 gene provides profound protection, although not absolute, against developing alcohol dependence.

---

and his epigenetic landscape, in which marbles were envisaged rolling down trajectories which were made increasingly irreversible due to the rising of longitudinal ridges, was a metaphor for the process of cellular differentiation by which different bodily tissues and organs develop (Goldberg et al., 2007). Molecular genetics has recycled these ideas to the study of vulnerability to disorders and behaviours. Epigenetics 'refers to modifications in gene expression that are brought about by heritable, but potentially reversible, changes in chromatin structure and/or DNA methylation' (Henikoff & Matzke, 1997). That is the addition of methyl groups, methylation, to particular sites on the DNA can silence gene expression as can changes in the configuration of the protein packaging of the DNA within the cell. More recently, non-protein products of the DNA, namely, non-coding RNAs (ncRNA), have also been shown to modulate gene expression. Such supra-DNA changes, being heritable and partially stable, may mediate the vulnerability to various behaviours, including addiction, and are readily studied in DNA extracts.

16.4.8   Gene–environment interaction

Genes do not act in isolation and much information may be lost, if gene–environment interactions over time are ignored, as occurs during the development of a condition. Indeed, such interactions may actually obscure and therefore hamper the current molecular genetic-orientated research. The best approach to untangle these complex interactions employs prospective longitudinal studies, combined with molecular genetic analysis, and the Dunedin longitudinal study is a fine example (Box 16.6).

Box 16.6   The Dunedin longitudinal study

This project continues to follow, at regular intervals, 1014 subjects born at the Queen Mary Maternity Hospital between April 1973 and March 1974. Thus far, almost 1000 publications have resulted including a paper indicating that cannabis exposure as a teenager may predispose to psychosis in those carrying a genetic predisposition (Caspi et al., 2005). This study suggested that cannabis use in adolescence is associated with an increased risk of developing a schizophreniform disorder in adulthood but only in those carrying a genetic variant in catechol-O-methyltransferase, particularly if they had two copies of the risk variant. In a different sample, Ducci and colleagues have reported that childhood sexual abuse is associated with higher rates of alcoholism and antisocial personality disorder in women carrying a low-activity variant of the monoamine oxidase A gene (Ducci et al., 2008). Whilst these studies need to be replicated, they demonstrate the usefulness of adopting a developmental approach, which permits the identification of gene–environment interactions.

The study of the hyphen in nature–nurture, which represents gene–environment interactions, is set to take a prominent role in this field and those who had the foresight to invest in longitudinal studies will be amply rewarded through the addition of a molecular genetics arm.

16.5   Why bother?

Identifying the genes that underpin the propensity for addiction will permit a better understanding of both the biological and environmental factors involved and their interaction. It may allow addiction to be divided into subtypes that may determine both treatment approaches and outcome. Furthermore, novel treatments may be developed and these, combined with those presently available, could be targeted and tailored to an individual, possibly aided by genetic information. Finally, genetic tests may also be used to refine a person's risk of developing addiction or to screen populations for vulnerable individuals. However, given the prediction that multiple genes will be involved, it is unlikely that screening and risk alteration will be feasible or cost-effective.

16.6   An addiction gene

The most likely outcome of this research is that multiple genes will be identified, of relatively small effect, which interact with environmental factors as addiction develops. Some genes will play a role across many addictive behaviours, whilst others will be substance or behaviour specific. Furthermore, some genes may exert their influence through several different mechanisms. This complex choreography will involve different genes throughout the different stages that comprise the natural history of addiction: from initiation, through regular use, tolerance, dependence, physical complications, psychological sequelae, treatment response, repeated relapse and hopefully recovery. Indeed, individuals will differ in the relative importance of both genetic and environmental factors in their progression through these stages. As a consequence, a gene that causes addictive behaviours will not be found; rather many genes will be identified that modulate vulnerability, either increasing or reducing risk, within the specific environmental setting. As such, these interactions, over time, will be active participants in the process of development that will modify the natural history of these conditions within the individual.

> **Box 16.7   Lethal genes**
>
> We may all carry lethal genes, which if they were not balanced by 'good' versions, would result in
> a failure to reproduce, through severe handicap or death. Such genes are called lethal equivalents
> and represent DNA variants that if present in both copies, that is the individual is a homozygote,
> would be lethal, or an equivalent combination of variants with less harmful effects. An estimate
> of the number of these can be gained by examining the increased mortality rates that occur in off-
> spring of consanguineous marriages. Alan Bittles and James Neel reviewed the published mortality
> rates in first cousin marriages, from seven countries, and included deaths from late miscarriages,
> premature births and stillbirths, with follow-up reported to an average age of 10 years (range
> 1 month to 30 years). These rates were compared with those reported in non-consanguineous
> marriages, and the average excess mortality was 4.4%. From these data they calculated, over the
> time course indicated, that the average individual carries 1.4 lethal equivalents that would result in
> death if they were not balanced by the other DNA they carry. This is likely to be an underestimate
> as early losses during pregnancy were not included due to the likelihood of inaccurate reporting;
> as such this period represents a high-risk time for the operation of lethal genes.

16.7   Ethics

Genetic research must be undertaken within the strict ethical guidelines described in Chapter 6, but
should also particularly consider how findings are disseminated, particularly if the genes studied have
direct clinical relevance. Certainly in the past, genetic improvement has been used to justify atrocities
such that it has been branded 'murderous science'. In truth, each of us is carrying on average 1.4
deleterious segments of DNA, termed lethal equivalents, which would not be compatible with life if
they were not balanced by 'good' DNA (Bittles & Neel, 1994) (Box 16.7).

Identifying the genes would have a profound impact on the way that addiction is viewed. By
supporting a medical model, it would endorse 'patient status' and elicit sympathy for those affected,
whilst perhaps influencing resource allocation. But suppose a gene of major effect is identified, would
those carrying it be absolved of all responsibility regarding their behaviour and could they sue their
parents for their unfortunate inheritance? Would possession of such a gene invoke a nihilistic attitude
to outcome both to, and by, the individual? Would those without the risky gene variant assume a
lifestyle based on a false assumption of invulnerability?

Finally, should the effect size of genes be so small that they are of little clinical relevance than
the cost/benefit of this research, and its applications will be high, and some have argued that
implementing public health measures of demonstrable efficacy represents better candidates for pri-
oritisation and funding.

16.8   Concluding remarks

There is convincing evidence from the natural experiments of family, twin and adoption studies that
genes are implicated in addiction. Given the continuing dramatic advances in molecular genetics, it
is now possible to chase these genes using the existing techniques of linkage and association. Linkage
is dependent on collecting samples from families, and therefore this is both labour intensive and
expensive. In addition, this approach may not be sensitive enough to identify the anticipated small
contribution of individual genes and initial findings have proved difficult to replicate. Association
studies are ideal for identifying these relatively small genetic contributions. They are cheap and it

is easy to establish a large DNA sample collection. However, it could be argued that the ease with which an association study can be 'piggybacked' onto another study, or established within a clinical setting, may be a weakness, as there is a temptation to undertake such studies 'on the cheap'; it is therefore vital that due effort is spent assessing the subjects and obtaining suitable controls. Indeed, the field is littered with non-robust, unreplicated genetic associations, and this will continue to be an issue as upwards of a million markers are examined in whole genome approaches. As such, the statistical 'sifting of the wheat from the chaff' represents a huge challenge. It is vital for the credibility of the field that individual findings should not be 'talked up' and such isolated associations, often celebrated in the media, are best considered with a healthy degree of initial scepticism. Furthermore, finding the genes, and their associated environmental factors, could have a profound effect on the management of addictive behaviours, and this has ethical implications that must be anticipated and widely debated.

Acknowledgement

Thanks to John Witton, Ian Craig, John Strang and Peter Miller for their very helpful comments on the script.

Note

1. See also Chapter 17, 'Animal Models'.

References

Agrawal, A. & Lynskey, M. T. (2008) Are there genetic influences on addiction: evidence from family, adoption and twin studies. *Addiction*, 103, 1069–1081.

Avery, O. T., MacLeod, C. M. & McCarty, M. (1944) Studies on the chemical nature of the substance inducing transformation of pneumococcal types. *Journal of Experimental Medicine*, 79, 158.

Bittles, A. H. & Neel, J. V. (1994) The costs of human inbreeding and their implications for variations at the DNA level. *Nature Genetics*, 8, 117–121.

Buckland, P. R. (2001) Genetic association studies of alcoholism–problems with the candidate gene approach. *Alcohol and Alcoholism*, 36, 99–103.

Caspi, A., Moffitt, T. E., Cannon, M., McClay, J., Murray, R., Harrington, H., Taylor, A., Arseneault, L., Williams, B., Braithwaite, A., Poulton, R. & Craig, I. W. (2005) Moderation of the effect of adolescent-onset cannabis use on adult psychosis by a functional polymorphism in the catechol-O-methyltransferase gene: longitudinal evidence of a gene X environment interaction. *Biological Psychiatry*, 57, 1117–1127.

Chen, Y. C., Lu, R. B., Peng, G. S., Wang, M. F., Wang, H. K., Ko, H. C., Chang, Y. C., Lu, J. J., Li, T. K. & Yin, S. J. (1999) Alcohol metabolism and cardiovascular response in an alcoholic patient homozygous for the ALDH2*2 variant gene allele. *Alcoholism, Clinical and Experimental Research*, 23, 1853–1860.

Dick, D. M., Rose, R. J. & Kaprio, J. (2006) The next challenge for psychiatric genetics: characterizing the risk associated with identified genes. *Annals of Clinical Psychiatry*, 18, 223–231.

Ducci, F., Enoch, M. A., Hodgkinson, C., Xu, K., Catena, M., Robin, R. W. & Goldman, D. (2008) Interaction between a functional MAOA locus and childhood sexual abuse predicts alcoholism and antisocial personality disorder in adult women. *Molecular Psychiatry*, 13, 334–347.

Farrer, L. & Cupples, L. A. (1998) Determining the genetic component of a disease. In: J. L. Haines & M. A. Pericak-Vance (eds) *Approaches to Gene Mapping in Complex Human Diseases*. New York: John Wiley & Sons, pp. 93–129.

Goldberg, A. D., Allis, C. D. & Bernstein, E. (2007) Epigenetics: a landscape takes shape. *Cell*, 128, 635–638.

Gottesman, I. I. & Gould, T. D. (2003) The endophenotype concept in psychiatry: etymology and strategic intentions. *American Journal of Psychiatry*, 160, 636–645.

Henikoff, S. & Matzke, M. A. (1997) Exploring and explaining epigenetic effects. *Trends in Genetics*, 13, 293–295.

Hesselbrock, V. (1995) The genetic epidemiology of alcoholism. In: H. Begleiter & B. Kissin (eds) *The Genetics of Alcoholism*. New York: Oxford University Press, pp. 17–39.

Higuchi, S., Matsushita, S., Masaki, T., Yokoyama, A., Kimura, M., Suzuki, G. & Mochizuki, H. (2004) Influence of genetic variations of ethanol-metabolizing enzymes on phenotypes of alcohol-related disorders. *Annals of the New York Academy of Science*, 1025, 472–480.

Kalsi, G., Prescott, C. A., Kendler, K. S. & Riley, B. P. (2008) Unraveling the molecular mechanisms of alcohol dependence. *Trends in Genetics*, 25(1), 49–55.

McElheny, V. K. (2003) *Watson and DNA : Making a Scientific Revolution*. Chichester, UK: Wiley.

McPherson, J. D., Marra, M., Hillier, L., Waterston, R. H., Chinwalla, A., Wallis, J., Sekhon, M., Wylie, K., Mardis, E. R., Wilson, R. K., Fulton, R., Kucaba, T. A., Wagner-McPherson, C., Barbazuk, W. B., Gregory, S. G., Humphray, S. J., French, L., Evans, R. S., Bethel, G., Whittaker, A., Holden, J. L., McCann, O. T., Dunham, A., Soderlund, C., Scott, C. E., Bentley, D. R., Schuler, G., Chen, H. C., Jang, W., Green, E. D., Idol, J. R., Maduro, V. V., Montgomery, K. T., Lee, E., Miller, A., Emerling, S., Kucherlapati, Gibbs, R., Scherer, S., Gorrell, J. H., Sodergren, E., Clerc-Blankenburg, K., Tabor, P., Naylor, S., Garcia, D., de Jong, P. J., Catanese, J. J., Nowak, N., Osoegawa, K., Qin, S., Rowen, L., Madan, A., Dors, M., Hood, L., Trask, B., Friedman, C., Massa, H., Cheung, V. G., Kirsch, I. R., Reid, T., Yonescu, R., Weissenbach, J., Bruls, T., Heilig, R., Branscomb, E., Olsen, A., Doggett, N., Cheng, J. F., Hawkins, T., Myers, R. M., Shang, J., Ramirez, L., Schmutz, J., Velasquez, O., Dixon, K., Stone, N. E., Cox, D. R., Haussler, D., Kent, W. J., Furey, T., Rogic, S., Kennedy, S., Jones, S., Rosenthal, A., Wen, G., Schilhabel, M., Gloeckner, G., Nyakatura, G., Siebert, R., Schlegelberger, B., Korenberg, J., Chen, X. N., Fujiyama, A., Hattori, M., Toyoda, A., Yada, T., Park, H. S., Sakaki, Y., Shimizu, N., Asakawa, S., Kawasaki, K., Sasaki, T., Shintani, A., Shimizu, A., Shibuya, K., Kudoh, J., Minoshima, S., Ramser, J., Seranski, P., Hoff, C., Poustka, A., Reinhardt, R. & Lehrach, H. (2001) A physical map of the human genome. *Nature*, 409, 934–941.

Mendel, G. J. (1866) Versuche über pflanzenhybriden. *Verhandlungen des Naturforschenden Vereines in Brünn*, 4, 3–47.

Newton, C. R., Graham, A. & Biochemical Society (1997) *PCR*, 2nd edn. Oxford, UK: BIOS Scientific Publishers.

Reich, T., Edenberg, H. J., Goate, A., Williams, J. T., Rice, J. P. & Van Eerdewegh, P., Foroud, T., Hesselbrock, V., Schuckit, M. A., Bucholz, K., Porjesz, B., Li, T. K., Conneally, P. M., Nurnberger, J. I., Jr, Tischfield, J. A., Crowe, R. R., Cloninger, C. R., Wu, W., Shears, S., Carr, K., Crose, C., Willig, C. & Begleiter, H. (1998) Genome-wide search for genes affecting the risk for alcohol dependence. *American Journal of Medical Genetics*, 81, 207–215.

Sanger, F. & Coulson, A. R. (1975) A rapid method for determining sequences in DNA by primed synthesis with DNA polymerase. *Journal of Molecular Biology*, 94, 441–448.

Tabakoff, B., Bhave, S. V. & Hoffman, P. L. (2003) Selective breeding, quantitative trait locus analysis, and gene arrays identify candidate genes for complex drug-related behaviors. *Journal of Neuroscience*, 23, 4491–4498.

Tabakoff, B. & Hoffman, P. L. (2000) Animal models in alcohol research. *Alcohol Research and Health*, 24, 77–84.

Venter, J. C., Adams, M. D., Myers, E. W., Li, P. W., Mural, R. J., Sutton, G. G., Smith, H. O., Yandell, M., Evans, C. A., Holt, R. A., Gocayne, J. D., Amanatides, P., Ballew, R. M., Huson, D. H., Wortman, J. R., Zhang, Q., Kodira, C. D., Zheng, X. H., Chen, L., Skupski, M., Subramanian, G., Thomas, P. D., Zhang, J., Gabor Miklos, G. L., Nelson, C., Broder, S., Clark, A. G., Nadeau, J., McKusick, V. A., Zinder, N., Levine, A. J., Roberts, R. J., Simon, M., Slayman, C., Hunkapiller, M., Bolanos, R., Delcher, A., Dew, I., Fasulo, D., Flanigan, M., Florea, L., Halpern, A., Hannenhalli, S., Kravitz, S., Levy, S., Mobarry, C., Reinert, K., Remington, K., bu-Threideh, J., Beasley, E., Biddick, K., Bonazzi, V., Brandon, R., Cargill, M., Chandramouliswaran, I., Charlab, R., Chaturvedi, K., Deng, Z., Di, F. V., Dunn, P., Eilbeck, K., Evangelista,

C., Gabrielian, A. E., Gan, W., Ge, W., Gong, F., Gu, Z., Guan, P., Heiman, T. J., Higgins, M. E., Ji, R. R., Ke, Z., Ketchum, K. A., Lai, Z., Lei, Y., Li, Z., Li, J., Liang, Y., Lin, X., Lu, F., Merkulov, G. V., Milshina, N., Moore, H. M., Naik, A. K., Narayan, V. A., Neelam, B., Nusskern, D., Rusch, D. B., Salzberg, S., Shao, W., Shue, B., Sun, J., Wang, Z., Wang, A., Wang, X., Wang, J., Wei, M., Wides, R., Xiao, C., Yan, C., Yao, A., Ye, J., Zhan, M., Zhang, W., Zhang, H., Zhao, Q., Zheng, L., Zhong, F., Zhong, W., Zhu, S., Zhao, S., Gilbert, D., Baumhueter, S., Spier, G., Carter, C., Cravchik, A., Woodage, T., Ali, F., An, H., Awe, A., Baldwin, D., Baden, H., Barnstead, M., Barrow, I., Beeson, K., Busam, D., Carver, A., Center, A., Cheng, M. L., Curry, L., Danaher, S., Davenport, L., Desilets, R., Dietz, S., Dodson, K., Doup, L., Ferriera, S., Garg, N., Gluecksmann, A., Hart, B., Haynes, J., Haynes, C., Heiner, C., Hladun, S., Hostin, D., Houck, J., Howland, T., Ibegwam, C., Johnson, J., Kalush, F., Kline, L., Koduru, S., Love, A., Mann, F., May, D., McCawley, S., McIntosh, T., McMullen, I., Moy, M., Moy, L., Murphy, B., Nelson, K., Pfannkoch, C., Pratts, E., Puri, V., Qureshi, H., Reardon, M., Rodriguez, R., Rogers, Y. H., Romblad, D., Ruhfel, B., Scott, R., Sitter, C., Smallwood, M., Stewart, E., Strong, R., Suh, E., Thomas, R., Tint, N. N., Tse, S., Vech, C., Wang, G., Wetter, J., Williams, S., Williams, M., Windsor, S., Winn-Deen, E., Wolfe, K., Zaveri, J., Zaveri, K., Abril, J. F., Guigo, R., Campbell, M. J., Sjolander, K. V., Karlak, B., Kejariwal, A., Mi, H., Lazareva, B., Hatton, T., Narechania, A., Diemer, K., Muruganujan, A., Guo, N., Sato, S., Bafna, V., Istrail, S., Lippert, R., Schwartz, R., Walenz, B., Yooseph, S., Allen, D., Basu, A., Baxendale, J., Blick, L., Caminha, M., Carnes-Stine, J., Caulk, P., Chiang, Y. H., Coyne, M., Dahlke, C., Mays, A., Dombroski, M., Donnelly, M., Ely, D., Esparham, S., Fosler, C., Gire, H., Glanowski, S., Glasser, K., Glodek, A., Gorokhov, M., Graham, K., Gropman, B., Harris, M., Heil, J., Henderson, S., Hoover, J., Jennings, D., Jordan, C., Jordan, J., Kasha, J., Kagan, L., Kraft, C., Levitsky, A., Lewis, M., Liu, X., Lopez, J., Ma, D., Majoros, W., McDaniel, J., Murphy, S., Newman, M., Nguyen, T., Nguyen, N. & Nodell, M. (2001) The sequence of the human genome. *Science*, 291, 1304–1351.

Watson, J. D. (1968) *The Double Helix: A Personal Account of the Discovery of the Structure of DNA*. London: Weidenfeld and Nicolson.

Wolff, P. H. (1972) Ethnic differences in alcohol sensitivity. *Science*, 175, 449–450.

Yin, S. J. & Agarwal, D. P. (2001) Functional polymorphism of ADH and ALDH. In: D. P. Agarwal & H. K. Seitz (eds) *Alcohol in Health and Disease*. New York: Marcel Dekker, pp. 1–26.

Chapter 17
ANIMAL MODELS

Leigh V. Panlilio, Charles W. Schindler and Steven R. Goldberg

17.1 Introduction

To understand many elements involved in addictive behaviour, sometimes science requires that researchers have the ability to control and manipulate the conditions that produce a phenomenon. However, there can be serious ethical and practical limitations to using experimental methods to study addiction in humans. On one hand, it would be unethical to induce addiction in drug-naive individuals. On the other hand, already addicted individuals come into the laboratory with a wide variety of prior drug experiences that cannot be controlled or even known with certainty. Due to difficulties such as these, as well as the fact that many neuroscience techniques can only be implemented in animals, the use of animal models plays an important role in the field of addiction.

Specific animal models have been developed to investigate most aspects of substance use and addiction. This approach is based on the implicit assumption that there are basic principles that guide behaviour, and that these principles are similar in humans and animals due to commonalities between human and animal brains. This application of animal models represents a specialised application of theories and techniques developed within a more general and comprehensive approach to the study of behaviour and the brain, now known as behavioural neuroscience. Historically, most of the basic procedures and the terminology used to describe these animal models come from the field of experimental psychology, especially the areas known as the experimental analysis of behaviour, which has a long tradition of studying interactions between behaviour and the environment, and behavioural pharmacology, which focuses on the behavioural effects of drugs. To understand the various ways that animal behaviour is used to model human drug abuse, it is especially important to become familiar with two specific principles of behaviour: reinforcement and the effects of environmental cues.

17.2 Basic principles of behaviour: Reinforcement

Addictive drugs function as rewards, much like natural rewards such as food and water. This reward process is known as *positive reinforcement*. When an action consistently produces a specific outcome, that outcome is said to be reinforcing if it makes the action more likely to be repeated in the future. The archetypal example of this principle is when a laboratory rat learns to press a lever that delivers food pellets. Many models of substance use are made possible by the fact that laboratory animals will also learn to press a lever that delivers intravenous injections of a drug such as heroin or cocaine. These *drug self-administration* procedures parallel human drug use, with the rat's lever-pressing response corresponding to a human action, such as inhaling tobacco smoke or injecting heroin intravenously, that is reinforced by the effects of the drug in the brain.

The ability of an outcome to have a reinforcing effect can vary from individual to individual, and from time to time in the same individual. The individual's current physiological state is an important factor that can determine whether an event will be reinforcing. For example, if the rat is not hungry, it will not press a lever that produces food. Similarly, a person maintained on methadone is less likely to take heroin. Nonetheless, virtually all addictive drugs are capable of producing reinforcing effects in both humans and animals, and testing a novel drug for reinforcing effects in animals is a highly reliable way to assess the abuse liability of the drug in humans.

If an event or situation is aversive, it can be reinforcing to avoid it or escape from it. *Negative reinforcement* is said to occur when removing or preventing something aversive increases the probability of a behaviour. For example, the action of taking heroin can be negatively reinforcing if it removes unpleasant withdrawal symptoms. Although there are animal models that have been developed to study the negative-reinforcement aspects of addiction, they have not been used as extensively as models based on positive reinforcement. This is because most evidence supports the theory that addiction results mainly from the rewarding effects of drugs, rather than the avoidance of withdrawal symptoms.

17.3　Basic principles of behaviour: Effects of environmental cues

A person's environment is composed of many individual stimuli. Some of these stimuli come to function as cues that indicate when a specific action will be reinforced. These environmental cues play a critical role in substance use by guiding the complex sequences of behaviour required to obtain, prepare and consume the drug. These cues can include the physical characteristics of specific people, places and things, such as the smell of tobacco smoke or the sight of a pack of cigarettes.

Drug-related cues can have several different functions, all of which can be modelled in the laboratory. A *discriminative stimulus* is a cue that signals when a response will be reinforced and that thereby gains control over the response. For example, if pressing a lever only produces a cocaine injection when a light is flashing above the lever, the rat will learn to respond on the lever when the light is flashing and stop when it is not.

When a cue has been associated with a drug's rewarding effects, the cue itself can become a *conditioned reinforcer*, capable of functioning as a reward. These conditioned reinforcing effects of a drug-associated cue are revealed if an action increases in probability when the only effect of the action is to produce the cue. Conditioned reinforcers can establish a completely new response or they can maintain an already established action over long periods when responding produces only the cue without the drug.

Drug-associated cues acquire these conditioned reinforcing effects through Pavlovian conditioning. These effects are analogous to the conditioned salivation exhibited by Pavlov's famous dogs when they were exposed to the ringing of a bell that had been associated with food. Stimuli that reliably predict the onset of a drug effect can become *conditioned stimuli* that elicit a reaction resembling the reaction to the drug itself. With drugs of abuse, this reaction often takes the form of general arousal and increased locomotor activity. This activity can be used as an animal model of the increased motivation to seek drugs, verbally expressed by human drug users as 'craving', which can be elicited by exposure to drug-related cues.

17.4　Drug self-administration: Simple schedules

Allowing animals to self-administer drugs under controlled laboratory conditions is the most direct way to model human drug abuse. This animal model exhibits a point-to-point correspondence with human behaviour, and this correspondence allows the basic procedure to be modified to focus on specific aspects of drug abuse. In general, these modifications involve manipulating the relationship between the self-administration response and delivery of the drug. This relationship, known as the *schedule of reinforcement*, specifies parameters such as what type of response is required (e.g. pressing a lever, pulling a chain), whether any cues are correlated with availability or delivery of the drug, how many responses are required for an injection, and how much time must pass before the next injection can be obtained.

Simple schedules of reinforcement require only a few responses for the delivery of each injection. These schedules provide a direct relationship between the rate of responding and the rate of drug injection, and are therefore well suited to studying factors that influence drug intake. Under this kind of schedule, animals typically develop a pattern of pausing for a certain amount of time after each injection. The duration of this pause is a direct function of the dose received with each injection, with higher doses producing longer pauses. As a result of this regular, dose-dependent pausing, the rate of drug intake over time is fairly constant. However, if the animal is allowed free access to the drug for extended periods, this behaviour can lose its regularity, and drug intake can escalate and become erratic; this *escalation* and *dysregulation* of drug intake is used as an animal model of the progression of substance use from casual, controlled use to uncontrolled addiction.

17.5 Drug self-administration: Using dose–effect curves to assess the effects of treatments

One important question that can be answered by using drug self-administration procedures is whether a novel compound is likely to be abused. Drugs that are self-administered by animals have a high abuse potential in humans. To determine whether a drug is an effective reinforcer in animals, a wide range of doses must be studied. Usually, one dose is offered for several sessions until the rate of responding stabilises, then another dose is offered, and so on. Then, the rate of responding is plotted as a function of dose to provide a *dose–effect function*. A dose is considered reinforcing if it maintains more responding than placebo injections of saline solution containing no drug.

The dose–effect functions obtained with self-administered drugs usually have an inverted U-shape. At low doses the drug is only marginally reinforcing, and might only maintain low rates of responding. At medium doses, the rate of self-administration is the highest; these doses are reinforcing, and the injections are taken in quick succession. At high doses, the drug has reinforcing effects, but there is a long pause after each injection, so the rate of self-administration is lower than under medium doses. These three respective parts of the dose–effect function seen under low, medium, and high doses are known as the ascending limb, peak, and descending limb of the curve.

Besides being useful for determining whether a drug will be self-administered, testing a range of doses and obtaining dose–effect functions are indispensable for determining how self-administration behaviour can be altered by an experimental treatment. Treatments might include a drug developed to have therapeutic effects, or a drug that selectively alters a specific brain process and is therefore used as a tool to study the role of that process in addiction (see Box 17.1).

17.6 Drug self-administration: Measuring the reinforcing effects of drugs

Shifts in the dose–effect function under simple schedules indicate changes in sensitivity to the drug, but they not do quantify the drug's strength as a reinforcer. Questions about a drug's ability to reinforce behaviour can take several forms. Is dose X of cocaine more reinforcing than dose Y of cocaine? Does a therapeutic treatment make dose X less reinforcing than when no treatment is

Box 17.1   Why dose–effect functions are important

Imagine that a new drug is designed to treat cocaine addiction. To test the new drug, rats are first trained to self-administer cocaine at a certain dose ('X'). Then, the new drug is given before a daily cocaine self-administration session, and it is found that it causes the rats to reduce their number of cocaine injections by half. Does this indicate that the new drug decreases the effects of cocaine? Unfortunately, since only dose X of cocaine was tested, it is impossible to tell whether the new drug increases or decreases the effects of cocaine. With the inverted U-shape of the cocaine dose–effect function, both lower and higher doses of cocaine might be self-administered at a lower rate than dose X. For this reason, it is essential to compare full dose–effect functions obtained with and without the treatment. If the treatment shifts the curve to the left, it increases sensitivity to the self-administered drug. If the treatment shifts the curve to the right, it reduces sensitivity to the self-administered drug. If the treatment shifts the curve downward, there is a reduction of self-administration at all doses; all else being equal (e.g. if side effects are minimal and the treatment drug itself is not liable to be abused), this is the most desirable effect for a potential drug abuse treatment in this kind of test (see Figure 17.1).

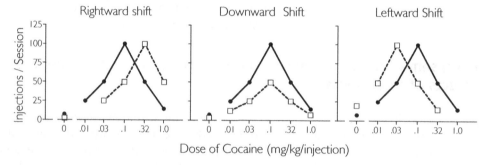

Figure 17.1 Shifts in dose–effect functions. These idealised curves show the number of intravenous self-injections of cocaine per session as a function of the dose delivered in each injection. Curves such as these are typically obtained when each response on a lever produces an injection, and the dose per injection is fixed within each session, but varied across sessions. It is customary to present pharmacological data with dose on a logarithmic axis. The *solid circles* represent the inverted U-shaped dose–effect curve usually seen with drug self-administration. The *open squares* in each panel represent the level of self-administration when the subjects are given a treatment drug prior to each cocaine self-administration session. In the *left panel*, the treatment has shifted the cocaine dose–effect curve to the right, indicating reduced sensitivity to cocaine; a higher dose of cocaine is required to achieve the same effect. This kind of effect would typically be produced by a low-to-moderate dose of a pre-treatment drug such as a dopamine receptor antagonist, which competitively blocks receptors involved in the reinforcing effects of cocaine. In the *centre panel*, the treatment has shifted the curve downward, reducing the rate of self-injection at all doses of cocaine. This kind of shift can be produced by treatments such as a higher dose of a dopamine antagonist (which more effectively blocks cocaine's reinforcing effects) or a drug-like amphetamine (which may produce a long-lasting, satiation-like effect). In the *right panel*, the treatment has shifted the curve to the left, indicating an increased sensitivity to cocaine; the same effects are now achieved with lower doses of cocaine. This kind of shift would typically be produced by a low-to-moderate dose of a reinforcing drug such as amphetamine. There is little or no responding under a zero dose of cocaine under most conditions, except in the right panel, where the cocaine-like effects of the treatment have produced a slight reinstatement of responding, even though the self-injections contain only saline. Note that in each panel, the treatment caused a 50% reduction in the rate of self-administration at the cocaine dose of 0.1 mg/kg; thus, if only that dose of cocaine had been studied, rather than a range of doses, the nature of the treatment effects would have been indeterminate. It should also be noted that to fully assess the effects of a treatment drug on drug self-administration, it is ideal to study a range of doses of not only the self-administered drug but also the treatment drug. (Adapted from Mello & Negus, 1996, by permission of Macmillan Publishers Ltd.)

given? Is dose X of cocaine more reinforcing than dose Z of amphetamine? Unfortunately, these questions cannot be answered by looking at response rates, because the response rate maintained by a specific dose of a drug does not equate with its strength as a reinforcer. Animals tend to pause for a long period after self-administering a high dose, and the reasons for this pausing (e.g. longer-lasting reinforcing effects, motor depression or the appearance of aversive side effects) may or may not be related to reinforcement. Therefore, dose–effect functions obtained with simple schedules of reinforcement cannot be used to answer these questions.

The strength of drug reinforcers can be measured by using more complex schedules of reinforcement and taking measures other than response rate. The most widely used of these procedures is the *progressive ratio schedule*, in which the number of responses required for each successive injection is increased in steps to find the response requirement at which the animal ceases to respond. In practice, a behavioural criterion is chosen to designate when responding has ceased during a session, such as 1 hour without a response. The highest response requirement that still maintains responding is termed the 'breakpoint', above which the response requirement exceeds the ability of the dose to maintain responding. In this procedure, breakpoint is considered a direct measure of a drug's reinforcing effect because a more reinforcing dose will produce a higher breakpoint even if the drug causes the animal to respond slowly or pause for a long time after each injection (see Figure 17.2).

Another strategy for assessing the effectiveness of drug reinforcers independently of the drug's effects on response rate is to use a *choice procedure*, in which the animal is allowed to choose between two or more options, such as a high dose versus a low dose, a high dose versus placebo or one drug versus another drug. The relative preferences for these options allow them to be rank ordered with respect to the strength of their reinforcing effects.

The value of drug reinforcers to the animal can also be assessed using *behavioural economics analysis*. This approach is based on microeconomic theory, considering the reinforcer as a commodity and the number of responses required for a given amount of drug as the unit price. A demand curve can be obtained by varying the unit price over a range of values and measuring the rate of intake. If intake varies little despite large changes in price, the demand for the drug is considered inelastic, indicating that the drug is highly valued. If the availability of another drug (e.g. methadone) increases the elasticity of the self-administered drug (e.g. causes heroin self-administration to cease when the cost is high), the other drug is said to substitute for that reinforcer. Thus, behavioural economics provides a sophisticated account of how behaviour is shaped by the available reinforcers. Choice and progressive ratio approaches can be considered specific applications of this more encompassing approach.

17.7 Drug self-administration: Modelling the effects of environmental cues with second-order schedules

Environmental cues can be incorporated into drug self-administration procedures in many ways. It is quite common to present a cue such as a brief tone or light each time the drug is injected, even when cues, per se, are not the focus of the experiment. This is done for practical purposes because the reinforcing effects of the drug are not immediate, and delayed reinforcers tend to have weak effects on behaviour. The immediate delivery of a drug-associated cue can have a conditioned reinforcing effect that essentially spans this gap in time, so the self-administration response is acquired and maintained more effectively. This procedure also makes the animal model more similar to human drug use, where cues (e.g. the multi-sensory experience of puffing a cigarette) are almost always associated with drug delivery.

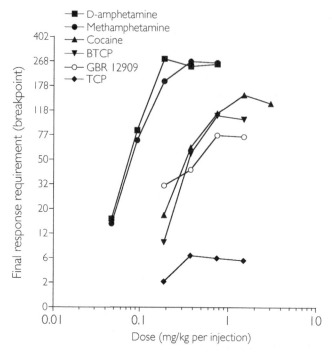

Figure 17.2 Progressive ratio drug self-administration, a procedure used to measure the strength of reinforcement. Dose–effect functions for several drugs were obtained in rats under a progressive ratio schedule of intravenous drug self-administration. The response requirement increased exponentially with each successive self-injection during a session until responding ceased. Each drug was studied over a range of doses, and the highest response requirement reached under the schedule before the responding ceased (i.e. the breakpoint) was plotted as a function of dose, using logarithmic axes for both measures. Higher breakpoints are considered an indication of greater effectiveness as a reinforcer. In general, the lowest dose was the weakest reinforcer, and the breaking-point curve increased as a function of dose over moderate doses, and then reached a plateau at the highest doses. Methamphetamine and D-amphetamine produced very similar effects to each other and also had similar potencies. Cocaine, BTCP (a phencyclidine derivative) and GBR 12909 (a selective dopamine uptake inhibitor) had fairly similar profiles to each other. Although the highest breakpoints for GBR 12909 and BTCP were slightly lower than the highest breakpoint for cocaine, the curves for all three of these drugs plateau at breakpoints lower than those obtained with methamphetamine and D-amphetamine, indicating that they were less effective as reinforcers. The fact that the maximum breakpoints in the cocaine, BTCP and GBR 12909 curves occurred at higher doses than in the methamphetamine and D-amphetamine curves simply indicates that the amphetamines have a higher potency. The reinforcing effects of TCP (a different phencyclidine derivative) were the weakest, failing to maintain responding when the response requirement was more than about six responses, a breakpoint much lower than seen with the other drugs. It should be noted that all these drugs did maintain self-administration responding when tested with a simple schedule. Thus, the differences in their efficacy as reinforcers were only revealed by testing them with the progressive ratio schedule. (Adapted from Richardson & Roberts, 1996, by permission of Elsevier.)

One of the most powerful demonstrations of how environmental cues can influence drug self-administration is seen with *second-order schedules*. In these procedures, the response produces a brief presentation of a cue, but the cue is only occasionally accompanied by a drug injection. For example, in one version of this schedule, every tenth response on a lever produces a coloured light for 2 seconds. Responding produces only these brief stimulus presentations until 60 minutes have passed, when the tenth response produces both the light and a drug injection. Under these conditions, the stimulus becomes a conditioned reinforcer and maintains a high rate of responding during the 60-minute period before the drug is received. If the cue presentations are discontinued, the number of responses is drastically reduced, even if the drug is still received when a response occurs at the end of the 60 minutes. What is more, presentations of a well-established cue sometimes maintain thousands of responses per day over many days when drug delivery is discontinued. Thus, the animal model resembles the human situation, in which environmental cues that have been associated with the reinforcing effects of a drug have powerful and persistent effects on behaviour.

Researchers often choose to use a second-order schedule instead of a simple schedule to achieve a closer approximation of how human behaviour is maintained in a substance use environment. Second-order schedules have also the advantage that the cue maintains a substantial amount of responding prior to the first drug injection. This is useful when the drug produces effects such as motor depression or hyperactivity that can greatly decrease or increase responding during the remainder of the session. Being able to study behaviour prior to the first injection also allows a distinction to be drawn between 'drug-seeking' behaviour maintained by the cue and 'drug-taking' behaviour maintained by the direct reinforcing effects of the drug. Using this technique, drug seeking and drug taking can be studied in relative isolation, and therapeutic interventions can be developed to target each of these processes.

17.8   Drug self-administration: Reinstatement

Relapse is one of the most important obstacles to treating addiction. The *reinstatement model* of relapse is one of the most widely used animal models of drug abuse. In this model, the animal learns to self-administer a drug during an initial training phase. Then, drug delivery (and sometimes the presentation of cues) is discontinued until the animal responds at very low levels; this *extinction* procedure typically takes several weeks. Finally, a test is performed in which drug delivery is still discontinued, but the animal is exposed to a treatment that can cause the drug-seeking response to resume.

There are three basic types of experimental treatment that are generally used to study reinstatement. First, *drug priming* involves injecting the animal with a drug just before the start of the test. Usually, this drug is the same one that was self-administered during training, but it could also be another drug of abuse, or a potentially therapeutic drug that is being tested to verify that it does not lead to relapse. Second, *cue-induced reinstatement* can be studied by re-instituting the presentation of a cue that was discontinued during extinction. This cue can be a response-contingent conditioned reinforcer that was associated with drug delivery during training, or it can be an experimenter-presented discriminative stimulus that signalled drug availability during training. Third, *stress-induced reinstatement* typically involves giving a series of mild, brief electric shocks through the floor of the training environment prior to the reinstatement test. These three basic reinstatement procedures model the major triggers of relapse in humans: re-exposure to the drug or a similar drug, re-exposure to drug-related cues and exposure to a stressful situation (see Figure 17.3).

17.9   Drug self-administration: Modelling the uncontrolled and compulsive nature of addiction

Even when it occurs frequently, drug use does not necessarily constitute addiction. The distinguishing characteristics of addiction are that drug use is uncontrolled or compulsive, and that it continues despite negative consequences and attempts to quit. In recent years, drug self-administration procedures have been developed to incorporate these aspects of addiction. The most prevalent technique

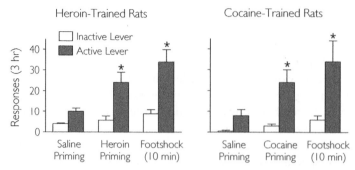

Figure 17.3 Reinstatement of drug self-administration responding after a period of abstinence, a procedure used to model relapse. Rats were first trained to self-administer heroin (*left panel*) or cocaine (*right panel*) intravenously by pressing a lever under a simple reinforcement schedule. As a control procedure to verify that responses on this lever were due to the reinforcing effects of the drug rather than drug-induced locomotor activity, there was also an 'inactive' lever, which had no effect when pressed. After 12 days, rats that reliably self-administered the drug were advanced to the extinction phase of the study, where abstinence was modelled by discontinuing drug delivery (i.e. substituting saline solution for the drug solution). Extinction training was continued for each rat until its rate of lever responding dropped to very low levels, which took about 1–2 weeks. Then, reinstatement tests were conducted by giving each rat either an intraperitoneal (i.p.) injection of saline solution (as a control condition), an i.p. injection of the training drug (to test for drug-induced priming), or a 10-minute period of stress, during which mild electric shocks were intermittently delivered through the floor of the training chamber. During the tests, drug delivery was still discontinued, and responses on the active (*solid bars*) and inactive (*white bars*) levers were recorded. The bars indicate the mean for each group, and the error bars indicate the standard error measurement (s.e.m.). The cocaine treatment and the stress treatment both caused a statistically significant reinstatement effect (as indicated by *asterisks*), increasing responding on the active lever. Responding on the inactive lever was not increased, indicating that the reinstatement of responding on the active lever represents a selective increase in drug 'seeking' an effect considered to be analogous to relapse in humans. (Adapted from Shaham et al., 2000, by permission of Elsevier.)

is to simply allow rats to have extended access to the drug. One result of this manipulation is that drug intake becomes uncontrolled (i.e. escalated or dysregulated). For example, if rats are allowed to self-administer cocaine for 1 hour per day, their rate of drug intake will stabilise at a certain level. But, if they are instead allowed access for 6 hours per day, their hourly rate of intake may escalate drastically over time (see Figure 17.4). They will also reach higher breakpoints under a progressive ratio schedule (indicating intensified reinforcing effects of cocaine), and they will have an increased likelihood of reinstatement after a period of abstinence. Rats given extended access to drugs also show signs of compulsivity, in that they will continue self-administering the drug even when their responding delivers electric footshock at an intensity that suppresses the responding of rats that have only limited drug access. Interestingly, certain rats appear to be predisposed to developing addiction-like behaviour, and the percentage of such rats (about 17%) is similar to the percentage of human cocaine users who become addicted (about 15%).

17.10   Intracranial drug self-administration and intracranial electrical self-stimulation

Addictive drugs are believed to produce their reinforcing effects by acting directly on the same brain mechanisms that are indirectly affected by natural reinforcers. Understanding these neural circuits is therefore critical for understanding addiction. One way to study this circuitry is to allow animals

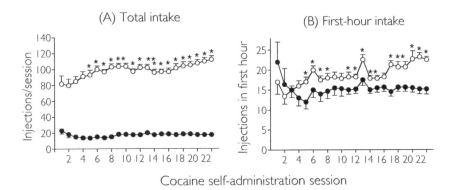

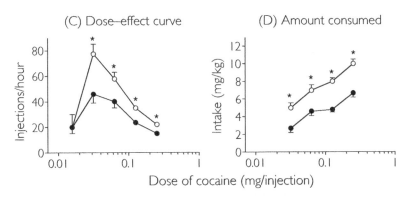

Figure 17.4 Escalated drug intake in rats given extended access to cocaine (6 hours/day), compared to rats given limited access (1 hour/day); a model of the addiction process. A cocaine dose of 0.25 mg was delivered in each intravenous self-injection under a simple reinforcement schedule (i.e. ~0.75–0.89 mg/kg per injection, depending on the body weight of the rat). All rats were originally trained to self-administer cocaine during daily 2-hour sessions, and then switched to 1-hour or 6-hour sessions. The circles indicate group means, and the error bars indicate the s.e.m. *Asterisks* indicate statistically significant differences between the two groups. *Panel A* shows that the number of self-injections per session began to escalate in long-access rats (*LgA; filled circles*) around the fifth day, but the number of injections per session remained stable throughout the 22 days of training in short-access rats (*ShA; open circles*). *Panel B* compares intake during just the first hour of each session. The first-hour intake was similar in the two groups during the first few sessions, but by the fifth session long-access rats consistently self-injected cocaine at a faster rate than short-access rats. During subsequent test sessions lasting 3 hours for both groups, the dose per injection was varied to obtain dose–effect functions (*lower panels*). The curves representing the rates of self-injection (*Panel C*) and cocaine intake (*Panel D*) were found to be shifted upwards in the long-access rats, indicating that their escalated intake was not simply the result of tolerance to cocaine, which would have produced a rightward shift. This kind of escalation has been demonstrated with a number of different drugs when rats are allowed extended access, and this escalated intake is associated with other indications of addiction-like behaviour analogous to that seen in humans, such as difficulty in achieving and maintaining abstinence, and persistence of use despite adverse consequences. (Adapted from Ahmed & Koob, 1998, by permission of American Association for the Advancement of Science.)

to self-administer extremely small quantities of a drug directly into a specific brain site, a technique known as *intracranial drug self-administration*. Specific brain circuits can also be activated directly by electrodes, and animals will readily perform a response such as lever pressing that electrically stimulates certain areas. Techniques have been developed to use this *intracranial self-stimulation* phenomenon to study the reinforcement-related effects of drugs of abuse. These procedures involve determining the threshold value for the frequency or intensity of the electrical impulse with versus without the drug. Certain drugs lower the thresholds for intracranial self-stimulation, and the ability of a drug to have this effect is a good predictor of its abuse liability. These procedures have the advantage of simultaneously focusing on both behaviour and its underlying brain circuitry.

17.11   Drug self-administration: Advantages and disadvantages

In our opinion, drug self-administration is the pre-eminent animal model of drug abuse. It is highly reliable and has strong face validity. It has also high predictive validity for assessing the abuse liability of novel compounds, and to a somewhat lesser extent with predicting the effects of treatments for drug abuse. The basic procedure is highly flexible, allowing it to be adapted as required to focus on specific aspects of drug abuse. However, drug self-administration does have several disadvantages. Compared with some other procedures (such as those described below), drug self-administration can be resource-intensive and technically difficult. Specialised equipment is required, and training sessions are relatively long, so that group sizes are often smaller than with other kinds of procedures. For intravenous drug delivery, animals must be implanted surgically with catheters. One of the largest obstacles to this kind of research is that catheters tend to last a few months at most in rodents. This makes it especially difficult to perform long-term studies or studies that require extensive training. For these reasons, procedures such as conditioned place preference and drug discrimination, which are both described below, are often used as screening procedures to detect promising treatments, which are then tested more intensively with drug self-administration procedures.

17.12   Conditioned place preference

Conditioned place preference is an alternative way to study the reinforcing effects of a drug. In this procedure, the training apparatus consists of two compartments that are easily distinguishable from each other. During training, the effects of a drug are associated with one of the compartments but not the other. For example, the following procedure would be typical. One compartment of the apparatus has white walls, and the other has black. On alternate days, a rat is injected with the drug before being confined in the white compartment for 15 minutes, or it is injected with placebo and confined in the dark component for 15 minutes. This continues until the drug's effects have been paired with the white side five times. Subsequently, administration of the training drug is discontinued, and testing is performed by placing the rat in the apparatus with a doorway open between the two compartments and measuring how much time it spends in each compartment. If the drug has reinforcing effects, the white walls of the drug-associated compartment should function as a conditioned reinforcer, and the rat should spend more time in the white compartment during testing.

   This procedure has the advantage of being simpler and faster than drug self-administration, which requires extensive training and the implantation and maintenance of intravenous catheters. In addition, this procedure can measure not only conditioned place preferences, but also conditioned place aversions, which occur when the drug has predominantly unpleasant effects. However, the conditioned place preference procedure cannot be modified as extensively as the drug self-administration procedure to focus on specific aspects of addiction. In addition, the conditioned place preference procedure often does not produce results that are clearly dose-dependent; instead of producing graded dose–effect curves such as those produced with drug self-administration, conditioned place preference curves are often flat over a wide range of doses, making it difficult to detect shifts in the curve that might indicate changes in reinforcement.

17.13 Drug discrimination

In *drug discrimination* procedures, animals are trained to detect whether they have received a certain drug. The interoceptive effects of the training drug are used as a discriminative stimulus for performing a food-reinforced response in a two-lever apparatus. During training, responding on one lever produces food pellets during sessions when the rat has been injected with the training drug, and responding on the other lever produces food pellets during sessions when the rat has been injected with placebo. Once the rat learns to consistently respond on the appropriate lever, a dose–effect function can be obtained for the training drug, and it can be determined whether experimental treatments shift this curve. For example, a treatment drug might be used to block or potentiate the effects of the training drug, shifting the curve to the right or left, respectively (see Figure 17.5). Other drugs can also be tested to determine whether they will cause the rat to respond on the drug-appropriate lever, indicating that the test drug has interoceptive effects that are similar in some way to those of the training drug. These are known as *generalisation tests*, because they determine the extent to which the rat generalises between the effects of the training dose and the effects of the test treatment. If the training drug is known to have reinforcing effects, the animal's choice of levers during the test might reflect these effects. However, this can only be inferred since the procedure does not directly measure reinforcement. Most addictive drugs have other effects in addition to their reinforcing effects, and test drugs that share these 'side effects' may not share the reinforcing effects. Despite the indirect nature of the drug discrimination approach, this procedure has the advantage that, once the rats are trained, a large number of test compounds can be quickly evaluated. Thus, the drug discrimination procedure is valuable as a screening technique and can be used to help choose candidate compounds for more extensive testing with other procedures, such as drug self-administration.

17.14 Locomotor activity

In studies of *locomotor activity*, a rat or mouse is injected with a drug and placed into an activity chamber where its movements are automatically recorded by an array of infrared photobeams. Locomotor activity is stimulated by many addictive drugs, including cocaine, amphetamine, heroin and nicotine. This reaction tends to increase in intensity with repeated exposure to the drug, an effect known as *behavioural sensitisation*. This behaviour is considered important because it may reflect increased sensitivity to reward-related effects of the drug and motivational effects of drug-associated stimuli, and this sensitisation has been proposed to be an underlying part of addiction.

Sensitisation to the locomotor-activating effects of drugs can be strongly influenced by environmental cues present in the activity chamber. For example, if rats are repeatedly given amphetamine in one environment and placebo in another environment during training, during subsequent testing they will only show a sensitised response to amphetamine in the drug-associated environment. In addition, the drug-associated environment can act as a conditioned stimulus, eliciting an increase in locomotor activity during a test when no drug is given. These effects, *conditioned locomotion* and *conditioned sensitisation*, respectively, can be used as animal models of conditioned drug effects.

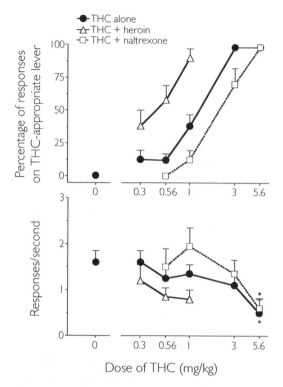

Figure 17.5 Drug discrimination, a procedure used to assess the subjective effects of drugs. Rats were trained to discriminate between the interoceptive effects of tetrahydrocannabinol (THC) (3 mg/kg) and its vehicle. An i.p. injection was given 15 minutes before each training session. Two levers were available in the training chamber, one that produced food only during sessions when the rat had received THC, and one that produced food only during sessions when the rat had received vehicle. Once the rats were well trained, generalisation tests were performed by giving different doses of THC (*solid circles*). All points in the figure indicate the mean for each condition, and the error bars indicate the s.e.m. The *upper panel* shows the generalisation curve, relating the mean percentage of responses on the drug-appropriate lever to the dose of THC. Note that, unlike the inverted U-shaped curves obtained with drug self-administration, generalisation curves obtained with drug discrimination procedures are typically sigmoidal (S-shaped). At the training dose and higher, rats responded 100% on the drug-appropriate lever. At doses from 0 to 0.56 mg/kg THC, rats responded mostly on the vehicle-appropriate lever. At 1 mg/kg of THC, the mean percentage of responding on the drug-appropriate lever was about 40%. However, when rats were treated with the opioid receptor antagonist, naltrexone (0.3 mg/kg, i.p., 15 minutes before THC; *open squares*), the THC curve was shifted to the right, such that higher doses of THC were required to achieve the same effects. In contrast, when rats were treated with the opioid receptor agonist, heroin (0.3 mg/kg, i.p., 15 minutes after THC; *open triangles*), the THC curve was shifted to the left, such that lower doses of THC were required to achieve the same effects. These shifts in the curve were quantified by calculating effective-dose 50 (ED_{50}) values, which indicate the dose of THC required to achieve 50% of responding on the drug-appropriate lever. The ED_{50} for THC alone was 1.22 mg/kg, but this was shifted to 2.48 by naltrexone and to 0.47 by THC. When reporting the results of drug discrimination experiments, it is customary to present both the generalisation curve and another curve showing response rates during the same sessions (see *lower panel*). It is important to consider the rate of responding because most drugs of interest in substance use research have the ability to disrupt behaviour if given in large enough doses. To properly interpret the generalisation curve, it is necessary to consider whether – and at what doses – such disruptive effects may have occurred. At doses where the disruptions are severe, the generalisation data may be uninterpretable. In addition, the effects of treatments on response rates are important in their own right, providing supplementary information about the general behavioural effects of the treatments. In this figure, it can be seen that THC caused a slight decrease in response rates at the highest dose, but naltrexone did not substantially alter this effect; as indicated by the *asterisks* in the lower panel, the decrease in

17.15   Adjunct procedures

Locomotor activity in the open field of an activity chamber is often used as an adjunct to other measures such as drug self-administration to learn more about the effects of a treatment. This can be a useful means of assessing general effects, such as sedation, that might alter drug self-administration through non-specific mechanisms, interfering with the motor response required for self-administration rather than affecting the reinforcing or motivational effects of the drug. In addition, since rats normally avoid open spaces and spend little time in the centre of the open field, the amount of activity that occurs in the centre of the activity chamber as opposed to near the walls can be used as a measure of anxiety. Changes in this behaviour provide a reasonable indicator of whether a treatment drug increases or decreases anxiety.

Another procedure that is not a model of substance use but that is often used to complement drug self-administration procedures is food-reinforced responding. Animals can be trained on a schedule of food reinforcement that is similar to the one used with drug reinforcement. By testing the treatment drug under both drug-reinforcement and food-reinforcement conditions, it is possible to determine whether a treatment drug has non-specific effects on behaviour, or whether it selectively alters drug-reinforced behaviour.

17.16   Integration of behavioural and neuroscience techniques

When the animal models described in this chapter are combined with the physiological techniques of neuroscience, researchers can study the relationships between behaviour and the underlying brain mechanisms involved in all stages of addiction. Some of the most important applications along these lines have included studying the behavioural effects of drugs that act as agonists or antagonists of specific neuroreceptors; studying the behavioural effects of lesioning or temporarily deactivating specific brain areas; measuring neurotransmitter release with in vivo microdialysis or measuring neural activity electrically during drug self-administration; using functional neuroimaging techniques to locate the brain areas that contribute to specific behavioural effects; and studying behaviour in animals genetically manipulated to have specific alterations in brain functions, such as a lack of a specific receptor or neurotransmitter. Through this multidisciplinary approach, much has been learnt about drugs, the brain and behaviour. The behavioural models and the physiological techniques they are combined with are continually modified as advances are made within not only the specialised area of addiction research but throughout the field of behavioural neuroscience.

Figure 17.5 (*Continued*) responding under the highest dose of THC was statistically significant both with and without naltrexone, but none of the other points in the figure differed from vehicle. Response rates were slightly decreased when heroin was given along with THC, but this change was not significant. Thus, the changes seen in the generalisation curve can be considered to reflect changes in lever choice, rather than a non-specific disruption of behaviour. Overall, these results indicate that THC's interoceptive effects can be modulated by the opioid system of the brain, with an opioid agonist increasing the effects of THC and an opioid antagonist decreasing the effects of THC. The information obtained with the drug discrimination procedure suggested directions for further research, using additional techniques to determine how the opioid system is involved in these presumably abuse-related effects of THC. (Adapted from Solinas & Goldberg, 2005.)

Acknowledgement

The preparation of this chapter was supported by the Intramural Research Program of the NIH, National Institute on Drug Abuse.

References for figures

Ahmed, S. H. & Koob, G. F. (1998) Transition from moderate to excessive drug intake: change in hedonic set point. *Science*, 282(5387), 298–300.

Mello, N. K. & Negus, S. S. (1996) Preclinical evaluation of pharmacotherapies for treatment of cocaine and opioid abuse using drug self-administration procedures. *Neuropsychopharmacology*, 14(6), 375–424.

Richardson, N. R. & Roberts, D. C. (1996) Progressive ratio schedules in drug self-administration studies in rats: a method to evaluate reinforcing efficacy. *Journal of Neuroscience Methods*, 66(1), 1–11.

Shaham, Y., Erb, S. & Stewart, J. (2000) Stress-induced relapse to heroin and cocaine seeking in rats: a review. *Brain Research Reviews*, 33(1), 13–33.

Solinas, M. & Goldberg, S. R. (2005) Involvement of mu-, delta- and kappa-opioid receptor subtypes in the discriminative-stimulus effects of delta-9-tetrahydrocannabinol (THC) in rats. *Psychopharmacology*, 179(4), 804–812.

References and recommended readings

Basic principles of behaviour: reinforcement and effects of environmental cues
Mazur, J. E. (2006) *Learning and Behavior*. Upper Saddle River, NJ: Prentice Hall.
– *A textbook covering the basic principles of behaviour, including reinforcement and the effects of environmental cues.*
Panlilio, L. V., Weiss, S. J. & Schindler, C. W. (2000) Effects of compounding drug-related stimuli: escalation of heroin self-administration. *Journal of the Experimental Analysis of Behavior*, 73(2), 211–224.
– *An example of the influence of environmental cues in an animal model of drug abuse.*
Poling, A. & Byrne, T. (2000) *Introduction to Behavioral Pharmacology*. Reno, NV: Context Press.
– *A textbook covering many of the issues related to the studies of drugs and behaviour.*

Drug self-administration: simple schedules
Lynch, W. J. & Carroll, M. E. (2001) Regulation of drug intake. *Experimental and Clinical Psychopharmacology*, 9(2), 131–143.
– *A review of potential mechanisms by which drug intake might be regulated.*

Drug self-administration: using dose–effect curves to assess the effects of treatments
Ator, N. A. & Griffiths, R. R. (2003) Principles of drug abuse liability assessment in laboratory animals. *Drug and Alcohol Dependence*, 70(3 Suppl.), S55–S72.
– *How to assess the abuse liability of novel compounds.*
Mello, N. K. & Negus, S. S. (1996) Preclinical evaluation of pharmacotherapies for treatment of cocaine and opioid abuse using drug self-administration procedures. *Neuropsychopharmacology*, 14(6), 375–424.
– *How to assess the effects of experimental treatments on drug self-administration.*

Drug self-administration: measuring the reinforcing effects of drugs
Bergman, J. & Paronis, C. A. (2006) Measuring the reinforcing strength of abused drugs. *Molecular Interventions*, 6(5), 273–283.

– *A review of the issues involved in measuring the effectiveness of drug reinforcers.*

DeGrandpre, R. J., Bickel, W. K., Hughes, J. R., Layng, M. P. & Badger, G. (1993) Unit price as a useful metric in analyzing effects of reinforcer magnitude. *Journal of the Experimental Analysis of Behavior*, 60(3), 641–666.

– *A review of behavioural economic analyses applied in drug self-administration studies.*

Negus, S. S. (2006) Choice between heroin and food in nondependent and heroin-dependent rhesus monkeys: effects of naloxone, buprenorphine, and methadone. *Journal of Pharmacology and Experimental Therapeutics*, 317(2), 711–723.

– *An example of the use of choice procedures to assess the strength of drug reinforcers.*

Richardson, N. R. & Roberts, D. C. (1996) Progressive ratio schedules in drug self-administration studies in rats: a method to evaluate reinforcing efficacy. *Journal of Neuroscience Methods*, 66(1), 1–11.

– *A review addressing the technical, statistical and theoretical issues related to the use of progressive ratio schedules.*

Drug self-administration: modelling the effects of environmental cues with second-order schedules

Schindler, C. W., Panlilio, L. V. & Goldberg, S. R. (2002) Second-order schedules of drug self-administration in animals. *Psychopharmacology*, 163(3–4), 327–344.

– *Discussion and examples of the effects of environmental cues in second-order schedules of drug self-administration.*

Drug self-administration: reinstatement

Shaham, Y., Shalev, U., Lu, L., De Wit, H. & Stewart, J. (2003) The reinstatement model of drug relapse: history, methodology and major findings. *Psychopharmacology*, 168(1–2), 3–20.

– *A review of reinstatement studies, including evidence that drug-, cue-, and stress-induced reinstatements have different underlying mechanisms.*

Drug self-administration: modelling the uncontrolled and compulsive nature of addiction

Deroche-Gamonet, V., Belin, D. & Piazza, P. V. (2004) Evidence for addiction-like behavior in the rat. *Science*, 305(5686), 1014–1017.

– *A study of individual differences in rats' propensity to develop addiction-like behaviour.*

Koob, G. F., Ahmed, S. H., Boutrel, B., Chen, S. A., Kenny, P. J., Markou, A., O'Dell, L. E., Parsons, L. H. & Sanna, P. P. (2004) Neurobiological mechanisms in the transition from drug use to drug dependence. *Neuroscience and Biobehavioral Reviews*, 27(8), 739–749.

– *A review of studies showing escalation of drug intake in rats given extended access to cocaine or heroin.*

Vanderschuren, L. J. & Everitt, B. J. (2005) Behavioral and neural mechanisms of compulsive drug seeking. *European Journal of Pharmacology*, 526(1–3), 77–88.

– *A review of studies that attempt to model loss of control over drug use.*

Intracranial drug self-administration and intracranial self-stimulation

Gardner, E. L. (2005) Brain-reward mechanisms. In: J. H. Lowinson, P. Ruiz, R. B. Millman & J. G. Langrod (eds) *Substance Abuse: A Comprehensive Textbook*, 4th edn. Philadelphia, PA: Lippincott Williams & Wilkins.

– *How intracranial self-stimulation studies are used to study drug abuse.*

McBride, W. J., Murphy, J. M. & Ikemoto, S. (1999) Localization of brain reinforcement mechanisms: intracranial self-administration and intracranial place-conditioning studies. *Neuroscience and Biobehavioral Reviews*, 101(2), 129–152.

– *A review of intracranial drug reinforcement studies.*

Conditioned place preference

Bardo, M. T. & Bevins, R. A. (2000) Conditioned place preference: what does it add to our preclinical understanding of drug reward? *Psychopharmacology*, 153(1), 31–43.

– An assessment of the strengths and weaknesses of conditioned place preference procedures.
Tzschentke, T. M. (1998) Measuring reward with the conditioned place preference paradigm: a comprehensive review of drug effects, progress and new issues. *Progress in Neurobiology*, 56(6), 613–672.
– An overview of recent findings from studies using conditioned place preference procedures.

Drug discrimination

Colpaert, F. C. (1999) Drug discrimination in neurobiology. *Pharmacology, Biochemistry and Behavior*, 64(2), 337–345.
– A discussion of theoretical issues related to drug discrimination research.
Solinas, M., Panlilio, L. V., Justinova, Z., Yasar, S. & Goldberg, S. R. (2006) Using drug-discrimination techniques to study the abuse-related effects of psychoactive drugs in rats. *Nature Protocols*, 1(3), 1194–1206.
– A discussion of practical issues related to drug discrimination research.

Locomotor activity

Robinson, T. E. & Berridge, K. C. (2001) Incentive-sensitization and addiction. *Addiction*, 96(1), 103–114.
– An update on Robinson and Berridge's influential theory relating addiction and sensitisation.
Vezina, P. (2004) Sensitization of midbrain dopamine neuron reactivity and the self-administration of psychomotor stimulant drugs. *Neuroscience and Biobehavioral Reviews*, 27(8), 827–839.
– A review of studies suggesting a direct relationship between sensitisation and excessive drug self-administration.

Section V
Specialist Methods

Chapter 18

UNDERSTANDING CONTEXTS: METHODS AND ANALYSIS IN ETHNOGRAPHIC RESEARCH ON DRUGS

Jeremy Northcote and David Moore

18.1 Introduction

As evidenced by the diverse chapters in this book, research on drugs encompasses many different methodologies. While these approaches provide invaluable insights into drug use – for example, its epidemiology, neurobiology and psychology – they sometimes neglect a critical dimension of drug use: how drug use is understood by drug users themselves. Ethnographic approaches to the study of drug use aim to provide rich descriptions of the 'cultural logics' constructed and enacted by drug users and the complex intersections between these cultural logics and wider social, economic and policy processes. Ethnography has made important contributions to the drug field through:

- explaining apparently 'irrational' or risky drug-related practices;
- documenting the negative impact of poorly designed policy on drug-related harm;
- providing important data on 'hidden populations';
- contributing to multidisciplinary research; and
- informing the design of drug policy that targets cultural and social contexts (Moore, 2005).

'Ethnography' refers both to a set of research methods (e.g. participant observation, observation, unstructured interviews) and to the textual products of such methods (e.g. published books and articles, documentary film). While ethnography shares some of the methods of qualitative research more generally, such as in-depth interviews, and also shares qualitative research's interest in explicating 'insider' perspectives, it can be distinguished by its principal reliance on interaction with drug users in situ, that is, as they go about their everyday activities. In the words of anthropologist Philippe Bourgois (1999, pp. 2158–2159, emphasis added):

> Anthropologists attempt to develop an *organic relationship* to a social setting where their presence only minimally distorts indigenous social interaction. They seek out a *legitimate social role within the social scene* they are studying in order to develop friendships (and sometimes enmities) that allow them (with informed consent) *directly* to observe behaviour in as unobtrusive a manner as possible. A major task of participant-observers is to put themselves 'in the shoes' of the people they study in order to *'see local realities' through local eyes*. [. . .] [C]ultural anthropologists try to get *as close as possible to indigenous street-based realities* without changing them. Their overall goal is to obtain a *holistic perspective on the internal logics and external constraints for the way processes unfold*.

The italicised phrases highlight the key methodological and analytical elements of ethnography: long-term interaction with drug users in natural settings in order to describe the lived experience, social processes and structural parameters of drug use.

In the remainder of this chapter, we provide a brief history of ethnographic drug research before considering issues of research design, access to the field, sampling, data collection, analysis and the production of ethnographic texts.

18.2 Tracing the history of ethnographic drug research

Ethnographic research on drug use has a long history, which overlaps with methodological and analytical developments in anthropology and sociology. In anthropology, the 'values and criteria of modern ethnography' were first outlined by Malinowski (1922), who advocated a systematic approach to data collection and analysis via long-term immersion in one's chosen field site. For Malinowski, the aim was to produce an insider account of a society and culture through detailed descriptions of social organisation, everyday practices and the 'native mentality'.

Although some have argued that drug ethnography can be traced back to nineteenth-century descriptions of opium use amongst the urban poor of England (Feldman & Aldrich, 1990; Singer, 1999), perhaps a better place to start is the ethnographic research conducted in the 1920s and 1930s by the 'Chicago School' sociologists. Embracing W.I. Thomas' dictum that 'if men define situations as real, they are real in their consequences' (Cuff & Payne, 1979, p. 104), these researchers emphasised the necessity of understanding the participants' 'definition of the situation'. This symbolic interactionist perspective, coupled with a combination of field-based, interview and documentary methods, inspired several ethnographies of drug use such as Dai's (1937) *Addiction in Chicago*. Chicago School ethnography sought to describe a particular 'community, group or situation' (Hammersley, 1992) as a means of appreciating the everyday context of lifestyles otherwise misunderstood or hidden from view. In the Chicago work, drug use, like other 'social problems' such as delinquency and gambling, was viewed as stemming from the 'social disorganisation' created by rapid industrialisation and urbanisation.

Building on the principles of symbolic interactionism, post-war ethnographies of drug use made substantial contributions to social explanations of drug use and addiction, to qualitative methodology and to theorising on 'deviance'. The clandestine nature of many drug 'subcultures' provided fertile ground for several classic ethnographic accounts of 'hidden' lifestyles (e.g. Sutter, 1966; Feldman, 1968; Spradley, 1970; Agar, 1973; Weppner, 1977). The authors of these works sought to counter popular and academic perceptions of drug users as passive, weak or deviant with alternative depictions of drug-user lifestyles as purposeful and active. A central theme in these studies was that dependent drug use was 'anything but an escape from life' since drug users 'actively engage in meaningful activities and relationships seven days a week', and their 'quest for heroin' may be interpreted as 'the quest for a meaningful life' (Preble & Casey, 1969, p. 2). Another key feature of these studies was that the life or behaviour under study 'becomes meaningful, reasonable and normal once you get close to it' (Goffman, 1961, p. ix). The symbolic interactionist tradition has continued to inform the use of ethnographic methods in drug research (e.g. Adler, 1985; Murphy, 1987; Sterk, 1999; Lalander, 2003).

From the 1990s onwards, epidemics of HIV infection among injecting drug users were associated with an increased receptivity in public health to ethnographic and other qualitative methods, particularly in mixed methods research (e.g. Connors, 1992; Grund, 1993; Koester, 1994; Clatts et al., 1999; Bourgois et al., 2006). While the primary reason for this greater acceptance may have been pragmatic – the need to better understand the social contexts of risk behaviour so as to control HIV transmission – it also reflected methodological and analytical interest in revisiting research paradigms capable of untangling the complex environments in which actions, diseases and policies interact (Rhodes & Moore, 2001). Agar (1997, p. 1166), for example, argued for an 'ethno-epidemiology' of drug use in which ethnography was viewed as an essential 'conceptual and theoretical means to a necessary epidemiological end'. He advocated a return to the nineteenth-century conception of epidemiology, which focused on the 'host' and 'environment' of ill health as well as the 'agent'.

A parallel development, in which there was less interest in combining qualitative and quantitative approaches, was the emergence of ethnographic analyses of drug use amongst populations marginalised on the basis of race/ethnicity, gender and/or social class (e.g. Bourgois, 1995; Maher, 1997; Maher & Dixon, 1999; Moore, 2004). While these accounts continued the earlier focus on participants' definitions of the situation – taking the reader into crack houses, shooting galleries and private homes – they are also reflexive in their conceptualisation of the relationship between ethnographers and subjects, attentive to the politics inherent in ethnographic representation and interested in how wider social forces (whether historical, structural or economic) shape the everyday realities lived by drug users.

18.3 Designing ethnographic research

One of the defining characteristics of ethnographic research is its emphasis on inductive design. Whereas most quantitative research tends to be deductive, defining the variables of interest a priori on the basis of pre-existing hypotheses and theoretical frameworks, inductive designs, while still employing particular theoretical positions (e.g. interactionist, materialist and post-structuralist), aim to construct interpretations on the basis of data as they emerge from participants' descriptions and practices (Agar, 1980). Whereas behavioural science research on drug use is construct-driven – reflected in its emphasis on hypothesis *testing* – and aims to produce objective measures, antecedents and correlates of drug use, ethnographic research on drug use is data driven, thus hypothesis *generating*, and aims to produce interpretations of the subjective meanings constructed through drug use. Ethnography is interpretive because the lived reality of people does not just present itself to be objectively recorded by researchers – it has to be reconstructed by the ethnographer using insights gained during fieldwork. Such immersion does not involve a straightforward 'reading' of the scene, but is characterised by a constant interplay between the field of study and the analyst's own representations. Consequently, while behavioural science research can be characterised as linear in conceptualisation and operationalisation, ethnographic research is iterative and cyclical, spiralling towards interpretation.

A second feature of ethnographic research design concerns its relationship to theory. In the view of some ethnographers, theory should emerge primarily through interpretation of research data. This approach is sometimes referred to as 'grounded theory', which simply means that theories are grounded in the field data. Grounded theory, as originally defined by Glaser and Strauss (1967), employs various coding and categorising techniques to elicit conceptual models during data analysis. Not all ethnographers employ the coding methods outlined by Glaser and Strauss, and so do not openly identify with grounded theory methodology, even if they subscribe to its general principles. Other ethnographers take a more theoretically informed approach, as outlined by Strauss and Corbin (2007) and Willis and Trondman (2000), where they have a special interest in a particular theoretical model or problem which shapes data collection and analysis.

A third feature of ethnographic research design is its emphasis on 'reflexivity' – that is, on identifying how the preconceptions and characteristics of the ethnographer shape both the field experience and the resulting interpretation. The tenets of inductive research encourage analyses grounded in the perspectives of participants, of which the researcher is one, and thus aim to make visible the subjective and intersubjective meanings of action (Rabinow, 1977; Agar, 1997). In adopting a different epistemological logic to interpretation and judgement than deductive approaches, inductive designs complement as well as challenge the assumed objectivity of commonsense understandings of drug use. Induction enables the discovery of plural – and sometimes competing – interpretations of drug use which often fall outside the more restricted interpretative frameworks championed by positivist and quantitative research. In other words, reflexivity involves critical awareness on the part of researchers that their perspective represents but one vantage point among many possible perspectives. This means that researchers' own conceptions of 'drug use', 'addiction' and 'dependence' are in part socially constructed by the paradigms, methods and findings of research (Moore, 1993). Ethnographic methods are, of course, not immune from this process (since all acts of research are forms of interaction and interpretation), but they aim to be reflexive about the process of interpretation and, most importantly, do not claim objectivity.

18.4   Getting started

18.4.1   Reviewing the literature

Most ethnographic research begins in the library. Previous ethnographic and other studies of drug-using practices, groups and settings can provide important information about the current state of knowledge, viable research topics, how to access suitable research sites and groups, and potential pitfalls. Reports issued by government agencies, local government authorities and other regulatory bodies may also provide insights into the policies and reforms that have shaped drug use in the proposed research setting, for example, what initiatives have recently been carried out by the police to curb drug dealing and drug use in the neighbourhood and what measures have the local council taken to regulate illicit activities in public areas?

18.4.2   Entering the field

Once the research topic and a possible field site have been identified, the next step is to make contact with people who use drugs. There are several different ways of making contact, each with their advantages and disadvantages. These approaches involve referral, cold canvassing, the use of field stations and peer research.

'Referral' describes a process where the ethnographer is introduced to potential participants by a mutual contact who is known both to the researcher (either directly or via someone else) and to the members of the target group. In some cases, this will be a member of the group to be studied; in other cases, the mutual contact may not be a drug user but someone who is known and trusted by the potential participants. This could be a community worker, a relative or another researcher. In both cases, the mutual contact acts as a cultural broker, helping to establish the legitimacy of the ethnographer and vouching for his/her good intentions. Where community workers or other service providers act as referrers, a potential drawback is that the ethnographer may also be misidentified as a 'worker' and possibly therefore as interested primarily in 'reforming' drug users. Choosing referrers therefore needs to be carefully thought through in terms of the impressions and expectations that they may create for potential participants.

A second common approach to contacting drug users is 'cold canvassing' or 'cold calling', which involves entering settings frequented by suitable participants without prior contact or the benefits of referral. The ethnographer visits locations frequented by drug users – street corners, pedestrian malls and bars – striking up conversations and attempting to establish relationships. In this way, the ethnographer is not reliant on a referrer (with the associated impressions and expectations), but it can also be time-consuming and requires considerable patience and perseverance.

Another way of contacting drug users, most common in US multidisciplinary drug research, is the ethnographic field station – a research site physically located in the community of interest (e.g. Goldstein et al., 1990). It provides researchers with a presence in the area, a base from which to recruit drug users, and a place to conduct interviews, administer surveys and develop relationships with key informants. The drawbacks include cost and the tendency to remain within the field station rather than interacting with drug users in natural settings, to develop a 9–5 mentality and to develop overly bureaucratic procedures.

Finally, peer research methods may be employed whereby participants are recruited as fieldworkers (e.g. Grace et al., 2009). This approach has several advantages: it avoids many of the issues and delays associated with becoming accepted by participants; peers have background information and inside knowledge that often improves understanding of observed events; and the self-consciousness of participants at being 'watched' is often reduced. Among its disadvantages are that peers may lack the formal expertise of trained researchers; be less-inclined to question the commonsense understandings that characterise their own way of life; find it difficult to interact with certain participants due to their social position or interpersonal history; and experience conflicts of interest while researching their friends and associates.

18.4.3   Informing participants

Once contact has been made with the target group, the next step is to explain the purpose of the study and gain permission from group members to carry it out. Gaining informed consent prior to data collection protects the rights to privacy of research participants and ensures that they understand and consent to any risk of harms that may result from the research. In previous times, some ethnographers delayed revealing their research purpose until they had successfully established a social presence within the target scene, only then explaining their intentions (e.g. Polsky, 1969).

18.4.4   Sampling

Because ethnographic research adopts a case study approach, sampling issues generally concern how to sample within cases, that is, 'where to observe and when, who to talk to and what to ask, [. . .] what to record and how' (Hammersley & Atkinson, 1995, p. 45). On the basis of a particular theoretical framework (e.g. a post-structuralist focus on drug discourse) or a specific research interest (e.g. in gender and drugs), 'theoretical' or 'purposive sampling' allows ethnographers to focus on particular geographical locations, times of the day and/or week, categories of drug user (e.g. on the basis of age, gender and experience), modes of drug use or types of event. For example, amongst recreational drug users, weekend drug use is likely to be the norm and so fieldwork would focus on the different settings frequented at this time (e.g. nightclubs and parties).

Sampling in ethnographic research is a gradual process of selecting appropriate locations and participants as the study unfolds and the researcher becomes familiar with the setting. Purposive sampling frames are sometimes designed following 'ethnographic mapping' (Clatts et al., 1995), which involves identifying the social and geographical locations of drug use and distribution, the sociodemographic characteristics of the drug-using population and broad patterns of drug use, in order to construct maps of drug markets and participant profiles. This means that the sample is more representative of the target population than self-selected samples or those drawn for surveys of the total population.

Field relationships are also relevant to sampling as identification with particular individuals within a group may facilitate access to specific events, people or activities. Alternatively, identification with particular individuals within a group can also serve to constrain research and may limit access if there are divisions or tensions within the network. Over time, the ethnographer may need to establish effective relationships with a number of network members in order to gain access to contrasting views and social action.

18.5 Collecting data

As part of its reflexive emphasis, ethnography places great importance on the interaction between researchers and participants in the collection of data. Without close personal relationships, conducting good ethnography is difficult. In most social research, participants are the focus of study, but in ethnography the 'participants' often become collaborators. Often, one or a small number of individuals become cultural guides, introducing the ethnographer to relevant people and helping to explain various aspects of the group or activity in question. Choosing appropriate guides can be very important, especially where the ethnographer is reliant on them for access to the community, because their goodwill, trust, status within the community and knowledge can improve the quality of data and help to maintain the confidence of participants.

Participant observation is the primary means of ethnographic data collection, usually supplemented by other methods such as in-depth interviews or visual recording. Participant observation involves the researcher spending extended periods interacting with drug users in their natural settings. It involves listening carefully to conversations, asking questions, observing and taking a social role in the group. The term 'participant observation' refers to the two aspects that are involved in this method – alternating between *participating* in the everyday life of the studied group and *observing* them.

When conducting participant observation, ethnographers typically record their observations in the form of field notes. While interacting with participants, some ethnographers keep a notebook handy in order to jot down 'condensed notes', which may consist of key words, phrases or other mnemonic devices. Other ethnographers wait until they have left the field setting to write 'expanded [or elaborated] notes', which involve a fuller narrative account of the day's or evening's events (Spradley, 1980). Field notes may also be audio-recorded for later transcription. In addition to empirical descriptions of people, places and activities, ethnographers may also write 'theoretical memos' – that is, more analytical notes that record initial interpretations about the possible meanings of particular events or activities. As part of the iterative research process, these may also inform future fieldwork. Some ethnographers also keep a fieldwork journal, which is reserved for recording personal ideas, feelings and concerns about the research experience.

In addition to participant observation, in-depth interviews are an important part of ethnography's toolkit. They are often employed to gain further insights into the settings being studied, gather data that is not always immediately apparent during everyday interactions (e.g. individual life histories) and to probe further into specific issues with key contacts. In-depth interviews may be relatively unstructured in form, allowing appropriate and relevant questions to emerge in response to issues raised in the unfolding conversation between ethnographers and drug users. More structured questioning, where the interview ranges over a set of predetermined topics, is useful in situations where key issues have already been identified and the researcher wishes to pursue specific insights relating to those issues.

Interview discussions tend to be recorded on audio devices or in notebooks. Audio devices are preferred by some ethnographers because of the advantage of being able to focus on the interviewee and the flow of interview discussion without the distraction of note taking. The accuracy of the data recorded is another distinct advantage of using such devices. In some situations, however, an audio device may be seen as too intrusive by participants, and this is particularly true of some drug-dealing networks where participants may feel uncomfortable in speaking freely about their illegal activity.

The recording of visual data, through digital photographic and video technology, is another method increasingly being used in drug ethnography. In particular, such data have been crucial in the description of injecting risk practices (e.g. Taylor et al., 2004). Visual data provide more accurate visual documentation of practices and settings than is possible by technologically unaided participants or ethnographers; enhance memory and analysis of past observations or experiences; reduce the possibility of premature inferences; reveal taken-for-granted, infrequent or background events; and enhance the description and analysis of interactions between bodies, drug-using practices and environments (Rhodes & Fitzgerald, 2006).

18.6 Analysing ethnographic data

The process of inductive analysis begins during fieldwork. Indeed, in ethnography, there is no rigid separation between data collection and analysis, but rather constant feedback in which preliminary interpretations are developed on the basis of observed behaviour and then tested in and used to guide further data collection. Formally, these ideas take the form of theoretical notes and memoranda; more informally, they are recorded as hunches and preliminary interpretations in field journals. Because ethnographic analysis is reflexive and iterative, aspects of the research design, research problem and other ideas may be transformed, adapted, revised or discarded during the research process.

Sometimes, ethnographers may take a break from data collection in order to begin some preliminary analysis, which allows them to identify gaps in the data and develop more targeted research questions that can guide further fieldwork. At some point, however, the fieldwork comes to a close, and the task of intensive analysis begins.

Once fieldwork has finished, the first step is to undertake a careful reading of the data. Researchers need to be very familiar with their field notes and other forms of collected data so that they can begin to identify patterns and formulate 'grounded' concepts and theories. Strauss and Corbin (2007) identify three stages in the coding process: open coding, axial coding and selective coding.

'Open coding' involves freely attaching classifications to the data during initial review. In this exploratory phase of the coding process, the idea is to identify the key issues that emerge in the data. These might include 'in vivo' codes, which refer to the categories of events and activities constructed by participants (Charmaz, 2006, pp. 55–57). Or codes might be developed on the basis of one's particular research objective – for example, coding data relating to 'drug overdose'. The ethnographer might also develop codes according to a particular theoretical perspective – for example, researchers working from a feminist perspective might use coding categories relating to the position and role of women, such as 'women and injection routine'.

The second stage in the coding process is 'axial coding', which refers to the identification of central themes in the data and how they relate to one another through the grouping of categories. An example is the way that drug-user activities such as buying drugs from trusted sources, testing small amounts of drugs before taking full doses and injecting in the company of others might be grouped together under the category of 'harm reduction strategies'. In the axial coding stage, it is often possible to create a hierarchical organisation of codes into main categories and subcategories, or 'category trees'.

The third stage in the coding process is 'selective coding'. This refers to the process of identifying cases that support the main findings. It is selective because, by this stage, the analysts know more or less what they are looking for in order to piece together the 'big picture'. The process of coding, as well as the management and storage of ethnographic data, has been greatly assisted by the development of computer software, such as Ethnograph, NVivo and Atlas.ti.

Some of the issues that drug ethnographers may focus on during analysis include the following:

1. Developing an adequate description and account of recurring drug-related practices and beliefs as enacted and understood by participants
2. Mapping the social relations that constitute the studied group or drug scene
3. Documenting 'speech acts' that identify important 'emic' (or insider-identified) categories, which can be contrasted with 'etic' (or observer-identified) categories
4. Identifying key practices or events that seem particularly important to participants, are puzzling or which deviate from normal participant activities
5. Exploring discrepancies between emic accounts of typical drug activity and observed practices
6. Examining variations in drug practices and emic accounts on the basis of age, gender, experience or other relevant categories
7. Considering how aspects of the wider context (legal, economic, social, historical) shape drug use
8. Comparing the findings to those discussed in previous studies of similar drug practices or groups.

Once a plausible explanation for the topic(s) of interest has been formulated, the next step is to assess its validity. While it is true that the work of ethnography is fundamentally interpretive, there are several ways of subjecting interpretations to some degree of testing. One such method is 'triangulation', which Glaser and Strauss (1967) describe as the 'constant comparative method'. Triangulation involves collecting and contrasting data on the same topic from different sources, such as comparing fieldwork observations with interview data, or seeking analytical input from participants. Having participants corroborate accounts and contribute to analysis can improve the empirical accuracy of field notes and their interpretation. Participants can correct or at least restrain the researcher from making fanciful generalisations from single incidents or from reading too much into what turns out to be relatively insignificant action. This involvement of participants in the translation of activity into field accounts is sometimes termed 'dialogical' (Clifford, 1986). Once they have gained confidence in their interpretations, ethnographers can then begin to compare them to those offered in the existing research literature or apply them to questions of drug policy and practice.

18.7   Producing ethnographic texts

The final stage is writing up the findings. However, to characterise this as the final stage is a little misleading, because just as data collection and analysis overlap in ethnographic research, so too do analysis and writing. Much of the writing is done during the collection and analysis stages – in the form of field notes and theoretical memoranda. But in the final 'write-up', these earlier textual forms become more formalised and abstract. What has been a sometimes difficult process, with interpretive dead ends, frustrations and a gradual attainment of analytical clarity, becomes, in the written version, an orderly account of a particular group, scene or form of drug use.

Different authors use various devices to create an orderly account: the 'natural history', chronological arrangement of events, or organisation under various topics or themes as defined by either the observer or the observed. The complexity of the research enterprise sometimes becomes lost in this final process, although there have been attempts to identify a more reflexive and dialogic writing style, which would allow some of these processes to become more explicit (e.g. Clifford & Marcus, 1986; Denzin, 1997).

Earlier, we noted that reflexivity is an important component of ethnographic work. With respect to writing, a reflexive approach highlights the role of the researcher-as-translator, and the ways in which the particular characteristics of the ethnographer (e.g. age, gender, research training and interpersonal style), and the social role adopted during fieldwork, shape the research findings and written account. Reflexivity acknowledges the crucial role of the researcher, rather than preserving the positivist fiction that research findings represent an unmediated glimpse into the world of research participants. Understanding how various research paradigms and methods produce their 'objects of inquiry', and being able to incorporate these understandings into analysis and the production of texts, remains a central challenge.

18.8 Conclusion

As a distinct approach in drug research, ethnography has many benefits:

1. It contributes valuable descriptive data
2. It furthers understanding of the contexts of drug use and their intersection with wider processes
3. It facilitates the process of theory construction
4. It has a high degree of 'ecological validity', in that natural settings are its focus
5. It is generalisable at the level of relationships between wider processes and specific scenes, groups or forms of drug use
6. It allows triangulation and various other checks on the research process.

Ethnography's disadvantages include it being:

1. time intensive;
2. unable to examine phenomena on a large scale like surveys (being better suited to microanalysis);
3. unable to generalise its findings to the wider population based on measures of statistical probability.

In summary, ethnography is best suited to understanding the 'how' and 'why' of social action at the everyday level. Why, for example, do injecting drug users share injecting equipment and therefore put themselves at risk of infection? How do poverty, racism and stigmatisation shape everyday lived experience? In what ways do drug users develop harm reduction strategies of their own? The outcome of a well-researched and well-written ethnography is a deeper understanding of the cultural logics and social processes of drug use, which can inform the design of quantitative research and the development of policy and interventions. To this end, the ethnographic study of drug use has a unique role to play in reducing the 'naïvity' factor that can creep into a research area where the world of its investigators is often far removed from the world of its subjects.

Acknowledgements

The authors acknowledge the support of Edith Cowan University and the National Drug Research Institute, which receives core funding from the Australian Government Department of Health and Ageing.

Excercises

The nature of ethnography means that it is difficult to do simple short exercises, but the tasks outlined below will provide you with some rudimentary insights into the challenges facing ethnographic researchers.

1. Find a friend, relative or classmate who smokes or enjoys an alcoholic drink, and conduct a 15-minute interview about the reasons they do so, recording their responses on a notepad. Be sure to ask them how often they smoke or drink, on what occasions (privately, at social gatherings, on special occasions), and whether their rate of smoking or drinking has fluctuated over time and why. Feel free to explore with them in some depth the circumstances in which they smoke or drink. Examine the data and see if habitual practices, life circumstances or social influences (or a combination) best make sense of their smoking or drinking practices. Write a one-page summary of your findings.
2. With a classmate, visit a local bar, club or university/college tavern and observe the spaces in which people smoke or drink alcohol over a 30-minute period. Pay attention to entry areas, seating areas, standing areas, dancing areas, toilets and outside areas. Are people smoking and drinking in equal proportion in the different spaces? Think about some of the factors that might account for any differences observed (e.g. activities such as dancing and eating, different social types preferring different areas, proximity to the bar or to open areas for smoking and level of group interaction). Write a one-page summary of your findings.

References

Adler, P. (1985) *Wheeling and Dealing: An Ethnography of an Upper-Level Drug Dealing and Smuggling Community*. New York: Columbia University Press.

Agar, M. (1973) *Ripping and Running: A Formal Ethnography of Urban Heroin Users*. New York: Academic Press.

Agar, M. (1980) *The Professional Stranger: An Informal Introduction to Ethnography*. New York: Academic Press.

Agar, M. (1997) Ethnography: an overview. *Substance Use and Misuse*, 32, 1155–1173.

Bourgois, P. (1995) *In Search of Respect: Selling Crack in El Barrio*. New York: Cambridge University Press.

Bourgois, P. (1999) Theory, method, and power in drug and HIV-prevention research: a participant observer's critique. *Substance Use and Misuse*, 34(14), 2155–2172.

Bourgois, P., Martinez, A., Kral, A., Edlin, B. R., Schonberg, J. & Ciccarone, D. (2006) Reinterpreting ethnic patterns among white and African American men who inject heroin: a social science of medicine approach. *PloS Medicine*, 3(10), e452.

Charmaz, K. (2006) *Constructing Grounded Theory: A Practical Guide through Qualitative Analysis*. London: Sage.

Clatts, M. C., Davis, W. R., & Atillasoy A. (1995) Hitting a moving target: the use of ethnographic methods in the development of sampling strategies for the evaluation of AIDS outreach programs for homeless youth in New York City. In: E. Y. Lambert, R. S. Ashery & R. H. Needle (eds) *Qualitative Methods in Drug Abuse and HIV Research*. Rockville, MD: National Institute on Drug Abuse, pp. 117–135.

Clatts, M. C., Heimer, R., Abdala, N., Goldsamt, L. A., Sotheran, J. L., Anderson, K. T., Gallo, T. M., Hoffer, L. D., Luciano, P. A. & Kyriakides, T. (1999) HIV-1 transmission in injection paraphernalia: heating drug solutions may inactivate HIV-1. *Journal of Acquired Immune Deficiency Syndromes*, 22, 194–199.

Clifford, J. (1986) Introduction: partial truths. In: J. Clifford & G. Marcus (eds) *Writing Culture: The Poetics and Politics of Ethnography*. Berkeley, CA: University of California Press, pp. 98–121.

Clifford, J. & Marcus, G. (eds) (1986) *Writing Culture: The Poetics and Politics of Ethnography*. Berkeley, CA: University of California Press.

Connors, M. M. (1992) Risk perception, risk taking and risk management among intravenous drug users: implications for AIDS prevention. *Social Science and Medicine*, 34(6), 591–601.

Cuff, E. C. & Payne, G. C. F. (1979) (eds) *Perspectives in Sociology*. London: George Allen and Unwin.

Dai, B. (1937) *Addiction in Chicago*. Montclair, NJ: Patterson Smith.

Denzin, N. K. (1997) *Interpretive Ethnography: Ethnographic Practices for the 21st Century*. Thousand Oaks, CA: Sage.

Feldman, H. W. (1968) Ideological supports to becoming and remaining a heroin addict. *Journal of Health and Social Behavior*, 9, 131–139.

Feldman, H. W. & Aldrich, M. (1990) The role of ethnography in substance abuse research and public policy. In: E. Y. Lambert (ed) *The Collection and Interpretation of Data from Hidden Populations*. Rockville, MD: National Institute on Drug Abuse, pp. 12–30.

Glaser, B. G. & Strauss, A. (1967) *The Discovery of Grounded Theory*. Chicago: Aldine.

Goffman, E. (1961) *Asylums*. London: Doubleday.

Goldstein, P. J., Spunt, B. J., Miller, T. & Bellucci, P. (1990) Ethnographic field stations. In: E. Y. Lambert (ed.) *The Collection and Interpretation of Data from Hidden Populations*. Rockville, MD: National Institute on Drug Abuse, pp. 80–95.

Grace, J., Moore, D. & Northcote, J. (2009) *Alcohol, Risk and Harm Reduction: Drinking among Young Adults in Recreational Settings in Perth*. Perth: National Drug Research Institute.

Grund, J-P. (1993) *Drug Use as a Social Ritual: Functionality, Symbolism and Determinants of Self-Regulation*. Rotterdam, the Netherlands: Instituut voor Verslavingsonderzoek.

Hammersley, M. (1992) *What's Wrong with Ethnography?* London: Routledge.

Hammersley, M. & Atkinson, P. (1995) *Ethnography: Principles in Practice*, 2nd edn. London: Routledge.

Koester, S. K. (1994) Copping, running, and paraphernalia laws: contextual variables and needle risk behavior among injection drug users in Denver. *Human Organization*, 53(3), 287–295.

Lalander, P. (2003) *Hooked on Heroin: Drugs and Drifters in a Globalized World*. Oxford: Berg.

Maher, L. (1997) *Sexed Work: Gender, Race, and Resistance in a Brooklyn Drug Market*. Oxford: Clarendon Press.

Maher, L. & Dixon, D. (1999) Policing and public health: law enforcement and harm minimization in a street-level drug market. *British Journal of Criminology* 39(4), 488–512.

Malinowski, B. (1922) *Argonauts of the Western Pacific*. London: Routledge & Kegan Paul.

Moore, D. (1993) Ethnography and illicit drug use: dispatches from an anthropologist in the 'field'. *Addiction Research*, 1(1), 11–25.

Moore, D. (2004) Governing street-based injecting drug users: a critique of heroin overdose prevention in Australia. *Social Science and Medicine*, 59(7), 1547–1557.

Moore, D. (2005) Key moments in the ethnography of drug-related harm: reality checks for policy makers? In: T. R. Stockwell, P. Gruenewald, J. Toumbourou & W. Loxley (eds) *Preventing Harmful Substance Use: The Evidence Base for Policy and Practice*. Chichester, UK: John Wiley & Sons, pp. 433–442.

Murphy, S. (1987) Intravenous drug use and AIDS: notes on the social economy of needle sharing. *Contemporary Drug Problems*, 14, 373–395.

Polsky, N. (1969) *Hustlers, Beats and Others*. Harmondsworth: Penguin.

Preble, E. & Casey, J. (1969) Taking care of business: the heroin user's life on the street. *International Journal of the Addictions*, 4, 1–24.

Rabinow, P. (1977) *Reflections on Fieldwork in Morocco*. Berkeley, CA: University of Chicago Press.

Rhodes, T. & Fitzgerald, J. (2006) Visual data in addictions research: seeing comes before words? *Addiction Research and Theory*, 14(4), 349–363.

Rhodes, T. & Moore, D. (2001) On the qualitative in drugs research. *Addiction Research and Theory*, 9(4), 279–299.

Singer, M. (1999) The ethnography of street drug use before AIDS: a historical review. In: P. L. Marshall, M. Singer & M. C. Clatts (eds) *Integrating Cultural, Observational, and Epidemiological Approaches in the Prevention of Drug Abuse and HIV/AIDS*. Bethesda, MD: National Institute on Drug Abuse, pp. 228–263.

Spradley, J. P. (1970) *You Owe Yourself a Drunk: An Ethnography of Urban Nomads*. Boston: Little, Brown.

Spradley, J. P. (1980) *Participant Observation*. New York: Holt, Rinehart & Winston.

Sterk, C. E. (1999) *Fast Lives: Women Who Use Crack Cocaine*. Philadelphia, PA: Temple University Press.

Strauss, A. & Corbin, J. (2007) *Basics of Qualitative Research: Techniques and Procedures for Developing Grounded Theory*, 2nd edn. Thousand Oaks, CA: Sage.

Sutter, A. (1966) The world of the righteous dope fiend. *Issues in Criminology*, 2, 177–222.

Taylor, A., Fleming, A., Rutherford, J. & Goldberg, D. (2004) *Examining the Injecting Practices of Injecting Drug Users in Scotland*. Glasgow: Scottish Executive Effectiveness Interventions Unit.

Weppner, R. S. (ed.) (1977) *Street Ethnography*. Beverly Hills, CA: Sage.

Willis, P. & Trondman, M. (2000) Manifesto for ethnography. *Ethnography*, 1(1), 5–16.

Recommended readings

Ethnographic accounts of drug use

Bourgois, P. (1995) *In Search of Respect: Selling Crack in El Barrio*. New York: Cambridge University Press.

Feldman, H. W. (1968) Ideological supports to becoming and remaining a heroin addict. *Journal of Health and Social Behavior*, 9, 131–139.

Koester, S. K. (1994) Copping, running, and paraphernalia laws: contextual variables and needle risk behavior among injection drug users in Denver. *Human Organization*, 53(3), 287–295.

Discussions of ethnographic method

Denzin, N. K. (1997) *Interpretive Ethnography: Ethnographic Practices for the 21st Century*. Thousand Oaks, CA: Sage.

Maher, L. (1997) Appendix: on reflexivity, reciprocity, and ethnographic research. *Sexed Work: Gender, Race, and Resistance in a Brooklyn Drug Market*, pp. 207–232. Oxford: Clarendon Press.

Rabinow, P. (1977) *Reflections on Fieldwork in Morocco*. Berkeley, CA: University of Chicago Press.

Chapter 19
EPIDEMIOLOGY

Mark Stoové and Paul Dietze

19.1 Introduction

In this chapter, we provide a short description of the origins of epidemiology and describe the fundamental approaches used in epidemiological research. We describe the basic units of measurement in epidemiology, using examples from the alcohol and other drug sector and explore some of the methodological challenges. Sources of error, particularly those relating to the epidemiology of alcohol and other drug use, are described, alongside the adoption of study designs and analysis strategies to minimise error and enhance the reliability of research findings.

19.2 Origins of epidemiology

Epidemiology is commonly understood as the study of the distribution and determinants of disease in human populations. The terms 'epidemic' and 'epidemiology' have their origins in the observations of Hippocrates who, more than 2400 years ago, used the term *epidemeion* (a verb meaning 'to visit') to differentiate diseases that 'visit' the community from those that reside within it. However, it is John Snow who is widely credited the first formal measurement and documentation of the distribution of disease in different populations during a cholera outbreak in nineteenth-century London. Before Snow's work, cholera was popularly thought to be spread through *miasma* (poisonous vapour identifiable by its nasty, foul smell). Snow kept detailed records of a cholera outbreak he observed around Broad Street in Soho in 1854. Through his records he showed that cholera was transmitted by contaminated water by linking cholera deaths that were clustered by time and place to particular water supplies. It was ultimately the removal of a handle from a public water pump that ended the outbreak. These events are traditionally seen as the birth of modern epidemiology. Not only had Snow been able to identify the source of the cholera outbreak by examining the distribution of disease in time and within subgroups of the population, he was able to isolate the determinants of cholera transmission (establishing a precedent that ultimately saved countless lives globally) and identify a simple public health intervention to prevent further disease.

19.3 Definitions and uses of epidemiology in alcohol and other drug research

Thus, epidemiology is the study of the distribution and determinants of disease in human populations. However, the measurement of patterns of disease implies that the absence of disease is also measured in epidemiology. In this context it is useful to think of outcome measures in modern applied epidemiology as indicators of states of health – a continuum from negative health states to positive health states, from death or severe morbidity to perfect health.

Measurement in epidemiology is based on people, place and time. When trying to understand the determinants of disease and health and developing ways to limit the former and promote the latter, we need to measure how disease and health are distributed across all three of these domains. We want to find out about the characteristics of the *people* affected by disease to examine intra- and inter-individual determinants, the *places* where disease is more or less likely to occur to examine the social and structural determinants, and also understand the distribution of disease across *time* to understand disease transmission or natural history of disease.

By measuring these parameters, the aim of epidemiology is to provide us with understandings of the causation and natural history of health and disease. In doing so, the products of epidemiological enquiry provide us with evidence to develop and evaluate strategies for the detection, management and prevention of disease.

19.3.1 Epidemiology and the alcohol and drug sector

Epidemiological investigations in the alcohol and other drug sector clearly involve the measurement and determinants of disease and health related to the use of drugs such as hepatitis C, HIV, alcoholic liver cirrhosis and mental health problems. Measurement of these diseases can be difficult, but the issues are similar to those evident in mainstream epidemiology. Alcohol and other drug epidemiology typically address a broad range of questions specifically related to drug use behaviours that in mainstream epidemiology would often be seen as an exposure or risk factor rather than an outcome in and of itself. Typical questions around drug use include: How prevalent is substance use and dependence? What are the determinants of different states of drug use – initiation, recreational use, dependence, abstinence? What are the patterns of substance use in different subpopulations and how does this relate to drug-related harms? What are the social and community determinants of changes in drug use trends?

There are significant challenges in measuring substance use in a robust and rigorous way. How do we measure substance use? By what criteria might we determine dependent or problematic drug use? What harms do we measure and are they directly or indirectly related to substance use? How do we sample populations that are likely to be substance dependent, considering the illicit nature of some substances, the social environments in which drug use occurs and the non-random distribution of substance use in a population? Responses to these have led to creative and innovative solutions in alcohol and other drug epidemiology.

19.4 Descriptive epidemiology

Much of the epidemiological work in the alcohol and other drug sector is descriptive in nature. The key descriptive terms are 'prevalence' and 'incidence', which are key to understanding the patterns and distribution of drug use and related harms across communities.

Prevalence defines the number of cases of a condition that exists in a defined population and a given point in time. The calculation of prevalence involves a denominator that defines the population at risk of the condition being measured and a numerator identifying all the people with the condition. For example, Vanichsenia et al. (2001) tested 3643 injecting drug users in Bangkok and found that 1089 were positive for HIV, providing a HIV prevalence in this group of:

$$1089/3643 = 0.2989 \text{ or } 29.8\,\%$$

Incidence refers to the frequency with which a condition occurs over a specified period. Whereas the numerator in calculating incidence is also the number of people with the condition, because we are interested how many people get a condition over time, the denominator is now a unit of time – the total time over which people are at risk. For example, Vanichsenia et al. (2001) also followed the group of injecting drug users that initially tested HIV negative and re-tested them to see how many seroconverted. Although the time over which individual study participants were followed varied considerably (4–40 months), the sum of the follow-up time for all participants amounted to the equivalent of 2308 person-years at risk. Over this time, 133 injecting drug users seroconverted, giving an overall HIV incidence of:

$$133/2308 = 0.057$$

This number would typically be multiplied by 100 to provide a more meaningful result – 5.7 per 100 person-years.

Although many factors affect prevalence, it is important to understand that both the frequency of occurrence of a condition (incidence) and the duration over which people are affected strongly influence prevalence. Obviously, the more people that are affected, the higher the prevalence of a given condition. However, even for commonly occurring diseases, prevalence will be low if the duration of disease is short. For example, short-duration curable conditions such as the common cold can have a high incidence but low prevalence, because many people get a cold each year, but few people actually have a cold at any given time. In these instances, prevalence is not a very useful indicator of health states.

19.5   Epidemiological research designs

Regardless of the study design used, epidemiology seeks to build evidence of relationships between exposures (e.g. risk factors such as dietary behaviours) and outcomes (e.g. mortality). There are two main classes of studies that seek to do this in epidemiology: observational and experimental studies. By far, the most common approach in epidemiology is observational.

Observational epidemiology involves investigators measuring risk exposures and their relationships with outcomes as they occur naturally in the population. Observational studies have made important contributions to our understanding of the relationship between risk and disease. The observational studies undertaken by Doll and Hill (1950, 1964) provided the first scientific observations of the causal relationship between tobacco use and lung cancer (see Box 19.1). Observational studies are commonly population or community based, where researchers collect information from a large number of people and aggregate the data to uncover relationships between exposures and outcomes. There are many specific epidemiological designs that adopt this approach and these are detailed later.

Experimental epidemiology involves the introduction of some sort of intervention (as an exposure) and seeks to understand the effect of this intervention on an outcome. Experimental epidemiology studies are most commonly conducted in clinical settings, the clinical trial. In this type of study, participants have been diagnosed with a specific condition or disease and the investigators assign participants to groups that receive a certain type of treatment. Typically, one group will receive no treatment or a standard treatment (the control group) and the other receives a treatment whose effectiveness is being assessed (the intervention group). By measuring indicators of disease in both groups before and after the treatment trial, researchers are able to measure the effect of the treatment on the disease.

Box 19.1 Doll and Hill's studies of smoking and lung cancer

When Richard Doll and Austin Hill instigated formal investigations in 1948, only very limited evidence existed of the link between smoking and lung cancer. Although some compelling associations between tobacco consumption and lung cancer mortality had emerged at a population level using ecological data (see Section 19.5.4 for limitations of ecological data), other potential factors such as concurrent increases in atmospheric pollutants from industry could also influence lung cancer mortality. Tobacco manufacturing had also developed into a lucrative industry with considerable political power, so more robust evidence beyond ecological data was needed in order to seriously advocate for public health solutions.

Between April 1948 and October 1949, Doll and Hill (1950) interviewed 709 lung cancer patients in 20 London hospitals alongside 709 non-cancer patients recruited from the same hospitals at the same time and matched by 5-year age groups and sex (a classic case-control study; see Section 19.5). Doll and Hill found that lung cancer cases tended to report higher levels of tobacco consumption compared to their matched controls. Doll and Hill were aware, however, that this type of study was not ideal for establishing a causal relationship. For example, cases may have over-reported tobacco consumption because they were aware of the possible link between lung cancer and cigarette smoking (recall bias; see Section 19.5). Or it was possible that non-cancer patients did not sufficiently match with cancer patients and that other environmental factors (confounding) may have explained the differences.

So in November 1951, Doll and Hill embarked on a larger, more ambitious study using a cohort study design – The British Doctor's Study. They sent questionnaires to all 60 000 people listed on the British medical register, of which 69% of men and 60% of women responded. Follow-up of these participants occurred via death registers and also a succession of mailed-out surveys to update data on tobacco consumption. Doll and Hill (1964) published the first 10-year follow-up of participants, and later publications reported on 20- and 40-year follow-up findings (Doll & Peto, 1976; Doll et al., 1994). Table 19.1 shows male lung cancer rates by cigarette consumption for the 10- and 40-year follow-up. These data show convincing evidence of the link between lung cancer and cigarette smoking. Not only are those that never smoked much less likely to die from lung cancer, but the chance of death increases as tobacco consumption increases (a dose–frequency response).

Table 19.1 Lung cancer mortality rates per 1000 population for British male doctors

Length of follow-up	Cigarette smokers (number per day)			
	Never smokers	1–14	5–24	25 or more
10 years	0.07	0.57	1.39	2.27
40 years	0.14	1.05	2.08	3.55

The British Doctor's Study also demonstrated similar results for other diseases, such as those related to respiratory and vascular functioning. They also showed that quitting smoking lowered mortality risk, and that longer periods of abstinence were associated with decreased risk. Alone, this study would be insufficient to establish a casual relationship between cigarette smoking and mortality. However, building on the work of Doll and Hill, many other researchers have established the same relationships across many different populations and settings. This evidence, combined with plausible biological pathways to explain the relationship, has resulted in the conclusion that tobacco consumption does, without any reasonable doubt, contribute to increased mortality.

Table 19.2　Study designs in epidemiology

Basic study design	Sampling	Specific study design
Observational	Populations	Routine/secondary data analysis
	Individuals	Ecological data analysis
	Outcomes	Cross-sectional
	Exposure	Case control
		Retrospective cohort
		Prospective cohort
Experimental	Patients	Clinical trial
	Populations	Preventive trial

In the hierarchy of 'evidence', the randomised clinical trial is considered the 'gold standard' study design. Issues of confounding and bias (see Section 19.8) are often cited as reasons for criticising findings of observational studies. It is often impossible, however, to examine relationships between exposures and outcomes using an experimental design. For example, it would be ethically fraught to assign non-smoking participants to a smoking group and compare lung cancer rates to a control group. Thus, studies of exposure and disease are often only possible using observational techniques. Fortunately, there are several prominent studies that have demonstrated high levels of consistency between findings of relationships between exposure and outcomes between randomised clinical trials and observational studies (e.g. Benson & Hartz, 2000; Concato et al., 2000; Ioannidis et al., 2001).

19.5.1　Specific epidemiological designs

So, how do we go about quantifying the association between exposures and health outcomes? How do we examine possible cause and effect relationships between exposures and outcomes? How can we assess the effect of an intervention on health outcomes? There are several specific study designs that can be adopted to answer these questions, presented in Table 19.2.

19.5.2　Descriptive epidemiology studies

Descriptive studies in epidemiology involve the measurement and comparison of health outcomes in populations, typically using the basic measurements of prevalence and incidence described earlier. It is useful to think of comparisons in epidemiology as largely involving comparing between people, place or time (or the interaction of two or more of these).

When comparing health outcomes between people, we usually compare across personal characteristics such as age, gender, ethnicity or socioeconomic status. For example, DeWit and colleagues (2000) found that age of first alcohol use was associated with alcohol dependence later in life. They compared the prevalence of alcohol dependence diagnoses 10 years after initiation between those who initiated alcohol consumption at ages 11–12 years, 13–14 years and 19 years and older. Alcohol dependence prevalence was 16, 9 and 1%, respectively, suggesting that the earlier the initiation of alcohol use, the higher the likelihood of alcohol dependence later in life.

When comparing health outcomes between places, we try to uncover what are the characteristics of place that influence health, such as income equality, sanitation or harm reduction approaches to substance use. For example, MacDonald and colleagues (2003) compared changes in HIV prevalence in 63 cities that introduced Needle and Syringe Programs compared to 36 that did not introduce Needle and Syringe Programs. They reported a mean annual increase in HIV prevalence of 8.1% in the former and a mean annual decrease in HIV prevalence of 18.6% in the latter.

Descriptive epidemiology also compares changes in health outcomes over time. These types of comparisons can be useful in determining seasonal changes or evaluating public health interventions by comparing health in populations before and after the introduction of the intervention. For example, Bauer and colleagues (2005) compared the prevalence of tobacco cessation from 1993 to 2001 among employees at workplaces that instigated smoking restriction policies. The prevalence of employees reporting quitting smoking over this time increased from 20 to 27 to 31% in workplaces that maintained unrestricted smoking policies, initiated smoke-free zones or initiated a ban on smoking, respectively.

19.5.3   Routine and secondary data analysis

Another commonly used approach in epidemiological studies is the use of routine and secondary data. *Secondary data* studies make use of routinely collected data such as mortality, hospitalisation or alcohol and other drug treatment data or data previously collected for other purposes. These data can be analysed on their own to provide overall descriptive data on, for example, the number of alcohol-related hospitalisations. Alternatively, secondary databases can be linked if there is a way of uniquely identifying people in each of the databases. The advantages of secondary data studies are that they are relatively low cost and usually the data they contain are reliable. The major disadvantage is that data are often not adequate for the purposes of the research. Important data on risk factors may not be included in the data or not adequately measured.

19.5.4   Ecological data analysis

Ecological approaches emphasise relations and interactions between individuals and their environment. In epidemiology, ecological studies compare health patterns between communities using aggregated population-level data, typically obtained from routine sources. For example, Ramstedt (2002) compared post-war trends in alcohol-related mortality and alcohol consumption in European Union member countries. Figure 19.1 shows a strong association between average per capita alcohol consumption and cirrhosis mortality aggregated by country.

Ecological studies are an effective way to provide an overview of health in different settings, can be suggestive of causative relationships between exposures and outcomes (that can be subsequently explored using more robust study designs), and usually involve data that can be obtained relatively quickly and cheaply. The disadvantages of ecological studies, however, are considerable. These studies are susceptible to confounding factors, in that different populations may have a large variety of characteristic differences that might influence results, differences that we cannot control for in this type of study (typically, because they are not measured). Another disadvantage of this study design is that whenever we analyse grouped or aggregated data in epidemiology, the potential for ecological fallacy exists. An *ecological fallacy* is the assumption that a relationship observed at a population-level will hold at an individual level (see Box 19.2).

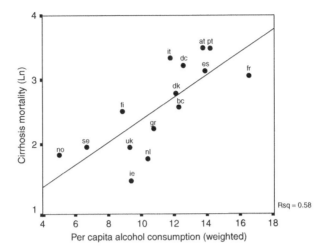

Figure 19.1 Relationship between alcohol consumption and cirrhosis mortality in European countries (Ramstedt, 2002).

19.5.5 Cross-sectional studies

One of the simplest types of observational studies is a cross-sectional survey. Cross-sectional studies can be thought of as a 'snapshot' in time. Information, including that related to exposures and health outcomes, is collected from a sample of a population at a given time. Cross-sectional studies are useful for measuring prevalence (of exposures and outcomes) and are also appropriate for assessing exposures that never change (e.g. genetics, hereditary factors). Cross-sectional studies are

---

Box 19.2 The ecological fallacy

The ecological fallacy refers to the assumption that a relationship that is observed at an ecological or aggregated group level will hold at an individual level. The notion of a stereotype can be considered a simple example of an ecological fallacy. A recent example of a potential ecological fallacy in substance use research can be found in Kozlowski and colleagues (2003) who analysed national health survey data since 1987 to suggest that the use of smokeless tobacco products (snuff, chewing tobacco or both), rather than being a potential 'gateway' behaviour to the smoking of cigarettes, may in fact be protective of cigarette smoking initiation. Their conclusion was based on data that showed higher prevalence of smokeless tobacco use in 23- to 26-year-old men compared to 31- to 34-year-old men, yet a lower prevalence of ever smoking in the younger group. Using these data to suggest that smokeless tobacco products are therefore protective against smoking ignores a number of other potentially confounding factors. First, that smoking prevalence is generally lower in younger age groups in the United States. Second, that the prevalence of smokeless tobacco use was lower among young men in the United States in the mid-1970s (when the older group was likely to have initiated smoking) compared to recent data, suggesting a higher likelihood of smoking initiation preceding smokeless tobacco initiation in the older group. It is therefore possible, if not likely, that the association between smokeless tobacco products and smoking behaviour is an artefact of historical and temporal relationships between tobacco use behaviour and age.

sometimes used to initially explore hypotheses and provide 'ball park' estimates of associations between exposures and outcomes.

Cross-sectional studies are not appropriate for measuring rare conditions or diseases of short duration. They are also clearly not suitable for measuring incidence, which requires repeated measurements over time.

One of the main disadvantages of cross-sectional studies is the problem of reliably establishing links between exposures and outcomes. Exposures may have occurred a considerable time in the past and with a long time lag to the occurrence of disease, so problems with the reliability of participant recall of past events can result in unreliable associations between possible exposures and health outcomes (recall bias, see Section 19.8). Indeed, problems with interpretation of timing between exposures and disease (i.e. which occurred first) mean that cross-sectional studies cannot reliably establish cause-and-effect relationships between exposures and outcomes.

19.5.6   Case-control studies

Case-control studies are distinct from all other epidemiological designs because they purposely sample participants according to an outcome. In this type of study, persons with the health outcome of interest (cases) and those without this condition (controls) are questioned in detail about possible past exposures. If participants with the condition more commonly report a particular exposure or risk factor compared to those without the condition, then a possible link between that exposure and an outcome is established.

Murphy and colleagues (2001) investigated risk factors for skin and soft tissue abscesses among injecting drug users by recruiting 151 injecting drug users treated for abscesses in an inpatient or emergency hospital setting (cases). Controls were 267 injectors recruited from the same setting without abscesses. Past clinical and interview data were compared between the two groups, and the researchers found that intramuscular (rather than intravenous) injection and injection of cocaine–heroin mixtures were more commonly reported by cases (risk factors for abscesses) and cleaning the skin with alcohol swabs prior to injection was more commonly reported by controls (protective factor against abscesses).

Case-control studies purposively sample people with particular conditions meaning that they are ideal for investigating rare diseases or outcomes that would require very large samples to detect in other types of study designs. Because data are collected cross-sectionally, case-control studies are relatively simple, cheap and quick – depending on the ability to easily recruit cases. However, as with cross-sectional studies, case-control studies involve data collection at a single time point, meaning that they cannot be used to measure incidence. Further, as exposures are typically measured on the basis of participants' recall of past events, case-control studies are particularly vulnerable to recall bias. In addition, cases and controls need to be carefully selected to ensure that they are recruited from similar or the same settings and display similar characteristics. Otherwise, unmeasured differences between groups may lead to spurious associations between exposures and outcomes (selection bias). Finally, case-control studies are not appropriate for identifying rare exposures (unless extremely large samples are used) and can usually only measure risk factors for one outcome at a time.

19.5.7   Case-crossover studies

One special example of the case-control study is the case-crossover study. In case-crossover studies, participants act as their own control. In a typical case-crossover study, cases are asked to recall their exposures prior to the occurrence of the outcome of interest. They are then asked to recall their exposures prior to another time where the event did not occur. Most famously applied to the question of mobile telephones and car accidents, where telephone records of crash victims were examined prior to the crash occurring and compared to similar times in the previous week (Redelmeier & Tibshirani, 1997), this study design is particularly suitable for examining transient changes in risk behaviours and their effects on health outcomes. Given this, the case crossover design has been recently applied to the study of a variety of outcomes related to alcohol and other drug use (Vinson et al., 1995; Mittleman et al., 2001; Borges et al., 2004; Dietze et al., 2005).

19.5.8 Cohort studies

Outside the controlled trial, the cohort study is considered the most powerful epidemiological design. *Cohort studies involve the identification and recruitment of a defined population that is followed-up over time.* Unlike the study designs described previously, incidence of health outcomes can be measured in cohort studies because people are examined over time. The most powerful cohort designs involve large random samples of the population. However, for the study of rare characteristics or behaviours such as those often of interest to alcohol and other drug epidemiology, cohorts are often selected on evidence of a characteristic or behaviour itself. For example, a specific cohort of injecting drug users may be recruited in order to study this rare behaviour that we know places people at higher risk of many adverse health outcomes. Recruitment of a specific cohort such as this allows for the assessment of incidence of specific outcomes in specific populations, such as the incidence of injection-related injuries in injectors who primarily inject pharmaceuticals compared to injectors who primarily inject heroin. In this latter example, we would consider a group as exposed or not exposed and compare the incidence of injection-related injuries in pharmaceutical injectors (exposed) and heroin injectors (unexposed).

Cohort studies have been particularly important in documenting some of the key adverse health consequences, such as mortality, associated with alcohol and other drug use. Bargagli and colleagues (2001) followed-up a cohort of 11 432 'problem drug users' (largely primary heroin injectors) recruited from drug treatment clinics in Rome between 1980 and 1995. In 1997, they linked the records of participants to a national death register to examine mortality in this cohort. They found 1734 deaths with cumulative person-years of follow-up of 80 787 years. Using the incidence formula presented earlier, this represented an overall mortality incidence rate of 21.5 per 1000 person-years, much higher than the rate for equivalently aged people in the general population. This type of study was also able to calculate changes in mortality incidence over time and was also able to calculate cause-specific mortality such as overdose mortality and AIDS-related mortality.

The fundamentals of following-up a cohort over time and measuring health outcomes appear straightforward. Cohort studies are of course subject to the same issues of bias and confounding depending on the rigour of measurement and sampling. However, there are specific issues with cohort studies that complicate design and analysis. For example, the definition of exposure can be related to time – if a drug user has a period of abstinence or infrequent use, should that period still be a part of the cumulative person-years that define a period of risk? Many of these issues are addressed in detail later in the chapter in relation to bias and confounding.

The cohort studies described above are called a **prospective cohort study** because people are followed up, prospectively, in time. However, the analytical tools can easily be applied to study participants retrospectively. In a **retrospective cohort study**, participants are identified through recorded information and traced backwards to examine their exposures to possible risk factors. This type of design is attractive because they can be relatively cheap and you do not have to wait years to begin getting study results. However, retrospective cohort studies are susceptible to recall bias, and sometimes records which are used to identify participants or trace risk exposures may be incomplete or missing for some participants.

19.6 Analysis of case-control and cohort studies

There are similarities in the ways in which case-control and cohort studies are analysed. Both studies are fundamentally concerned with measuring the chance of an outcome occurring and, when comparing across exposure groups, we are concerned with comparative chance. The basic distinction between the analysis and interpretation of results in these studies can be seen in Figure 19.2. This figure shows a schematic of a case-control study and a cohort study, both designed to measure the effect of benzodiazepine use on the chance of experiencing overdose among heroin injectors. Although the hypothesis is the same, the resultant statistics used to test the hypothesis are different and need to be interpreted differently.

In the case-control study example detailed in Figure 19.2, we have purposively sampled according to the outcome of interest-heroin injectors that experienced an overdose and those that did not. Basic results are expressed as odds – the number of times the outcome occurs relative to the number of times it did not. In this example, we first want to know what the odds are that participants who

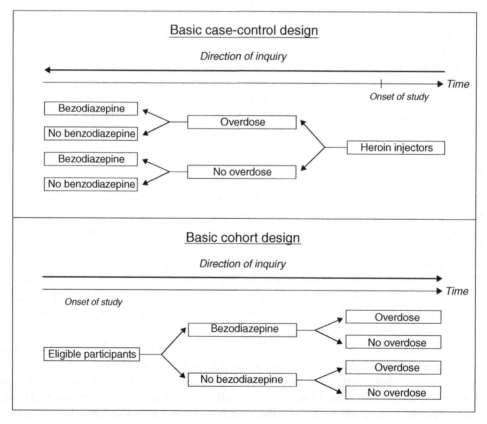

Figure 19.2 A hypothetical basic design for a case-control and a cohort studies.

Table 19.3 Display of data from the case-control and cohort studies

Exposure	Outcome		Total
	Overdose	No overdose	
Benzodiazepine	40	30	70
No benzodiazepine	80	140	220
Total	120	170	290

overdosed reported benzodiazepine use. We then need to know the odds that participants who did not overdose reported benzodiazepine use. The difference between the two odds is called the odds ratio – the basic statistic generated through case-control studies.

The **odds ratio** is traditionally generated using two-by-two tables. Table 19.3 displays hypothetical data from the case-control study described in Figure 19.2.

Table 19.3 shows that we have a total of 290 heroin injectors participating – 120 cases (experienced an overdose) and 170 controls (had not experienced an overdose). Of the overdose cases, 40 reported using benzodiazepines prior to overdosing and 80 reported not using benzodiazepines. Of the controls, 30 reported using benzodiazepines prior to their last injecting drug use session and 140 reported not using benzodiazepines.

We calculate benzodiazepine use odds in cases as: 40/80 = 0.50.

We calculate benzodiazepine use odds in controls as: 30/140 = 0.21.

We calculate the odds ratio as: 0.50/0.21 = 2.38.

We interpret an odds ratio (and risk ratios in cohort studies, see below) as follows:

$>1.0 \Rightarrow$ greater risk in the exposed
$\approx 1.0 \Rightarrow$ no association, no risk or protective effect from exposure
$<1.0 \Rightarrow$ lower risk in the exposed, protective effect

As such, we can interpret this result as suggesting that using benzodiazepines more than doubles (138% increase in comparative odds) the odds of an overdose among heroin injectors.

In the hypothetical cohort study presented in Figure 19.2, we have recruited a sample of heroin injectors, followed up them over time and recorded, among other things, their experience of overdose and the substances they have injected. In a cohort study design, basic results are expressed as risk. First, we can describe the risk of experiencing an overdose during follow-up among participants reporting benzodiazepine use. We can also determine the risk of overdose for those who do not report using benzodiazepines. The difference between the two risk estimates (the comparative chance) is called the **risk ratio** – the basic statistic generated through cohort studies.

Two-by-two tables are also used to generate risk ratios when analysing cohort study data. In the cohort study presented in Table 19.3, a total of 290 heroin injectors were recruited and interviewed every 3 months for 12 months. In this time, 120 participants reported experiencing at least one overdose and 170 did not. Of those reporting an overdose, 40 also reported using benzodiazepines during follow-up and 80 did not. Of those not reporting an overdose during follow-up, 30 reported using benzodiazepines during follow-up and 140 did not. The calculation of risk uses the same numbers to record outcomes as those used in the case-control example (numerator) but a different denominator.

We calculate the risk of overdose among benzodiazepine users as the number reporting an overdose out of all benzodiazepine users: 40/70 = 0.57.

We calculate the risk of overdose among non-benzodiazepine users as the number reporting an overdose out of all non-benzodiazepine users: 80/220 = 0.36.

We calculate the risk ratio as: 0.57/0.36 = 1.57.

The locations of risk ratios around 1.0 (>, ≈, and <) are interpreted in the same way as for odds ratios presented above. As such, we can interpret this result as suggesting that benzodiazepine use increases the risk of an overdose among heroin injectors by 57%.

19.6.1   Risk ratios versus odds ratios

As we have seen, both odds and risk measure the chance of an outcome occurring. But we can also see that the same data obtained from a case control and that obtained from a cohort study can produce markedly different ratios. Both estimates indicated that the use of benzodiazepines increased the chance of overdose among heroin injectors, but the magnitude of the chance was markedly different, dependent on which statistic is selected. So, which figure, the odds ratio or the risk ratio, is appropriate?

People generally think of chances of developing disease or some other outcome in terms of risk (i.e. what is the increased risk of overdose for benzodiazepine users?). Odds are less meaningful when thinking about health outcomes (i.e. what are the odds of an overdose if a person uses benzodiazepines?).

Of course, the risk ratios (the relative risk) cannot be calculated from all study designs. Odds ratios are a good approximation of risk in these circumstances, but are prone to overestimate risk when outcomes are more common (e.g. occurring among greater than 10% of an unexposed population). In our example, overdose prevalence in the non-benzodiazepine group (unexposed) exceeded one-third, and in this case the odds ratio should be considered an overestimate of risk.

19.7   Experimental study designs

There are two types of experimental designs used in epidemiology. In *clinical trials*, patients with a clinical condition receive either an intervention or no intervention (or some standard intervention). In this design, markers of patients' clinical condition are measured and compared between groups. In *preventive trials* (sometimes called community or community intervention trials), interventions are applied to a group of people (as opposed to a single patient) and the effectiveness of the intervention to prevent disease or enhance health is measured and compared to a group of people that do not receive the intervention.

In reality, preventive trials are rare in alcohol and other drug research. One type of intervention that does lend itself to evaluation through a preventive trial framework is school-based health and well-being interventions. These invariably involve components that aim to directly or indirectly influence substance use. For example, Hawthorne and colleagues (Hawthorne et al., 1995; Hawthorne, 1996) compared alcohol, smoking and analgesic use behaviours among students in a group of Australian schools that received Life Education with students in schools that did not receive the programme. Controversially, Hawthorne found that, not only did Life Education not prevent the use of these substances in the short term, but that students exposed to the programme were slightly more likely to use these substances.

19.8   Potential sources of error in epidemiology

Regardless of the time, resources and expertise of those involved, no research is perfect. All research is subject to some sort of error; it is simply that the best research within particular design parameters tries to limit this error as much as possible. So, what do we mean by error in epidemiology? When trying to understand error in epidemiology, it is perhaps most useful to think of epidemiology as simply an endeavour in measurement – largely of exposures and outcomes. Say, we wanted to estimate the incidence of psychotic events among recent amphetamine users in a given population. We can imagine that there is a true value for this outcome, but unless we followed up the entire population in question over time, prospectively recording and observing amphetamine consumption and episodes of psychosis, we cannot know exactly what this incidence value is. Instead, research will seek to estimate the true value by taking measures from a sample of the population. Research that produces a value that is close to the true value can be considered to have little error. Research that produces a value that is substantially different from the true value can be considered as having considerable error. Of course, because we do not know what the correct incidence is, we also cannot know exactly how much the estimated incidence differs from the true incidence. However, it is the job of the epidemiologist to adopt a research design that produces high-quality measurement and allows for reliable estimates of the association between exposures and outcomes. Such a design ultimately minimises the number of potential error sources, which can be thought of as random or systematic. Random error is really nothing more than an artefact of natural variability in data, whereas systematic error occurs as a result of the study design and execution.

19.8.1   Random error

Random error is related to probabilities and chance. As described in the above example, we cannot prove or definitively answer a research question unless we are able to take 'true' measures from entire populations. Regardless of how robust and methodically we take a sample from the population we are studying, there is a chance that we may simply have lucked upon a sample with certain characteristics that are not representative of the population and which produce results that are not therefore generalisable. It is not the poor execution of the study that is at fault here, but simply the natural variation to participant characteristics and bad luck.

It is beyond the scope of this chapter to delve deeply into the concept of random error. But readers should be aware that the best ways to control random error in studies are twofold:

1. Recruit a *sufficiently sized sample* to enhance the prospects that the group recruited reflects the natural variation of characteristics of the population (also enhanced through good sampling methods which are elaborated below when we discuss sampling bias).
2. Use *appropriate statistical techniques* which allow you to estimate the natural variability in data measurement and provide an indication as to how precise our approximations are.

19.8.2   Sample size and precision

The precision of an estimate of incidence for example is largely affected by two things: **variability** and **sample size**. Clearly, if the frequency of the outcome we are attempting to measure varies considerably in a population (e.g. across individual characteristics), it will be difficult to reliably measure incidence. However, if we recruit a sample of sufficient size, we hope to include in our sample enough variation in individual characteristics that our estimate will more precisely reflect what is happening in the true population. For example, the true probability of tails occurring when tossing a coin should be 0.5 (half the time). However, it would not be unexpected that if we tossed a coin 10 times, that tails might come up seven times, providing us with a probability estimate of 0.7 – in this result, random error would be said to be large. If, however, we tossed a coin 1000 times, the natural variability in heads and tails should mean that a closer approximation of the real probability of 0.5 emerges. Even if we ended up with 550 tails, our estimated probability of 0.55 much more closely estimates the true value.

The most commonly used estimate of precision readers will come across in epidemiology is the **confidence interval**, typically, a 95% confidence interval. Where possible, *all estimates produced in epidemiology should be accompanied by confidence intervals*. We can think of the actual estimate produced as almost like a best guess of the true value, but we accompany this best guess with a number below the estimate (lower confidence limit) and above the estimate (upper confidence limit) between which we are very confident the true value lies. Statistically, a 95% confidence interval is a set of numbers between which, if we replicated the data collection and analysis repeatedly, the true value of what we are measuring would occur 95% of the time. It is useful here to point out that research never 'proves' a hypothesis or provides perfectly accurate results, but simply indicates what is highly likely to be the truth.

19.8.3   Systematic error

Systematic error is also called **bias**. Although most people might think of bias as being an attribute of an individual, such as when a person is biased towards umpiring decisions that favour their own football team, bias can also refer to an attribute of a study. A study can be biased because of the way in which a sample is recruited (**sample bias**), or the way variables are measured in a study (**measurement bias**), or because not all things that potentially affect the results of a study have been measured and taken account of (**confounding**). Each of these sources of bias will be briefly described in the context of alcohol and other drug epidemiology.

19.8.4   Sample bias

Sampling bias occurs when procedures used to select participants or other factors that affect the likelihood of someone participating in a study result in a study sample that is not representative of the population being investigated. **Random sampling** (whereby every member of the target population should have the same chance of being recruited to a study) is held up as the gold standard method by which study recruitment should occur. However, this type of sampling is not often possible in alcohol and other drug research.

The clearest example of the difficulties associated with sampling bias occurs with low-prevalence illegal drug-using behaviours. If we take heroin injectors for example, there are characteristics of this population that would make true random sampling impossible:

1. Heroin injectors make up a small minority of the population and usually cluster within particular geographic locations in a community. A random population sample would need an enormous sample size to recruit enough heroin users for an effective study with reliable and generalisable findings.
2. Heroin injectors are often highly mobile, have higher rates of homelessness and incarceration. These factors make household or telephone sampling unreliable. These factors mean that not all members of the population would have the same chance of being sampled.

3. Heroin injectors engage in socially stigmatised and often illegal behaviours which they may attempt to conceal to minimise adverse legal or social consequences. As such, even if we could reach large proportions of this population and invite them into the study, many would not consent to participate due to fear regarding the disclosure of sensitive information.

Consequently, sampling of drug users is often done through service providers, but this would bias any study towards those that are more likely to use services and under-represent users not in touch with services, for whom adverse outcomes might be subsequently more prevalent. Sampling of drug users also often uses 'snowball' methods whereby new participants are obtained through the social networks of people already recruited to the study. This is again a method not without considerable potential for bias, although the development of more sophisticated snowballing methods such as **respondent-driven sampling** (see Salganik & Heckathorn, 2004; Abdul-Quader et al., 2006) have been proposed to minimise such bias.

19.8.5 Measurement bias

There are different types of measurement bias, but all relate to inaccuracies in the ways in which data are collected that result in incorrect reflections of reality, and which can produce erroneous research conclusions.

Misclassification bias occurs when an error is made when assigning a person to a particular group. For example, consider an investigation of adverse health outcomes between dependent and occasional users of analgesics. Based on self-reported analgesic use, participants are assigned to either a dependent or an occasional user group. If, however, people under-report (either consciously or unconsciously) their analgesic use, then some participants who should be classified as dependent are actually analysed as part of the occasional user group. This type of misclassification would potentially overestimate adverse health consequences in the occasional group and diminish our estimate of the differences in poor health outcomes between the groups.

Recall bias occurs when participants incorrectly recall past events in a survey or interview. Case-control and retrospective cohort studies are particularly prone to this type of error because they rely heavily on participants recalling past exposures. Consider an example of an investigation of the effect of cannabis use on psychosis using a case-control design. Because of their experience of psychotic episodes, cases have an additional stimulus to recall potential exposures that may have caused their illness. This may result in an overestimation of cannabis consumption in this group. Controls with no condition, or a condition not potentially associated with cannabis exposure, are more likely to blithely recall past patterns of cannabis consumption, and be more likely than among cases to be an underestimate. In this circumstance, association between cannabis consumption and later psychosis will be overestimated.

19.8.6 Confounding

Confounding is a fundamental consideration in epidemiology and a central issue in any study design. Confounding can be best thought of in terms of the simple examination of a single exposure and its effect on a single outcome. In this case, a third factor may be important in explaining the relationship between the exposure and the outcome. This factor is called a **confounding variable**. For instance, we have good reason to believe that heroin use leads to increased morbidity. However, we also know that heroin users are often socioeconomically disadvantaged and more likely to have poor nutrition. Poor nutrition also has an influence on our morbidity outcome – the confounding variable is related to both the exposure and the outcome. The problem of the confounding variable here is untangling how much morbidity is caused directly by heroin use and how much is caused by poor nutrition. The problem, of course, is actually much more complicated than this because we know that there are many more potential exposures that relate to heroin use and which will influence morbidity – homelessness, incarceration, dental hygiene, unemployment, social isolation and social capital, and a myriad of other factors which are all intertwined.

19.8.7   Controlling confounding

So, how do we go about controlling for confounding factors? Before we go into this, we need to confess that not all confounding can be controlled for. The assessment of confounders is done through a priori knowledge of relationships between variables and by observed relationships in the data we have. The first point is susceptible to flaws in previous research and theoretical suppositions, while the latter (which is in part informed by prior knowledge and thus susceptible to the same issues) is limited by the data that have been collected. We cannot, of course, assess the influence of a confounding factor that we either have not suspected as a confounder or have not measured. These points lead us to one way of trying to control confounding factors in the study design phase – assiduous background reading and thinking to ensure that data on as many possible confounders as possible are collected.

Confounding can also be limited in the study design phase through the randomisation of groups in an experimental design or by matching groups in an observational design. Even then, random error and bad luck could still influence an uneven distribution of confounding factors between groups. The problem here is that groups can only feasibly be matched on a limited number of factors and only those that researchers are able to measure. Many unknown or pragmatically not considered factors could still influence findings.

Confounding is also commonly controlled using advanced statistical methods such as modelling and regression techniques. In these types of analyses, the across sample data variability of multiple measures are considered simultaneously and controlled for. In this way, so-called pure relationships between two variables emerge. This type of result is often called a **standardised coefficient** because the coefficient (a measure of the association between variables) is standardised according to the other variables in the statistical model. This method is somewhat limited, however, by the number of variables a researcher might want to control for and the size of the study sample (controlling for more variables requires larger sample sizes). In addition, this method is also limited to the data the researcher has collected. Unknown or not measured factors can clearly not be controlled for statistically because the data are not there to do so.

19.9   Summary

Epidemiology is the study of the distribution and determinants of health across people, place and time. A central component of epidemiology is therefore the development and application of methods to measure health and exposures that influence health outcomes. Although alcohol and other drug epidemiology also involves the measurement of health, this field of epidemiology commonly measures the distribution and determinants of substance use as an outcome – a behaviour that, in mainstream epidemiology, might traditionally be perceived as an exposure that influences health.

The basic descriptive measurement approaches and research designs in alcohol and other drug epidemiology are consistent with more traditional areas of epidemiological enquiry. Measurements, such as the prevalence and incidence of substance use, are used to establish the scope of substance use behaviours, and exposures are measured to establish potential determinants of these outcomes. Most alcohol and other drug epidemiology is observational, with traditional epidemiological research designs such as cross-sectional surveys and cohort studies, establishing a hierarchy for the reliability of research findings.

The challenges associated with reliable and valid measurement in epidemiology, however, are compounded in alcohol and other drug epidemiology by the nature of substance use. Factors such as the low population prevalence and non-random distribution of certain types of substance use, the illicit nature of some drugs, and the stigma associated with certain substance-using behaviours, makes alcohol and other drug epidemiology particularly complex. To design and conduct good epidemiology studies in substance use, researchers require a thorough understanding of traditional epidemiological approaches and potential sources of bias and confounding in measurement, in addition to an appreciation of the complex social and behavioural context of substance use.

Exercises

1. Measurement in epidemiology is based on people, place and time. Construct a list of potential factors we might want to measure within each of these measurement domains to help us understand the possible determinants of:
   (a) Drug use initiation
   (b) Alcohol-related traffic accidents
   (c) Alcohol and other drug treatment demand
2. Calculate prevalence in each of the following examples:
   (a) An examination of coronial records from 1234 heroin overdose deaths found that 346 cases also had alcohol detected in their blood. What is the prevalence of heroin overdose deaths in which alcohol was also implicated?
   (b) Among 2678 secondary school students who completed a telephone survey, 658 reported recent (past 6 months) use of cannabis. What is the prevalence of recent cannabis consumption in this study?
   (c) In 1 year, 1347 prison receptions were tested for hepatitis C. Among 721 of these, hepatitis C antibodies (a marker of hepatitis C virus exposure) were detected and 285 were PCR positive (a marker of chronic hepatitis C infection). What is the prevalence of hepatitis C exposure and chronic hepatitis C infection in this prison entry sample? In this sample, what is the prevalence of chronic hepatitis C among those exposed to the hepatitis C virus?
3. If a study recruited 345 adolescents and followed-up them for 3.5 years, what would the total person-years of follow-up be? What descriptive epidemiological measurement would we calculate with this unit of time?
4. In the above study, 67 adolescents reported initiating tobacco smoking and 17 reported initiating ecstasy use. What is the incidence of initiation of tobacco smoking and ecstasy use in this sample (be sure to convert your answer into an appropriate and meaningful unit)?
5. Critique the following statement:

   We have found in several countries a strong association between the prevalence of amyl and Viagra consumption reported in surveys of gay communities and incident rates for HIV among gay men. This demonstrates clearly that the consumption of these types of drugs is contributing to increased transmission of HIV in gay men.

6. A case-control study aimed at investigating possible links between depression and the use of amphetamines recruited 150 outpatient participants with depression from a hospital clinic and 150 participants not previously diagnosed with depression from nearby workplaces. All participants completed a detailed survey that asked them about previous exposures, including

substance use. Outline the limitations of this research design in the light of potential sources of bias and confounding.

7. A research team wishes to investigate a possible causal relationship between the injection of pharmaceuticals and endocarditis – a relatively rare and potentially fatal cardiac condition affecting the function of heart valves. Provide a schematic description of this investigation using a prospective cohort and a case-control design. Which of these research designs would be most appropriate for this research question and why?

8. Using data from a case–control study of regular cannabis users presented in the following table, calculate the appropriate statistics to describe the association between the mode of cannabis consumption and occurrence of upper respiratory tract infections. Provide a written interpretation of your final result.

	Outcome		
Exposure	Upper respiratory tract infection	No upper respiratory tract infection	Total
Primary 'bong' smoker	139	274	375
Primary 'joint' smoker	59	174	233
Total	198	410	608

9. A prospective cohort study followed-up a group of hepatitis C negative regular injectors over a 4-year period to investigate factors associated with subsequent hepatitis C infection. The following table describes data on hepatitis C seroconversion according the high-versus-low injecting frequency. Using these data, calculate the appropriate statistics to describe the association between the frequency of injecting and hepatitis C seroconversion. Provide a written interpretation of your final result.

	Outcome		
Exposure	HCV seroconversion	HCV negative	Total
Inject daily or more often	318	173	491
Inject less than daily but more than weekly	281	328	609
Total	599	501	1100

10. Accounting for participant losses over time, the follow-up of the cohort study described above accounted for a total of 3213 person-years of follow-up – 1301 person-years for the daily or more injectors and 1912 person-years for the less than weekly, more than daily injectors. Calculate the hepatitis C incident rate for the whole cohort and for each frequency of injecting group (again, be sure to convert your answer into an appropriate and meaningful unit).

11. Critique the following research design:

Khat is a stimulant-type substance primarily cultivated in East Africa and the Middle East. Although Khat consumption is not common in Western populations, there have been reports of increasing popularity within some drug-using subcultures such at dance parties and raves. In addition, the cultural attachment with Khat means that its consumption remains popular within Middle Eastern and African communities that have settled in Western countries.

> *Because we believe that Khat consumption is not high, we aim to survey a large number of respondents in order to get a more reliable and accurate estimate of the prevalence of Khat consumption. We propose to place research assistants at three major metropolitan train stations during peak-hour services to determine the prevalence of lifetime and recent consumption of Khat in a sample of 5000 respondents.*

12. Discuss the potential sources of systematic bias in the following research design:

> *A case-control study is investigating associations between early initiation of substance use and cognitive disorders in adulthood. All patients diagnosed with cognitive disorders using standard thinking and reasoning tests in four major outpatient clinics between 1996 and 2001 were invited to participate in the study. Of 2670 diagnoses, 1231 participants consented to completing a standardised survey and an interview with a trained clinician designed to explore developmental factors reasoned to influence the occurrence of cognitive disorders.*

References

Abdul-Quader, A. S., Heckathorn, D. D., McKnight, C., Bramson, H., Nemeth, C., Sabin, K., Gallagher, K. & Des Jarlais, D. C. (2006) Effectiveness of respondent-driven sampling for recruiting drug users in New York city: findings from a pilot study. *Journal of Urban Health*, 83(3), 459–476.

Bargagli, A. M., Sperati, A., Davoli, M., Forastiere, F. & Perucci, C. A. (2001) Mortality among problem drug users in Rome: an 18-year follow-up study, 1980–1997. *Addiction*, 96, 1455–1463.

Bauer, J. E., Hyland, A., Li, Q., Steger, C. & Cummings, K. M. (2005) A longitudinal assessment of the impact of smoke-free worksite policies on tobacco use. *American Journal of Public Health*, 95(6), 1024–1029.

Benson, K. & Hartz, A. J. (2000) A comparison of observational studies and randomized, controlled trials. *New England Journal of Medicine*, 342(25), 1878–1886.

Borges, G., Cherpital, C. & Mittleman, M. A. (2004) Risk of injury after alcohol consumption: a case-crossover study in the emergency department. *Social Science and Medicine*, 58(6), 1191–1200.

Concato, J., Shah, N. & Horwitz, R. I. (2000) Randomized, controlled trials, observational studies, and the hierarchy of research designs. *New England Journal of Medicine*, 342, 1887–1892.

DeWit, D. J., Adlaf, E. M., Offord, D. R. & Ogborne, A. C. (2000) Age at first alcohol use: a risk factor for the development of alcohol disorders. *American Journal of Psychiatry*, 157, 745–750.

Dietze, P., Jolley, D., Fry, C. & Bammer, G. (2005) Transient changes in behaviour lead to heroin overdose: results from a case-crossover study of non-fatal overdose. *Addiction*, 100(5), 636–642.

Doll, R. & Hill, A. B. (1950) Smoking and carcinoma of the lung. Preliminary report. *British Medical Journal*, ii, 739–748.

Doll, R. & Hill, A. B. (1964) Mortality in relation to smoking: ten years' observations of British doctors. *British Medical Journal*, i, 1399–1410, 1460–1467.

Doll, R. & Peto, R. (1976) Mortality in relation to smoking: 20 years' observation on male British doctors. *British Medical Journal*, ii, 1525–1536.

Doll, R., Peto, R., Wheatley, K., Gray, R. & Sutherland, I. (1994) Mortality in relation to smoking: 40 years' observations of male British doctors. *British Medical Journal*, 309, 901–911.

Hawthorne, G. (1996) The social impact of Life Education: estimating drug use prevalence among Victorian primary school students and the statewide effect of the Life Education programme. *Addiction*, 91, 1151–1159.

Hawthorne, G., Garrard, J. & Dunt, D. (1995) Does Life Education's drug education programme have a public health benefit? *Addiction*, 90, 205–215.

Ioannidis, J. P., Haidich, A. B. & Lau, J. (2001) Any casualties in the clash of randomised and observational evidence? *British Medical Journal*, 322, 879–880.

Kozlowski, L. T., O'Connor, R. J., Edwards, B. Q. & Flaherty, B. P. (2003) Most smokeless tobacco use is not a causal gateway to cigarettes: using order of product use to evaluate causation in a national US sample. *Addiction*, 98, 1077–1085.

MacDonald, M., Law, M., Kaldor, J., Hales, J. & Dore, G. J. (2003) Effectiveness of needle and syringe programmes for preventing HIV transmission. *International Journal of Drug Policy*, 14, 353–357.

Mittleman, M. A., Lewis, R. A., Maclure, M., Sherwood, J. B. & Muller, J. E. (2001) Triggering myocardial infarction by marijuana. *Circulation*, 103(23), 2805–2809.

Murphy, W. L., DeVita, D., Liu, H., Vittinghoff, E., Leung, P., Ciccarone, D. H., & Edlin, B. R. (2001) Risk factors for skin and soft-tissue abscesses among injection drug users: a case-control study. *The Journal of Infectious Diseases*, 33, 35–40.

Ramstedt, M. (2002) Alcohol-related mortality in 15 European countries in the postwar period. *European Journal of Population*, 18, 307–323.

Redelmeier, D. A. & Tibshirani, R. J. (1997) Association between cellular-telephone calls and motor vehicle collisions. *New England Journal of Medicine*, 336, 453–458.

Salganik, M. J. & Heckathorn, D. D. (2004) Sampling and estimation in hidden populations using respondent-driven sampling. *Sociological Methodology*, 34, 193–239.

Vanichsenia, S., Kitayapornb, D., Mastrob, T., Mock, P., Rakthama, S., Des Jarlais, D., Sujarita, S., Srisuwanvilai, L., Young, N. L., Wasi, C., Subbarao, S., Heyward, W. L., Esparza, J. & Choopanya, K. (2001) Continued high HIV-1 incidence in a vaccine trial preparatory cohort of injection drug users in Bangkok, Thailand. *AIDS*, 15, 397–405.

Vinson, D. C., Mabe, N., Leonard, L. L., Alexander, J., Becker, J., Boyer, J. & Moll, J. (1995) Alcohol and injury: a case-crossover study. *Archives of Family Medicine*, 4, 505–511.

Recommended websites

http://www.openepi.com/menu/openEpiMenu.htm
OpenEpi
This website contains free, open source, online access to software for epidemiological analyses.

http://www.emcdda.europa.eu/html.cfm/index190EN.html
The European Monitoring Centre for Drugs and Drug Addiction (EMCDDA)
The EMCDDA is the European hub for drug-related information. The EMCDDA website contains dozens of epidemiology, surveillance and research reports relating to drug use at European national and multinational levels.

http://ndarc.med.unsw.edu.au/
The Australian National Drug and Alcohol Research Centre (NDARC)
The NDARC at the University of New South Wales coordinates many key epidemiological and surveillance projects to monitor substance use in Australia. The NDARC website contains excellent examples of technical reports and papers covering a range of substance use epidemiology topics.

http://www.unodc.org/unodc/en/data-and-analysis/WDR.html
United Nations Office of Drugs and Crime (UNODC) World Drug Report
This UNODC website contains the annual World Drug Reports dating back to 1997. These reports collate epidemiological data from around the world to describe a range of drug-related issues including the prevalence of consumption, trafficking and production of licit and illicit drugs.

http://www.wiley.com/bw/journal.asp?ref=0965-2140&site=1
Peer-reviewed journal – *Addiction*
This journal is the top-ranked (impact factor) journal in the substance use field and routinely publishes epidemiological studies on substance use and associated behaviours.

http://www.sciencedirect.com/science/journal/03768716
Peer-reviewed journal – *Drug and Alcohol Dependence*
This journal is the second-ranked (impact factor) journal in the substance use field. *Drug and Alcohol Dependence* publishes research on a wide range disciplinary approaches to substance use, including epidemiology.

Chapter 20

META-ANALYSIS: SUMMARISING FINDINGS ON ADDICTION INTERVENTION EFFECTS

John W. Finney and Anne Moyer

20.1   Introduction

Consider a hypothetical practice guideline panel that is charged with making a recommendation about a treatment that has been shown to be significantly better than a comparison condition in 10 studies, but produced results indistinguishable from the comparison condition in 8 other studies. Not only have these 18 relevant studies produced different findings, they have also used different outcome measures, sampled research participants from different populations and used different treatments as a comparison condition. How can the guideline panel or anyone else make sense out of that body of research? In situations like these, meta-analytic techniques are especially useful in synthesising results across studies and identifying factors that explain differences in results.

'Meta-analysis', a term first coined by Glass (1976), refers to systematic techniques that quantitatively combine findings from multiple studies. An index of the size of the effect from each study is calculated and then these 'effect sizes' are aggregated. In the addiction field, meta-analyses have been used to summarise findings on a wide range of topics, including the psychometric characteristics of an alcohol-screening instrument (e.g. Berner et al., 2007), cognitive factors that predict ecstasy use (Peters et al., 2008), the link between smoking and developing cancer at various sites (Gandini et al., 2008), and how short-term and long-term methamphetamine use affects the central nervous system (Scott et al., 2007). In this chapter, we focus on meta-analyses of addiction, including substance misuse, and intervention effects.

20.2   Overview of meta-analytic methods

The goals in conducting a meta-analysis of intervention effects are typically similar to those of a primary intervention study. Primary intervention studies usually focus on how well an intervention 'works' relative to a comparison condition. In a meta-analysis, a reviewer wants to determine across multiple studies the magnitude of the effect of an intervention versus a comparison condition. In a primary intervention study, an investigator may also attempt to explain variation in effects among research participants: Are individuals who smoke more cigarettes each day more likely to respond to a medication than those who smoke fewer? Likewise, a meta-analyst may ask: Is the effect of a particular intervention stronger in studies depending on the proportion of high-volume smokers in the samples?

In conducting a meta-analysis, a research question is first formulated. Then, rigorous search procedures help to identify and obtain reports of studies meeting eligibility criteria. Information is abstracted from the reports so that (a) relationships or intervention effects of interest can be calculated and (b) relevant characteristics of the studies can be codified. The data are then analysed and the results are interpreted. Thorough documentation of procedures means that meta-analytic reviews can be scrutinised and replicated, just as primary studies can.

Research questions amenable to such syntheses are those for which a number of prior quantitative studies have amassed. In addition to providing clear summaries of the results of prior studies, a meta-analysis can provide 'synthesis-generated' evidence by examining the relationships between study-level 'moderator variables' and effect sizes. A 'moderator' variable is one that is linked to differences in the magnitude and even the direction of a relationship between two other variables (e.g. that between intervention/comparison condition status and outcome). For example, effect sizes for a medication (versus placebo) for alcohol use disorders might vary across studies depending on the alcohol use disorder severity (a moderator) of the studies' samples.

In addition to sample characteristics (such as severity or gender composition), other common moderator variables examined to explain variation in effect sizes across studies include type of intervention, type of outcome variable and/or how outcomes were assessed, and research design (e.g. randomised controlled trial versus naturalistic study). By examining moderator variables, research syntheses can address questions that have not been directly investigated in primary studies. For instance, a meta-analysis of 72 clinical trials examining motivational interviewing to alter alcohol use and other behaviours found that *un*manualised as opposed to manualised interventions had significantly more positive outcomes and noted that no primary study addressed this question (Hettema et al., 2005). Research syntheses can also point to areas for additional research or theory development. For example, Hettema et al.'s meta-analysis found variation in motivational interviewing effect sizes across providers, populations, target problems and settings, indicating that this intervention's mechanisms of action are not well understood and should be the focus of future inquiry.

20.2.1   Research question(s) and study eligibility criteria

One research question involved in synthesising addiction intervention research is usually straightforward: What is the magnitude of the effect of the intervention (vs a comparison condition) on outcome? Other research questions might involve moderator variables. For example, how does the effect of an intervention vary by aggregated recipient characteristics (e.g. severity of addiction or gender composition) across studies?

In most cases, the research questions will need further specification, which occurs during the formulation of study eligibility criteria, for instance:

- What are the parameters of the intervention(s) to be included (e.g. cognitive–behavioural therapy, more broadly, social skills training, more specifically)?
- What is the relevant population of research participants (e.g. persons with unhealthy drinking, but not alcohol dependence; persons with diagnoses of opioid dependence)?
- What outcome variable(s) will be included (e.g. continuous abstinence from smoking; number of cigarettes smoked)?
- Will both randomised and 'naturalistic' or quasi-experimental trials be included?
- Will reports that have not been published in peer-reviewed journals be included?

The eligibility criteria can also encompass 'demographic' features of studies (i.e. year of publication, language of report).

20.2.2   Identifying relevant studies

Once the research questions and eligibility criteria have been formulated, a comprehensive literature search is performed and reports are examined to determine the studies that meet the specified eligibility criteria. Comprehensive literature searches typically involve multiple channels, such as bibliographic databases, reference sections of retrieved primary study reports and review articles, and select journal tables of contents. In addition, trial registries (e.g. http://clinicaltrials.gov), conference proceedings and researchers working in the field of interest are sources of relevant unpublished studies (White, 2009).

Depending on the intended scope of the synthesis, the eligibility criteria may be more or less inclusive. For instance, a meta-analysis examining the efficacy of cognitive–behavioural relapse prevention for substance use (Irvin et al., 1999) took a broad approach, including published and unpublished studies reported from 1978 to 1995 that investigated interventions directed at alcohol use disorders, substance use disorders and smoking, and that used varying types of comparison conditions; this strategy identified 26 relevant studies. In contrast, a meta-analysis with a narrower scope examined the efficacy of the relatively new medication naltrexone in preventing relapse among alcohol-dependent individuals and focused only on randomised, placebo-controlled trials (Streeton & Whelan, 2001); this strategy identified seven relevant studies.

20.2.3   Coding study characteristics

Studies are then coded to provide information on their features. The number of variables coded can vary, depending on the scope and goals of the synthesis. Extracted information is recorded on coding forms guided by a coding manual (see Lipsey & Wilson, 2001, for an example of each). Some coded information is at the study level and can be included on a single form (e.g. participant characteristics, type of research design). Other information, such as data on different outcomes variables assessed at different follow-up points that are used in calculating specific effect sizes, can be coded on separate forms and linked to the study-level information by a study ID number. This multi-level information can then be entered into a relational database.

Coding decisions in meta-analyses are not always straightforward. Thus, intercoder reliability is typically evaluated by having at least two raters independently code a sample of project reports. Reliability of coding can be expressed in a variety of ways, such as per cent agreement between coders, an intra-class correlation coefficient or a kappa coefficient (see Orwin & Vevea, 2009). If a large number of studies is to be coded, it can be valuable to also evaluate intracoder reliability to determine if there is coding 'drift' over time. Regular meetings in which coding decisions are discussed can help maintain between- and within-coder consistency.

20.2.4   Calculating effect sizes within studies

Quantitative summaries of diverse literatures reporting different outcomes are made possible by expressing each outcome to be synthesised in a 'common currency'. The most frequently used effect sizes in meta-analyses are the standardised mean difference, the odds ratio and the correlation coefficient. The **standardised mean difference** is the difference between the means on a continuous outcome variable for an intervention and a comparison condition, typically divided by the pooled standard deviation of the two groups. This **effect size** indicates by how many standard deviations, or by what proportion of a standard deviation, the intervention group is functioning better than the comparison condition. Hedges and Olkin (1985) demonstrated that the standardised mean difference

---

Box 20.1　Calculating odds ratios

	Living	Deceased	Odds of mortality at follow-up	Likelihood of mortality at follow-up	Odds ratio – treatment vs no treatment	Likelihood of mortality ratio – treatment vs no treatment
Treatment	144	16	16/144 = 0.11	16/160 = 0.10	0.11/0.25 = 0.44	0.10/0.20 = 0.50
No treatment	128	32	32/128 = 0.25	32/160 = 0.20		

The example of the outcomes of 160 individuals receiving treatment and 160 individuals receiving no treatment, with respect to their odds and likelihood (probability) of mortality at a follow-up.

---

estimator of effect sizes in studies with small samples is upwardly biased (tends to be too large). Consequently, most meta-analysts use the effect size developed by Hedges and Olkin that adjusts for this bias.

Odds ratios can be used to calculate effect sizes for truly dichotomous outcomes (e.g. mortality status). An odds ratio of 1.00 indicates no difference between a treatment and a comparison conditions on a dichotomous outcome. 'Odds' are the probability of something happening divided by the probability of it not happening. Thus, if 10% of the individuals in a treatment group had died by at an extended follow-up point, the odds of mortality for that group would be 0.10/0.90 or 0.11. If 20% of the individuals in a no-treatment comparison condition were deceased at follow-up, the odds of mortality for that group would be 0.20/0.80 or 0.25. An 'odds ratio' is the odds for one group divided by the odds for another group. In our example, the odds ratio of mortality for the treatment group relative to the control group would be 0.11/0.25 or 0.44. Note, however, that treatment group members are not 0.44 times as likely to die as control group members, but are 0.5 times as likely (0.10 in the treatment group vs 0.20 in the control group). See also the calculations in Box 20.1.

Some dichotomous outcomes in addiction intervention studies can be conceptualised as having an underlying continuous distribution. For example, 'relapsed to heavy drinking' (Y/N) is a dichotomised form of a continuous alcohol use dimension. For such dichotomous outcome variables, the d_{Probit} estimate can be used to yield relatively unbiased estimates of the effect size for the underlying continuous outcome with either normal or skewed distributions (see Sanchez-Meca et al., 2003). As a further check, one should determine if continuous versus dichotomised continuous outcome is a moderator of effect sizes (Lipsey & Wilson, 2001). If effect sizes do differ by type of outcome measure, the meta-analysis should be conducted separately for each type.

Finally, a **correlation coefficient** (r, transformed to Fisher's Z scores for analyses) can be used to express the relationship between a continuous intervention dimension and an outcome. Typically, 'intervention' is not a continuous variable in addiction studies, but there are exceptions. For example, Tonigan et al. (1996) used r as the effect size to examine the relationship between amount of Alcoholics Anonymous involvement (a continuous variable) and drinking outcomes. Correlation coefficients can usually be converted into standardised between-group mean effect sizes (but see McGrath & Meyer, 2006).

Study reports do not always provide the information (e.g. the means and standard deviations on a continuous outcome for the intervention and comparison groups) needed to calculate effect sizes directly. If results of statistical tests are reported, those can often be used to estimate effect sizes (but see Ray & Shadish, 1996). For example, the value of a t-test can be readily converted into a standardised mean difference effect size. Software programmes are listed in 'Technical assistance' section at the end of the chapter that compute effect sizes from the results of various statistical tests.

Typically, in calculating effect sizes, scores on 'negative' outcomes variables, such as problems associated with drug use, are reverse-scored so that higher scores on both negative and positive outcomes (e.g. per cent days abstinent) indicate better functioning at follow-up. This process allows effect sizes for positive and negative outcomes from a study to be combined and yield a meaningful overall study effect size. Another convention is for a positive effect size to indicate that the intervention was more beneficial than the comparison condition. Effect sizes for multiple outcomes in a given domain (e.g. smoking behaviour) are aggregated (usually averaged) so that there is a single effect size for each study for that outcome domain.

20.2.5   Calculating aggregated effect sizes across studies

Effect sizes derived from individual studies need to be synthesised to arrive at some estimate of the magnitude of the pooled effect size across studies and to determine if this aggregated effect size differs significantly from zero. These calculations can be made with a 'fixed-effects' or a 'random-effects' model. The **fixed-effects** approach assumes that the error in estimating the population effect size stems only from random factors associated with subject-level sampling error, whereas random-effects approaches assume that there is study-level sampling error in addition to subject-level sampling error (see Lipsey & Wilson, 2001, p. 117). '**Random-effects** models treat the effect size parameters as if they were a random sample from a population of effect parameters and estimate hyperparameters (usually just the mean and variance), describing this population of effect parameters...' (Hedges & Vevea, 1998, p. 486). Thus, a random-effects model allows inferences about effect sizes to be generalised beyond the specific sample of studies examined, whereas for a fixed-effects analysis, conclusions are limited to the set of studies examined (Hedges & Vevea, 1998). Typically, a random-effects model is preferred. However, a fixed-effect model has more statistical power (Hedges & Pigott, 2001), so with a small number of relevant studies, a meta-analyst may be willing to trade increased power for reduced generalisability.

It is sometimes suggested that the results of a '**homogeneity test**' (discussed below) should drive the decision of whether a random- or fixed-effects model is used. However, Hedges and Vevea (1998) argue convincingly that the choice of a model should depend on the inferences the meta-analyst wishes to make from the results of the analysis. Usually, the greater generalisability afforded by a random-effects analysis is desirable. Regardless of which approach is used, effect sizes from studies with larger sample sizes (Ns) are more precise (have less variance across studies) and are given greater weight in calculating the overall effect size using an inverse variance formula (Hedges & Olkin, 1985). Weighting effect size estimates across studies, computing the weighted summary effect size and testing whether the summary effect size differs significantly from zero in either a random- or fixed-effects analyses can be done using specific programmes for meta-analyses or by using routines and macros in standard statistical analysis software (see 'Technical assistance' section at the end of the chapter).

20.2.6   Analysing moderator variables

Another goal of many meta-analyses is to explain variation in study-level effect sizes by examining potential moderator variables (e.g. different interventions, participant sample characteristics or methods across studies). First, however, a meta-analyst will determine if effect sizes vary more than one would expect from subject-level sampling fluctuations in a fixed-effect model or more than subject-level sampling fluctuations and an additional study-level random factor in a random-effects model. In other words, is there additional variation in effect sizes that might be explained by moderator variables? A 'homogeneity test' (a Q test; Hedges & Olkin, 1985; Viechtbauer, 2007) is used to determine whether such 'excess variation' is present. It is also useful to calculate the I^2 index (Higgins & Thompson, 2002; Huedo-Medina et al., 2006) to estimate the proportion of the total variation in effect sizes due to 'heterogeneity' across studies.

To determine the extent to which moderator variables account for excess variation in study effect sizes, meta-analysts typically use analogues of analysis of variance and regression analysis techniques (Hedges & Olkin, 1985). For analysing the effects of a dichotomous moderator variable (e.g. Intervention A vs Intervention B as compared to a control condition), the between- and within-category homogeneity tests described in Hedges and Olkin (1985) can be used. The between-category test determines if a moderator variable is significantly related to variation in the magnitude of effect sizes. The within-category test determines if the variation remaining within categories of the moderator variable following the between-category test exceeds that which would be expected from sampling fluctuations. If significant, it indicates that still other study features may account for the remaining variation in effect sizes. For example, a between-category analysis may indicate that the effect sizes for Intervention A (in comparison to a control condition) are significantly larger than those for Intervention B (in comparison to the same control condition), but the within-category (i.e. within the group of studies for Intervention A and for Intervention B) homogeneity test could indicate that there was still additional variation in, say, post-intervention drinking behaviour that might be explained by one or more additional moderator variables.

Regression analyses (see Hedges & Olkin, 1985) can be used to determine how well a single continuous moderator variable (e.g. length of intervention) or a set of moderator variables accounts for variation in effect sizes. With multiple moderator variables, the independent 'effect' of each can be estimated. Product terms, in which a score on one moderator variable is multiplied by that on another moderator variable for each study, can be included in the regression analysis to determine if the moderator variables interact in a linear way to explain effect sizes. For example, the interaction between type of outcome variable and research design might explain more of the variance in intervention effect sizes than the additive or main effects of those two moderator variables.

20.2.7 Statistical power of meta-analytic techniques

Like that for many of the statistical procedures used in primary intervention studies, the *a priori* power of the meta-analytic techniques described above can be calculated. Hedges and Pigott (2001) discuss calculating the power of fixed- and random-effects model analyses to estimate pooled effect sizes. Just as sample size is influential in determining the statistical power of primary intervention studies to detect significant effects, the power of meta-analytic procedures is driven heavily by the N of studies. An aggregated effect size that is not significantly different from zero in an underpowered meta-analysis is weak evidence of a lack of an intervention effect in the population(s) of studies (Hedges & Pigott, 2001).

Tests for interaction effects (e.g. the patient by type of treatment interactions in accounting for patient outcomes) in primary studies have less power than tests for main effects (e.g. of treatment). Likewise, tests of moderator variables in meta-analyses generally have less power than do tests of the summary effect sizes in meta-analyses (Hedges & Pigott, 2004). Awareness of the power of moderator variable analyses is important because it may be used to rule out study characteristics (e.g. participant characteristics) as factors that are linked to effect sizes variation across studies. If a moderator test has low power and the result is non-significant, the mistaken impression can be conveyed that the moderator variable is not linked to different magnitudes of effect sizes. Low-power moderator tests should either not be conducted in the first place, or if they are conducted, their low power should be reported (Hedges & Pigott, 2004). On the other hand, if the test of a variable's ability to account for heterogeneity in effect sizes has high power, a failure to find a significant moderating effect can be interpreted with some confidence as indicating that the moderator variable does not 'explain' variation in between-study effect sizes. Meta-analytic reports should provide information on the *a priori* statistical power of the analyses presented.

20.2.8 Evaluating publication bias

Even with a rigorous literature search process, a meta-analyst is unlikely to locate every study that has been conducted on the topic of interest. Published reports of studies are more readily found than are unpublished reports. 'Publication bias' refers to the tendency of studies with significant findings to be more likely to be published than studies with non-significant results. Although publication bias is often thought of in terms of the tendency for journals not to publish submitted manuscripts unless they report significant results, researchers terminating studies that are not yielding significant results, or not submitting a report with non-significant results, also contribute to publication bias (Kraemer et al., 1998).

To probe for publication bias, meta-analysts often generate 'funnel plots' that graphically depict the relationship between studies' effect sizes and sample sizes. Effect sizes from smaller studies will have more variation than effect sizes from larger studies, so the plot usually will resemble an upside-down funnel. If there is no publication bias, the funnel plot should be laterally symmetrical (see Figure 20.1). An asymmetrical funnel plot in which larger effect sizes tend to come from smaller studies (more likely in early published results) can signal publication bias.

In addition to visual inspection of funnel plots, statistical methods have been developed to evaluate asymmetry in funnel plots (see Rothstein et al., 2005). However, Sutton and Higgins (2008) note that 'unfortunately, there is still widespread lack of appreciation that funnel plot asymmetry can be due to causes other than publication bias; any influential covariate that is related to precision (or sample

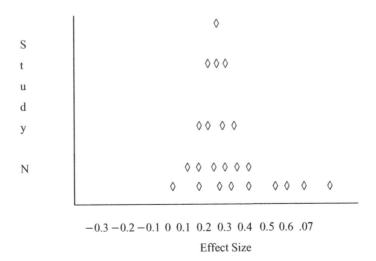

Figure 20.1 A funnel plot of hypothetical data on study sample sizes and effect sizes.

size) can induce such a pattern through confounding' (p. 632). Kraemer et al. (1998) have suggested that the influence of publication bias could be substantially reduced if only studies that had a priori statistical power to detect a 'critical effect size', that is 'one that conveys the researcher's threshold of clinical or policy significance' (p. 26), were included in a meta-analysis. Lipsey and Wilson (2001) argue that this proposal counteracts the advantage of meta-analyses to achieve sufficient power by aggregating results from multiple underpowered studies. However, aggregation of findings from a few early published studies would likely yield upwardly biased estimates of effect sizes.

Some meta-analysts use the 'trim and fill' method developed by Duval and Tweedie (2000; see also Peters et al., 2007) to conduct sensitivity analyses to explore whether adjusting for 'missing studies' alters aggregate effect size estimates. First, the number of 'missing studies' is estimated (see Duval & Tweedie, 2000, or Peters et al., 2007, for formulae for different approaches to estimating the number of missing studies). The assumption is that effect sizes for 'missing studies' would not be included in the lower left side of the asymmetrical funnel because of publication bias. Next, the effect sizes for that estimated number of studies are deleted (trimmed) from the lower right side of the funnel (i.e. effect sizes for published studies with small samples and large effect sizes) and the aggregated effect size of the more symmetrical set of remaining studies is calculated. That new aggregated effect size estimate is then used to calculate a new estimate of the number of missing studies and which are then trimmed. This process is repeated until the estimate of the number of missing studies is stable. At that point, all the previously trimmed effect sizes are re-inserted and mirror-image counterparts of them are placed (filled) on the left size of the funnel plot, after which the 'final' adjusted estimate of the pooled effect size is calculated.

20.2.9 Reporting findings

Like the CONSORT statement for reporting primary randomised clinical trials (RCTs) (Altman et al., 2001), the QUOROM checklist (Moher et al., 1999) guides the reporting of meta-analyses of RCTs. It provides recommendations for the information to be included in the abstract, introduction, methods, results and discussion sections of meta-analytic reports. It also includes recommendations for presenting information on the numbers of RCTs identified, included and excluded, as well as the reasons for excluding trials in a flow diagram.

Reports of meta-analyses often present results on effect sizes across studies in a 'forest plot' (Figure 20.2). Forest plots convey a great deal of information. Varying magnitudes of effect sizes are arrayed

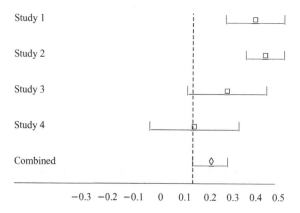

Figure 20.2 A forest plot of four hypothetical studies comparing an intervention and a control condition.

along the horizontal axis. A zero effect size (intervention no better or worse than the comparison condition) sometimes is indicated by a vertical line. The plot gives the effect size for each study (indicated in Figure 20.2 by a '□'), along with a horizontal line indicating the 95% confidence interval for that effect size. The width of the confidence interval succinctly conveys the relative sample sizes of each study (larger studies have narrower confidence intervals). The final row in the forest plot usually presents the summary effect size across studies (indicated by a '◇' in Figure 20.2) and its confidence interval. If the confidence interval for an effect size for a particular study or the pooled effect size across studies does not subsume zero, it indicates that the effect size is significantly different from zero.

To convey results to audiences for which differences in standard deviation units have little meaning, effect sizes sometimes are converted to a metric that will be more clinically meaningful. For example, the 'binomial effect size display' (Rosenthal & Rubin, 1982) converts effect sizes to a difference in success rates for intervention and comparison conditions (Hsu, 2004, suggests the binomial effect size display overestimates differences in success rates; see also Thompson & Schumacker, 1997). The 'number needed to treat' (Laupacis et al., 1988) refers to the number of individuals that would need to receive the intervention in order to have one more individual with a positive outcome (e.g. abstinence) relative to the comparison condition. Thus, a number needed to treat of ten indicates that ten people would need to be treated in order to have one more abstinent person than would be found if the ten persons had received the comparison condition.

A forest plot provides a great deal of important information about one of the main goals of most meta-analyses, effects sizes within and across studies. Usually, information about moderator variables is presented in tables and in the narrative of a meta-analysis report. However, Ogilvie et al. (2008) suggest a 'harvest plot' can be useful in succinctly and visually conveying more complex findings on moderator variables, multiple outcomes and other study features (e.g. methodological quality).

20.3 Issues in meta-analyses of addiction interventions

In this section, we consider issues that arise commonly in research syntheses in this field, although they are not unique to meta-analyses of findings on addiction intervention effects.

20.3.1 Participant characteristics as moderator variables

Consumers of meta-analyses want to be able to make some estimate of the population to which the results can generalise and whether interventions have different effects for different populations. If narrow, clearly specified study participant characteristics are used as inclusion criteria in selecting studies for the meta-analysis, then the population to which findings generalise may be straightforward. With a broader selection of studies, sample compositions may vary more and participant characteristics become potentially important moderator variables to examine.

For example, in a meta-analysis by Moyer et al. (2002), brief interventions for alcohol misuse provided mainly to patients in medical settings had a significant effect size at follow-ups of 3+ to 6 months for those studies in which individuals with alcohol dependence (as opposed to risky or hazardous drinking) had been excluded, but not otherwise. If studies of different interventions involved different populations, a comparison of their relative efficacy or effectiveness can be misleading. Unfortunately, poor reporting of participant characteristics in study reports (e.g. Swearingen et al., 2003) is a common challenge in meta-analyses.

Examining participant characteristics as moderator variables in meta-analyses of intervention effects corresponds somewhat to identifying recipient–intervention interactions in primary studies. However, participant-level and study-level analyses are clearly different. The 'ecological fallacy' (whereby inferences about the nature of individuals are based solely on aggregate statistics collected for the groups to which those individuals belong; Robinson, 1950) applies in interpreting meta-analytic results. The constructs being assessed and the confounders present at the study level may differ from those at the participant level. For example, a meta-analytic finding that Intervention A is more effective than Intervention B when provided to samples that have larger proportions of women is not the same as finding an interaction between gender and response to Intervention A versus Intervention B in a primary study (see Berlin et al., 2002). However, study-level findings could suggest issues that could then be addressed at the participant level in future primary studies.

20.3.2   Comparison conditions

The comparison captured in effect sizes should be commensurate across studies in order to be meaningful and interpretable. A set of studies with commensurate comparisons can be achieved either through the initial selection of studies or through identifying subgroups of studies in moderator variable analyses. Accordingly, one would generally not want to combine findings from studies of two alternative interventions with studies of one or the other of those interventions versus no-intervention control conditions (e.g. a waitlist control group). Effect sizes for intervention–intervention comparisons are usually smaller than those for intervention–control comparisons, with intervention–placebo comparisons typically falling somewhere in-between (Grissom, 1996). For ethical reasons, most multiple-condition studies in the addictions field are intervention–intervention comparisons, rather than comparisons of one or more interventions with no- or minimal-intervention control conditions. For example, Swearingen et al. (2003) found that only 35% of 404 comparative alcohol treatment studies included a no- or minimal-treatment control condition.

If the effect sizes for quite different pairs of interventions and comparison conditions have been included in a standard meta-analysis, it is difficult to make sense of the results (e.g. Agosti, 1995). Some techniques have been developed to 'chain together' and indirectly estimate intervention effects from studies of different pairs of interventions (e.g. Intervention A versus Intervention B, Intervention B versus Intervention C; Bucher et al., 1997; Lumley, 2002; Psaty et al., 2003; Song et al., 2003; Lu & Ades, 2004). 'Limited evidence suggests that, when the individual studies are similar and of good quality, and intervention effects are consistent over a variety of comparators, adjusted indirect comparisons usually agree with results of head-to-head comparisons if intervention effects are similar across studies . . .' (Santaguida et al., 2005; see also Baker & Kramer, 2002). Given these restrictions and the limited evidence available on indirect methods, we believe that meta-analyses are currently best conducted for well-specified pairs of intervention and comparison conditions. That can be achieved by only including studies comparing the same two conditions (e.g. naltrexone versus placebo for alcohol dependence), or by examining through moderator variable analyses two or more interventions (e.g. different medications for alcohol dependence) whose studies have a similar comparison condition (e.g. placebo).

20.3.3   Individual- and group-administered interventions

Interventions in the addictions field are sometimes administered to groups of participants rather than to individual participants. Most statistical techniques, as well as the standard calculation of effect sizes, assume independence of observations, an assumption that is violated when an intervention is administered to groups of research participants. The lack of independence of assessments (see Herzog et al., 2002, as an example) can increase **Type I error** (rejecting the null hypothesis of no intervention effect when none exists in the population). Baldwin et al. (2005) found that none of 33 studies with group administration of psychotherapy properly analysed its data. After applying corrections assuming different levels of dependency in the data, they concluded that only 12.4–68.2% of the originally significant results remained significant. Depending on assumptions regarding the degree of data dependence, 6–19 of the 33 studies no longer had significant results after a correction was imposed.

The same issue arises in a meta-analysis when groups or clusters of participants (e.g. treatment centres) are randomised to intervention and comparison conditions in some studies, whereas randomisation is at the individual (e.g. patient) level in others. Effect sizes from studies of individually and group-administered interventions, or from studies using individual and cluster randomisation, should not be combined without some correction of the 'grouped' results to estimate an individual-level effect size (see Rooney & Murray, 1996, for an example of a meta-analysis of smoking cessation intervention studies that addressed this issue and Hedges, 2007, for a more recent technical article).

20.3.4 Multiple outcome variables

If multiple outcome variables are assessed in the same study, they should be combined into a single effect size so that the effect sizes in the aggregated (cross-study) analysis are independent. It may be that more than one outcome domain is assessed in a study (e.g. substance use variables, employment status and legal problems). Aggregated within-study effect sizes should be calculated for each of the different outcome domains and examined separately in cross-study meta-analyses. Statistical approaches are available for combining effect sizes on multiple outcome variables within a study (e.g. Arends et al., 2003), but they require information on the interrelationships (covariance) among the outcome variables (which often needs to be imputed from findings of other studies) and are complicated to implement. As a result, many meta-analysts simply average within-study effect sizes for outcome variables in the same domain.

20.3.5 Follow-up point at which outcomes are assessed

The effects of treatments or interventions often decay over time. For example, Moyer et al. (2002) and Finney and Moos (1996) found larger, statistically significant effect sizes for brief interventions versus routine medical care, and for inpatient/residential treatment versus outpatient treatment for alcohol use disorder, respectively, at earlier but not at later follow-ups (also see Hettema et al., 2005; cf. Stanton & Shadish, 1997). Thus, it does not make sense to evaluate effects sizes for an intervention versus control condition, or an intervention–intervention comparison, and ignore the points at which outcomes have been assessed. Follow-up points should be examined as a potential moderators of intervention effect sizes.

20.3.6 Between- and within-group effect sizes

Although the typical effect sizes reported in meta-analyses of intervention effects are drawn from outcome comparisons between groups, effect sizes indexing the difference between the participant functioning before and after intervention can also be calculated and analysed. Becker (1988) has described a technique for calculating such within-group effect sizes (but see Morris, 2000). A meta-analysis focusing solely on change scores across studies should pay attention to similarity across studies of baseline and follow-up functioning measures, as well as the length of time between baseline and follow-up assessment, or the interval between the end of intervention and follow-up. In any event, between- and within-group effect sizes are not commensurate and should not be mixed in the same meta-analysis (cf. Marsch, 1998), unless some explicit approach is used to combine them into a common metric (see Morris & DeShon, 2002).

20.3.7 Attrition during and after intervention

Two types of attrition can occur during the course of an intervention trial: research participants can drop out before or during the intervention or they can be lost to follow-up after the intervention has ended. Variation in intervention compliance can affect primary study results; individuals who receive a 'sufficient' dose of treatment may have better outcomes. Likewise, in meta-analyses, treatment dropout can be examined as a moderator variable. Alternatively, Stanton and Shadish (1997) corrected effect sizes for dropout from treatment in a meta-analysis of family–couples therapy for addiction to illicit drugs.

Regardless of variation in intervention compliance, the primary recommended approach for assessing intervention effects in randomised trials is an 'intent-to-treat' (ITT) analysis, in which persons randomly assigned to intervention and comparison conditions are included regardless of how much of the intervention or the alternative they received. Study variation in the use of ITT analysis may moderate intervention effect sizes.

Whether an ITT or some other form of analysis is performed in individual intervention trials, not all participants are likely to have been successfully followed up. Some, even among those who completed the intervention, will likely have missing data on outcome variables. Methods have been developed for imputing outcome scores for persons with missing data (e.g. Schafer & Graham, 2002). Actual follow-up rate and whether missing data were imputed (and the interaction of follow-up rate and imputation of missing data) could be moderators that account for variation in intervention effect sizes.

20.3.8 Methodological quality and research design

Taking study quality into account is important in meta-analyses. Two approaches for factoring in quality are (1) to include only studies deemed to be of acceptably high quality or (2) to include studies varying in their quality and then examine the effect of coded (aspects of) quality in moderator analyses. Among the challenges to implementing these goals are the numerous scales and instruments that have been developed to assess quality, the lack of consensus on what factors should be focal and the difficulty in accurately coding quality, given variation in the completeness and clarity of study reporting. Only factors related to 'internal validity' (the level of confidence one has that intervention/comparison status caused the outcome difference) or level of bias in effect sizes are useful for weighting or adjusting effect sizes. However, separate assessments of external validity (generalisability), adherence to ethical standards, and completeness and cogency of reporting can help to qualify the conclusions of investigations and can be used to describe and compare different areas of study (Moyer & Finney, 2005).

A significant determinant of a study's methodological quality is its research design. Various comparative research designs are used in addiction intervention studies, including RCTs and naturalistic or 'non-equivalent control groups' designs (Cook & Campbell, 1979) in which participants either self-select or are allocated to different intervention/control conditions in a non-random, non-systematic way. Of course, randomised trials provide the strongest basis for inferring causal intervention effects. If varied comparative designs are included in a meta-analysis, research design should be examined as a moderator variable to determine if effect sizes vary as a function of design.

20.4 Limitations

One of the most frequently voiced criticisms of meta-analysis is that one cannot meaningfully synthesise findings from dissimilar studies, or the 'apples and oranges' problem. We hope we have demonstrated that meta-analyses, given a sufficient number of studies, can examine variation in participant populations, outcome measures, research design and other moderator variables that may 'explain' differences in intervention effects across studies.

Another criticism is that meta-analyses mix studies of varying methodological quality, or the 'garbage in, garbage out' problem. We have noted that measures of methodological quality can be used as eligibility criteria to restrict studies to only those of high quality or as a moderator variable to examine the relationship between methodological quality and effect sizes. Nevertheless, a reader of a meta-analytic report needs to make a determination about the extent to which methodological features, particularly those not examined as moderator variables, might account for some of the observed variation in effect sizes.

Just as findings from primary intervention studies can be biased by missing data, missing data in meta-analyses can bias estimates of intervention effect sizes and of relationships between moderator variables and effect sizes. For example, information needed to calculate effect sizes for some or all of the outcome variables and/or information needed to code moderator variables may not be reported, and may not be obtainable. However, some methods, including multiple imputation methods, have been developed to handle missing data in meta-analyses (Pigott, 2001, 2009).

One needs to keep in mind that even a meta-analysis of findings only from RCTs is an 'observational' (non-experimental) study. One should approach the conduct of a meta-analysis or read a meta-analytic report the same way one would conduct or read a report of a primary observational study. What important variables were not assessed that might explain variation in effect sizes? What variables were assessed but not examined? Is there overlap or confounding among moderator variables? The fact that a moderator variable accounts for some variation in effect sizes does not rule out the possibility that another moderator variable (assessed or not assessed in studies) might also account for much of the same variation. For example, differences in methodological features might account for some of the observed variation in effect sizes across studies that may have been attributed to other substantive moderator variables (e.g. different types of interventions; variation in sample composition – see Wilson & Lipsey, 2001).

A single study, even an RCT, is not typically accepted as solid evidence of the efficacy or effectiveness of a particular intervention. This maxim generalises to meta-analyses. Intervention effect sizes can change over time. For example, publication bias can result in upwardly biased effect sizes in early results; effect sizes may decline or change in other ways as more studies accumulate (see Kraemer et al., 1998; Trikalinos et al., 2004; Feinn & Kranzler, 2005; Gehr et al., 2006). Cumulative meta-analyses (Wetterslev et al., 2008), as are done by the Cochrane Collaboration (Moher et al., 2008), can examine changes in effect sizes over time and determine when results reach a 'steady state.'

20.5 Conclusion

The exponential growth of meta-analyses attests to their perceived value (Sutton & Higgins, 2008). For those inspired to embark on a meta-analysis of their own, particularly individuals early in their careers, there are several benefits (Boynton, 2008). First, if the number of relevant studies is relatively small and the number of variables to be coded is limited, this type of 'research about research' does not necessarily require external funding, because the required resources (i.e. access to bibliographic search engines and statistical software; coding time) are minimal. Second, data collection does not involve research participants. Third, conducting a meta-analytic review can help one build a deeper understanding of a research area and make an important contribution to the literature. In the future, the accumulation of knowledge surely will continue to accelerate, fuelling the need to synthesise and make sense of research relevant to interventions for addictions and other conditions. Indeed, the increasing emphasis on evidence-based interventions means that clinicians, policy makers and researchers will be ever more reliant on the guidance of those who can synthesise complex literatures using meta-analytic skills.

Acknowledgements

Preparation of this chapter was supported by the U.S. Department of Veterans Affairs, Veterans Health Administration, Health Services Research and Development Service for the first author and by start-up funding from Stony Brook University for the second author. The views expressed are those of authors and do not necessarily represent the views of the Department of Veterans Affairs or Stony Brook University. We thank Keith Humphreys for his comments on an earlier draft of this chapter.

Exercises

It can be instructive to compare the results of a 'box-score' review, based on the proportion of studies with significant findings, with those of a meta-analysis with effect sizes. It is usually not possible to find an example of each type of review that uses the same set of studies. However, Finney et al. (1996) conducted a box-score review of inpatient/residential versus outpatient treatment for alcohol use disorders. Finney and Moos (1996) then secured unpublished data needed to conduct a meta-analysis of findings from the same studies. Read each review and see if you get a different sense of magnitude or strength of the inpatient/residential versus outpatient treatment effect and of how enduring it is. How do you view the relative strengths and weaknesses of the two reviews?

References

Agosti, V. (1995) The efficacy of treatments in reducing alcohol consumption: a meta-analysis. *International Journal of the Addictions*, 30, 1067–1077.

Altman, D. G., Schulz, K. F., Moher, D., Egger, M., Davidoff, F., Elbourne, D., Gøtzsche, P. C. & Lang, T., for the CONSORT Group (Consolidated Standards of Reporting Trials) (2001) The revised CONSORT statement for reporting randomized trials: explanation and elaboration. *Annals of Internal Medicine*, 134, 663–694.

Arends, L. R., Voko, Z. & Stijnen, T. (2003) Combining multiple outcome measures in a meta-analysis: an application. *Statistics in Medicine*, 22, 1335–1353.

Baker, S. G. & Kramer, B. S. (2002) The transitive fallacy for randomized trials: if A bests B and B bests C in separate trials, is A better than C? *BMC Medical Research Methodology*, 2(13).

Baldwin, S. A., Murray, D. M. & Shadish, W. R. (2005) Empirically supported treatments or type I errors? Problems with the analysis of data from group-administered treatments. *Journal of Consulting and Clinical Psychology*, 73, 924–935.

Becker, B. J. (1988) Synthesizing standardized mean-change measures. *British Journal of Mathematical and Statistical Psychology*, 41, 257–278.

Berlin, J. A., Santanna, J., Schmid, C. H., Szczech, L. A., Feldman, H. I. & the Anti-Lymphocyte Antibody Induction Therapy Study Group. (2002) Individual patient-versus group-level data meta-regressions for the investigation of treatment effect modifiers: ecological bias rears its ugly head. *Statistics in Medicine*, 21, 371–387.

Berner, M. M., Kriston, L., Bentele, M. & Harter, M. (2007) The Alcohol Use Disorders Identification Test for detecting at-risk drinking: a systematic review and meta-analysis. *Journal of Studies on Alcohol and Drugs*, 63, 461–473.

Boynton, M. H. (2008) Top ten tips for graduate students who want to conduct a meta-analysis. *Psychological Science Agenda*, 22(4). Available online: http://www.apa.org/science/psa/apr08ssc.html (accessed 6 October 2009).

Bucher, H. C., Guyatt, G. H., Griffith, L. E. & Walter, S. D. (1997) The results of direct and indirect treatment comparisons in meta-analysis of randomized controlled trials. *Clinical Epidemiology*, 50, 683–691.

Cook, T. D. & Campbell, D. T. (1979) *Quasi-Experimentation: Design and Analysis Issues for Field Settings*. Chicago: Rand McNally.

Duval, S. & Tweedie, R. (2000) Trim and fill: a simple funnel-plot-based method of testing and adjusting for publication bias in meta-analysis. *Biometrics*, 56, 455–463.

Feinn, R. & Kranzler, H. R. (2005) Does effect size in naltrexone trials for alcohol dependence differ for single-site vs. multiple-center studies? *Alcoholism: Clinical and Experimental Research*, 29, 983–988.

Finney, J. W., Hahn, A. C. & Moos, R. H. (1996) The effectiveness of inpatient and outpatient treatment for alcohol abuse: the need to focus on mediators and moderators of setting effects. *Addiction*, 91, 1773–1796.

Finney, J. W. & Moos, R. H. (1996) The effectiveness of inpatient and outpatient treatment for alcohol abuse: effect sizes, research design issues, and explanatory mechanisms [Response to commentaries]. *Addiction*, 91, 1813–1820.

Gandini, S., Botteri, E., Iodice, S., Boniol, M., Lowenfels, A. B., Maisonneuve, P. & Boyle, P. (2008) Tobacco smoking and cancer: a meta-analysis. *International Journal of Cancer*, 122, 155–164.

Gehr, B. T., Weiss, C. & Porzsolt, F. (2006) The fading of reported effectiveness: a meta-analysis of randomised controlled trials. *BMC Medical Research Methodology*, 6(25).

Glass, G. V. (1976) Primary, secondary and meta-analysis of research. *Educational Researcher*, 10, 3–8.

Grissom, R. J. (1996) The magical number .7 ± .2: meta-meta-analysis of the probability of superior outcomes in comparison involving therapy, placebo, and control. *Journal of Consulting and Clinical Psychology*, 64, 973–982.

Hedges, L. V. (2007) Effect sizes in cluster-randomized designs. *Journal of Educational and Behavioral Statistics*, 32, 341–370.

Hedges, L. V. & Olkin, I. (1985) *Statistical Methods for Meta-analysis*. New York: Academic Press.

Hedges, L. V. & Pigott, T. D. (2001) The power of statistical tests in meta-analysis. *Psychological Methods*, 6, 203–217.

Hedges, L. V. & Pigott, T. D. (2004) The power of statistical tests for moderators in meta-analysis. *Psychological Methods*, 9, 426–445.

Hedges, L. V. & Vevea, J. L. (1998) Fixed- and random-effects models in meta-analysis. *Psychological Methods*, 3, 486–504.

Herzog, T. A., Lazev, A. B., Irvin, J. E., Juliano, L. M., Greenbaum, P. E. & Brandon, T. H. (2002) Testing for group membership effects during and after treatment: the example of group therapy for smoking cessation. *Behavior Therapy*, 33, 29–43.

Hettema, J., Steele, J. & Miller, W. R. (2005) Motivational interviewing. *Annual Review of Clinical Psychology*, 1, 91–111.

Higgins, J. P. T. & Thompson, G. S. (2002) Quantifying heterogeneity in a meta-analysis. *Statistics in Medicine*, 21, 1539–1558.

Hsu, L. M. (2004) Biases of success rate differences shown in binomial effect size displays. *Psychological Methods*, 9, 183–197.

Huedo-Medina, T. B., Sánchez-Meca, J., Marín-Martínez, F. & Botella, J. (2006) Assessing heterogeneity in meta-analysis: Q statistic or I^2 index? *Psychological Methods*, 11, 193–206.

Irvin, J. E., Bowers, C. A., Dunn, M. E. & Wang, M. C. (1999) Efficacy of relapse prevention: a meta-analytic review. *Journal of Consulting and Clinical Psychology*, 67, 563–570.

Kraemer, H. C., Gardner, C., Brooks, J. O. & Yesavage, J. A. (1998) Advantages of excluding underpowered studies in meta-analysis: inclusionist versus exclusionist viewpoints. *Psychological Methods*, 3, 23–31.

Laupacis, A., Sackett, D. L. & Roberts, R. S. (1988) An assessment of clinically useful measures of the consequences of treatment. *New England Journal of Medicine*, 3318, 1728–1733.

Lipsey, M. W. & Wilson, D. B. (2001) *Practical Meta-analysis*. Thousand Oaks, CA: Sage.

Lu, G. & Ades, A. E. (2004) Combination of direct and indirect evidence in mixed treatment comparison. *Statistics in Medicine*, 23, 3105–3124.

Lumley, T. (2002) Network meta-analysis for indirect treatment comparisons. *Statistics in Medicine*, 21, 2313–2324.

Marsch, L. A. (1998) The efficacy of methadone maintenance interventions in reducing illicit opiate use, HIV risk behavior and criminality: a meta-analysis. *Addiction*, 93, 515–532.

McGrath, R. E. & Meyer, G. J. (2006) When effect sizes disagree: the case of r and d. *Psychological Methods*, 11, 386–401.

Moher, D., Cook, D. J., Eastwood, S., Olkin, I., Rennie, D. & Stroup, D. F. (1999) Improving the quality of reports of meta-analyses of randomised controlled trials: the QUOROM statement. Quality of reporting of meta-analyses. *Lancet*, 354, 1896–1900.

Moher, D., Tsertsvadze, A., Tricco, A. C., Eccles, M., Grimshaw, J., Sampson, M. & Barrowman, N. (2008) When and how to update systematic reviews. *Cochrane Database of Systematic Reviews, January*, 23(1), MR000023.

Morris, S. B. (2000) Distribution of standardized mean change effect size for meta-analysis on repeated measures. *British Journal of Mathematical and Statistical Psychology*, 53, 17–29.

Morris, S. B. & DeShon, R. P. (2002) Combining effect size estimates in meta-analysis with repeated measures and independent-groups designs. *Psychological Methods*, 7, 105–125.

Moyer, A. & Finney, J. W. (2005) Rating methodological quality: toward improved assessment and investigation. *Accountability in Research*, 12, 299–313.

Moyer, A., Finney, J. W., Swearingen, C. E. & Vergun, P. (2002) Brief interventions for alcohol problems: a meta-analytic review of controlled investigations in treatment-seeking and non-treatment-seeking populations. *Addiction*, 97, 279–292.

Ogilvie, D., Fayter, D., Petticrew, M., Sowden, A., Thomas, S., Whitehead, M. & Worthy, G. (2008) The harvest plot: a method for synthesising evidence about the differential effects of interventions. *BMC Medical Research Methodology*, 8(8).

Orwin, R. G. & Vevea, J. L. (2009) Evaluating coding decisions. In: H. Cooper, L. V. Hedges & J. C. Valentine (eds) *The Handbook of Research Synthesis and Meta-Analysis*. New York: Russell Sage Foundation, pp. 173–203.

Peters, G. J., Kok, G. & Abraham, C. (2008) Social cognitive determinants of ecstasy use to target in evidence-based interventions: a meta-analytical review. *Addiction*, 103, 109–118.

Peters, J. L., Sutton, A. J., Jones, D. R., Abrams, K. R. & Rushton, L. (2007) Performance of the trim and fill method in the presence of publication bias and between-study heterogeneity. *Statistics in Medicine*, 26, 4544–4562.

Pigott, T. D. (2001) Missing predictors in models of effect size. *Evaluation and the Health Professions*, 24, 277–307.

Pigott, T. D. (2009) Handling missing data. In: H. Cooper, L. V. Hedges & J. C. Valentine (eds) *The Handbook of Research Synthesis and Meta-Analysis*. New York: Russell Sage Foundation, pp. 399–416.

Psaty, B. M., Lumley, T., Furberg, C. D., Schellenbaum, G., Pahor, M., Alderman, M. H. & Weiss, N. H. (2003) Health outcomes associated with various hypertensive therapies used as first-line agents: a network meta-analysis. *JAMA: The Journal of the American Medical Association*, 289, 2534–2544.

Ray, J. W. & Shadish, W. R. (1996) How interchangeable are different estimators of effect size? *Journal of Consulting and Clinical Psychology*, 64(6), 1316–1325.

Robinson, W. (1950) Ecological correlations and the behavior of individuals. *American Sociological Review*, 15, 351–357.

Rooney, B. L. & Murray, D. M. (1996) A meta-analysis of smoking prevention programs after adjustment for errors in the unit of analysis. *Health Education Quarterly*, 23, 48–64.

Rosenthal, R. & Rubin, D. B. (1982) A simple, general purpose display of magnitude of experimental effect. *Journal of Educational Psychology*, 74, 166–169.

Rothstein, H. R., Sutton, A. J. & Borenstein, M. (eds) (2005) *Publication Bias in Meta-analysis: Prevention, Assessment and Adjustments*. Chichester: John Wiley.

Sanchez-Meca, J., Marin-Martinez, F. & Chacon-Moscoso, S. (2003) Effect-size indices for dichotomized outcomes in meta-analysis. *Psychological Methods*, 8, 448–467.

Santaguida, P. L., Helfand, M. & Raina, P. (2005) Challenges in systematic reviews that evaluate drug efficacy or effectiveness. *Annals of Internal Medicine*, 142, 1006–1072.

Schafer, J. L. & Graham, J. W. (2002) Missing data: our view of the state of the art. *Psychological Methods*, 7, 147–177.

Scott, J. C., Woods, S. P., Matt, G. E., Meyer, R. A., Heaton, R. K., Atkinson, J. H. & Grant, I. (2007) Neurocognitive effects of methamphetamine: a critical review and meta-analysis. *Neuropsychology Review*, 17, 275–297.

Song, F., Altman, D. G., Glenny, A. M. & Deeks, J. J. (2003) Validity of indirect comparison for estimating efficacy of competing interventions: empirical evidence from published meta-analyses. *British Medical Journal*, 326, 472.

Stanton, M. D. & Shadish, W. R. (1997) Outcome, attrition and family-couples treatment for drug abuse: a meta-analysis and review of the controlled, comparative studies. *Psychological Bulletin*, 122, 170–191.

Streeton, C. & Whelan, G. (2001) Naltreone, a relapse prevention maintenance treatment of alcohol dependence: a meta-analysis of randomized controlled trials. *Alcohol and Alcoholism*, 36, 544–552.

Sutton, A. J. & Higgins, J. P. (2008) Recent developments in meta-analysis. *Statistics in Medicine*, 27, 625–650.

Swearingen, C. E., Moyer, A. & Finney, J. W. (2003) Alcoholism treatment outcome studies, 1970–1998: an expanded look at the nature of the research. *Addictive Behaviors*, 28, 415–436.

Thompson, K. N. & Schumacker, R. E. (1997) An evaluation of Rosenthal and Rubin's binomial effect size display. *Journal of Educational and Behavioral Statistics*, 22, 109–117.

Tonigan, J. S., Toscova, R. & Miller, W. R. (1996) Meta-analysis of the literature on Alcoholic Anonymous: sample and study characteristics moderate findings. *Journal of Studies on Alcohol*, 57, 65–72.

Trikalinos, T. A., Churchill, R., Ferri, M., Leucht, S., Tuunainen, A., Wahlbeck, K. & Ioannidis, J. P. A., for the EU-PSI Project (2004) Effect sizes in cumulative meta-analyses of mental health randomized trials evolved over time. *Journal of Clinical Epidemiology*, 57, 1124–1130.

Viechtbauer, W. (2007) Hypothesis tests for population heterogeneity in meta-analysis. *British Journal of Mathematical and Statistical Psychology*, 60, 29–60.

Wetterslev, J., Thorlund, K., Brok, J. & Gluud, C. (2008) Trial sequential analysis may establish when firm evidence is reached in cumulative meta-analysis. *Journal of Clinical Epidemiology*, 61, 64–75.

White, H. (2009) Scientific communication and literature retrieval. In: H. Cooper, L. V. Hedges & J. C. Valentine (eds) *The Handbook of Research Synthesis and Meta-Analysis*. New York: Russell Sage Foundation, pp. 51–71.

Wilson, D. B. & Lipsey, M. W. (2001) The role of method in treatment effectiveness research: evidence from meta-analysis. *Psychological Methods*, 6, 413–429.

Recommended readings

Borenstein, M., Hedges, L. V., Higgins, J. P. T. & Rothstein, H. R. (2009) *Introduction to Meta-analysis (Statistics in Practice)*. Hoboken, NJ: John Wiley & Sons.

Cooper, H., Hedges, L. V. & Valentine, J. C. (eds) (2009). *The Handbook of Research Synthesis and Meta-analysis*, 2nd edn. New York: Russell Sage Foundation.

Higgins, J. P. T. & Green, S. (eds) (2009) *Cochrane Handbook for Systematic Reviews of Interventions*, Version 5.0.2 [updated September 2009]. The Cochrane Collaboration. Available online: www.cochrane-handbook.org (accessed 6 October 2009).

Lipsey, M. W. & Wilson, D. B. (2001) *Practical Meta-analysis*. Thousand Oaks, CA: Sage.

Technological assistance

Bax, L., Yu, L. M., Ikeda, N., Tsuruta, N. & Moons, K. G. M. (2006) *MIX: Comprehensive Free Software for Meta-analysis of Causal Research Data*, Version 1.7. Available online: http://www.mix-for-meta-analysis.info (accessed 6 October 2009).

Borenstein, M., Hedges, L. V., Higgins, J. & Rothstein, H. (2005) *Comprehensive Meta-analysis*, Version 2. Englewood, NJ: Biostat.

Shadish, W. R., Robinson, L. & Lu, C. (1999) *ES: Effect Size Calculator*. St Paul, MN: Assessment Systems Corp. Available online: http://www.assess.com/xcart/product.php?productid=226&cat=0&page=1 (accessed 6 October 2009).

Wilson, D. B. (2009) Macros for use with SPSS software and effect size calculation software. Available online: http://mason.gmu.edu/-dwilsonb/ma.html (accessed 6 October 2009).

Chapter 21
DRUG TREND MONITORING

Paul Griffiths and Jane Mounteney

21.1   Introduction

From the beginning of the modern debate on drugs and their control, arguments about the size, nature and consequences of the phenomena have been key concerns (Musto, 1973). As a result the use and misuse of statistics has informed, and misinformed, the policy discussion since its earliest days. Influential first measures to promote drug control in the United Sates were based on highly inflated estimates of the problem (Musto & Sloboda, 2003) and even today some would argue that the global debate on drugs is positioned on figures whose exactitude is so questionable that they may mislead as much as inform (Rossi, 2002). Nonetheless, a strong commitment to monitoring can still be found in the rhetoric of the global debate on drugs, and although the picture is geographically diverse, monitoring systems are to be found in most parts of the developed world and some parts of the developing and transitional world (see 'Recommended websites' at the end of this chapter). These systems have been shaped by the methodological challenges of monitoring a diverse set of behaviours that are highly stigmatised and engaged in by individuals who have often good reasons for not wishing to be identified (Hartnoll, 2004). The existence of a number of textbooks and university courses on the topic of drug epidemiology would suggest that methods in this area have now developed to an extent to which they may even be considered a distinct discipline (Bull on Narcotics, 2003, 2006; Sloboda, 2005). This chapter provides an overview of the approaches that have been developed in an attempt to provide policy makers with what they claim to need most for guiding their actions: a sound understanding of the nature, scale and dynamic of the drug problem.

21.2   Point of departure – divergent policy perspectives, difficulties in definition and temporal relevance

Before embarking on a discussion of the methodological evolution of drug monitoring, it is worth noting three issues that have a direct bearing on how drug monitoring systems have developed.

The first of these is the nature of the subject itself. Few areas of scientific inquiry are faced with such a highly politicised and sensitive topic matter. Moreover, since monitoring activities are intended to inform a debate on appropriate actions and their impact, a risk always exists that the messengers' message may not be welcome. The driving engines for monitoring illicit drug use have been both concerns about drug control (e.g. interdiction efforts against production, trafficking and use) and public health issues (e.g. treating drug dependence and preventing HIV transmission through injecting drug use). As such, much of the data available on illicit drug trends stem from law enforcement efforts to control illicit drugs (e.g. arrests for drug use and drug seizure data) as well as its consequences (e.g. demand for drug treatment, morbidity and mortality data). Historically, drug control objectives were generally more important for the establishment of drug monitoring systems, but a growing public health agenda since the 1970s onwards, and growing concerns about the risks of HIV infection in particular, has seen public health approaches become more important and they now take dominance in many systems. Public health and drug control concerns do not always make good bedfellows, and information on the failings in the control system or the negative impact of drug use is important for both those wishing to argue for more restrictive or more liberal policy perspectives. One consequence of this is that information systems can find themselves dependent on information providers who may sometimes be ambivalent or even hostile to providing data that may subsequently be used to undermine or attack them. Local, national and international efforts to monitor drug problems have faced this problem, and this is why concerns about the development of networks, reporting structures and feedback mechanisms have played such an important role in work in this area (Bergeron & Griffiths, 2006).

The second problem is conceptual rather than political in nature. Put simply, it is not easy to decide exactly what should be measured, and what is possible to measure is rarely what is optimally required. Definitional problems and the practical difficulties of monitoring drug use mean that most monitoring systems are based on a multi-indicator approach in which any one indicator only provides a partial, and often distorted, part of the whole. If currently collected data provide a mirror on patterns and trends in drug use, it is a broken one, where individual pieces offer only a glimpse of the underlying form. How systems have attempted to put this image back together is a topic we return to later.

The third and arguably most intractable issue for drug monitoring systems to address is the need for temporal relevance. Information systems are as much about understanding future problems as learning from historical trends. The policy debate is preoccupied with the potential for new threats and the desire to see how current initiatives may be impacting on the situation. Information systems are faced with the problem that the collection and reporting of data is often a time-consuming business. There has been considerable interest in developing approaches that are both sensitive to changes and that can report rapidly, a simple objective to state, but one that presents considerable conceptual, methodological and practical challenges to those who would attempt to achieve it.

21.3   International, national and local drug monitoring mechanisms

Historically, the main engine driving drug monitoring was the need to assess the effectiveness of supply reduction measures, keep track of addicts and control the prescribing of physicians and pharmacists, and at the international level, assess the adherence of signatories to the international drug control conventions (Courtwrite, 1992). For example, this can be seen in the United Kingdoms Addicts Index where the Home Office required physicians to register those they suspected of being addicted to narcotic substances (Mott, 1994).

As noted already, this drug control perspective has become increasingly joined by public health concerns. At the international level, an outcome of this transition can be seen in the range of bodies: the United Nations Office on Drugs and Crime (UNODC), the International Narcotics Control Board (INCB), as well as the World Health Organization (WHO) and United Nations Program on HIV/AIDS (UNAIDS). Indeed, the number of international bodies collecting information on aspects of drug use has prompted calls for more system-wide coherence on this issue.

At the regional level, the Inter-American Drug Abuse Control Commission (CICAD) plays an important role in monitoring drug use in the Americas through a multi-evaluation mechanism. The European Monitoring Centre for Drugs and Drug Addiction (EMCDDA) is responsible for collecting data and reporting on drug use in Europe (Griffiths et al., 2008). UNODC also supports a number of initiatives such as the ACCORD network in Asia (UNODC, 2006) and has attempted previously to establish regional systems elsewhere.

A number of important national systems also exist. Of particular note, simply because of the resources at its disposal, is the National Institute on Drug Abuse (NIDA) in the United States, which supports scientific research and dissemination of information, as well as data collection, and the U.S. Community Epidemiological Working Group (CEWG) has been particularly influential, with its approach has imitated and adopted elsewhere (Sloboda & Kozel, 1999; Sloboda & Kozel, 1999). Australia has also invested resources in developing national sentinel monitoring systems, such as the Illicit Drug Reporting System. In South Africa, SACENDU (South African Community Epidemiology Network on Drug Use) (Parry et al., 2004) is probably the best example of a long-standing and successful monitoring programme in the developing world although attempts to extend this model into neighbouring countries have been less successful.

Drug monitoring systems also operate at the local and city level. The Dutch Antenna project is perhaps the most long-standing, having provided annual updates on the youth and drug scene in Amsterdam since 1993 (Korf & Nabben, 2000).The German city of Frankfurt has the MoSyd system for monitoring drug trends, comprising an open scene survey, a school survey and a trend scout panel in order to monitor the city drug scene (Kemmesies & Hess, 2001). The Norwegian BEWS system has been reporting on trends in the city of Bergen since 2002 using routine data, key informants and media monitoring (Mounteney & Leirvåg, 2004; Mounteney & Haugland, 2009).

In some respects, although they seem very different and the information they provide is used for different purposes, the fundamental issues for drug monitoring systems are broadly similar be they working at local, national, regional or international level (Box 21.1).

21.4 Challenges in monitoring illicit drug use

A number of problems hamper any discussions of illicit drug trends. A large part of uncovering the public health aspect of illicit drug trends involves appreciation of the nuances involved regarding which substances are classified as drugs, what constitutes drug use, and when drug use becomes 'drug abuse' or problematic. Ideally, for monitoring purposes, applying diagnostic criteria such as those provided by DSM and ICD diagnostic systems to those experiencing problems with their drug use would be appropriate. However, this is difficult to do in practice although some surveys try. Moreover, drug use encompasses a complex set of behaviours that are usually found at low prevalence and tend to be stigmatised and well hidden. For practical and methodological reasons, monitoring the extent of drug use is typically restricted to simple behavioural measures of drug use within a temporal reference period. Currently, the most common measures used for monitoring purposes are the lifetime prevalence of specified drug, past year prevalence, past month prevalence and, if available, the number of days the drug was used in the past month. There has been increasing recognition of the need to adapt current approaches to be more sensitive to polydrug use, although the complex and dynamic consumption pattern of many drug users makes this objective a challenging one. To date, the most common approach here has been to look at what are considered important drug combinations.

Even defining which psychoactive substances fall under the general heading of illicit drug use can be problematic. Illicit drugs are scheduled by the United Nations and national governments according to their perceived degree of harm as well as other considerations. However, not all drugs that are prohibited at a national level necessarily fall under international control. *Khat*, for

Box 21.1   A local level case study – the Bergen earlier warning system (BEWS)

The Bergen earlier warning system (BEWS) has been monitoring drug trends in Norway's second largest city, Bergen, since 2002 (Mounteney & Leirvåg, 2004). BEWS was established with the aim of providing an earlier warning of emerging trends in drug and alcohol use, with a view to facilitating early intervention by policy makers and practitioners. BEWS operates by collecting and analysing drug-related data from approximately 50 data sources and reporting on a six-monthly basis on patterns and trends in drug consumption in the city. Both quantitative and qualitative data are utilised including a schools panel and survey, secondary data such as police arrests, seizures, treatment demand data and alcohol sales, as well as a media monitoring element, which follows local newspapers, youth and drug professional publications and drug user websites (see Figure 21.1). Few routine data sources provide information on drug use in nightlife settings, and therefore to fill this information gap, a key informant panel was established as a central component of the system.

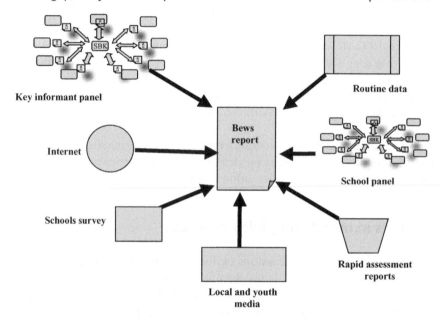

Figure 21.1   Overview of information sources used by BEWS.

BEWS multi-method, multi-indicator approach has proved effective for the rapid reporting of emerging drug trends at a city level (Mounteney & Leirvåg, 2004). In addition, the model proved adept at identifying has been used in combination with rapid assessment methodologies to explore in-depth emerging drug phenomena, including an increase in the number of young opiate users in the city.

example, is currently prohibited in some countries but freely available elsewhere, and is not subject to international control in its natural plant form (Anderson et al., 2007).

Drug problems can also occur through the misuse of diverted medicines intended for therapeutic or pharmaceutical purposes, or by imbibing household or industrial products that contain psychoactive chemicals. The innovative nature of the contemporary synthetic drug market also lends itself to discovery of new psychoactive substances which do not fall under current international drug control conventions.

Classification of drug types is a further concern when monitoring global illicit drug trends. Some countries still classify drugs as being 'narcotics' or 'psychotropics' according to whether they fall under the 1961 Single Convention on Narcotic Drugs (including cocaine, heroin and cannabis), or the later conventions on psychotropic substances, which cover a range of synthetic drugs (United Nations, 1961, 1971, 1988). The most problematic area in terms of drug classification is the nomenclature used to describe various types of synthetic drugs, where drug market conditions can preclude monitoring-specific substances (e.g. the use or marketing of pills containing a combination of illicit psychoactive ingredients).

One of the most fundamental challenges of monitoring drug use is posed by the methodological and practical difficulties of sampling in this area. Many forms of drug use occur at very low frequency and the behaviour is unlikely to be evenly distributed within the general population. Moreover, the stigmatised and hidden nature of drug use means that the possibility of both response and non-response bias have to be carefully considered. Drawing up sampling frames that allow a credible random probability sample is often very difficult. These issues are dealt with in more detail in Chapter 3. It is worth noting that with sensitive approaches, cannabis and other high-prevalence drug use can be assessed to some extent using survey approaches; however, more innovate sampling techniques are required for other drugs. Assessing levels of opioid use and drug injecting are particularly challenging, and some complex statistical approaches have been developed in this area that seek to calculate the size of the non-observable population. A review of these approaches as well as a more general discussion of sampling issues in drug monitoring can be found in Taylor and Griffiths (2005) and in EMCDDA (2001).

21.5   An overview of common information sources and some of their limitations

Drug trend monitoring usually involves imperfect information – it is common to use indicators, proxy or surrogate measures, which tell us something about consumption trends, populations, etc., but do not provide the whole picture. There exist a number of comprehensive reviews of the indicators most commonly used in drug monitoring systems (Hartnoll et al., 1989, 1998; Sloboda & Kozel, 2003; Degenhardt & Dietze, 2005). The main focus has been on routine data sets and quantitative sources, with less written on the use of qualitative sources.

A range of data sources, usually referred to as indicators are available, all of which are deficient in some respects and require careful interpretation. However, when they are taken together they can nonetheless provide an image of the phenomenon. By using a variety of indicators in combination, none of which is sufficient on its own, they can provide a more accurate picture of drug use in a given population and allow changes over time to be identified. This is most commonly done under the banner of 'triangulation' (Denzin, 1978). Certain methods are often more appropriate than others for measuring specific types of drug use, depending on general prevalence in the population, degree of hidden use and stigmatisation, and cost-effectiveness.

The main indicators used to monitor illicit drug use can be found in the United Nations Annual Reports Questionnaire. At an international level, the Lisbon consensus statement forms a basis for agreements on drug monitoring standards. A central issue is that of finding a balance between the need for comparable data and the need to develop data collection methods that are sensitive to local cultures and contexts. There has been international agreement to focus on a core data set – a limited number of indicators to be developed and included in monitoring systems: drug consumption among the general population, drug consumption among the youth population, high-risk drug abuse, service utilisation for drug problems, drug-related morbidity and drug-related mortality. In a European context, the EU action plan on drugs calls for member states to provide reliable and comparable information on five key epidemiological indicators (Hartnoll, 2003; http://www.emcdda.europa.eu/?nnodeid=1380, EMCDDA, 2001):

- Prevalence and patterns of drug use among the **general population** (population surveys)
- Prevalence and patterns of **problem drug use** (statistical prevalence/incidence estimates and surveys among drug users)
- **Drug-related infectious diseases** (prevalence and incidence rates of HIV, hepatitis B and C in injecting drug users)
- **Drug-related deaths and mortality** of drug users (general population mortality, special registers for statistics, and mortality cohort studies among drug users)
- Demand for **drug treatment** (statistics from drug treatment centres on clients starting treatment)

The most common sources used in drug trend monitoring systems are prevalence surveys and routine or secondary data sets, whilst systems focusing on emerging trends also utilise more sensitive sources such as key informants and youth media.

21.5.1 School surveys

The most comprehensive and comparable global data set on illicit drug use arises from school surveys on drug use, which are inexpensive and easy to conduct. These surveys are particularly useful because they target adolescents, who are a high-risk group for drug use (Hibell et al., 2004). At the global level, questions on cannabis use are included in the WHO survey on Health Behavior in School-Aged Children. In the United States, the Monitoring the Future annual survey of 8th, 10th, and 12th graders represents one the most developed and largest survey exercises, running since 1975. In Europe, the ESPAD study group (European School Survey Project on Alcohol and Other Drugs) reports on drug use among 15- to 16-year-olds in over 30 countries every 4 years and which has recently reported its fourth round of data collection (Hibell et al., 2007).

Problems of bias related to non-responses and dishonest responses can be a difficulty for any survey, but they present a particular challenge when surveying illicit drug use. Techniques have been developed to ensure confidence in anonymity, in order to improve the honesty and accuracy of responses. Notably, these include the use of a dummy drug category in order to check the number of school children who are misreporting use. School surveys face additional problems: in many countries, whereby the children most at risk of using drugs do not attend school for various reasons, while in the developing world, education is not often universal, or is limited to the early years of schooling. Therefore, generalisations from the results of school surveys to the wider population of young people need to be made with some caution. Similarly, interpreting trends from school survey data are complicated by the fact that prevalence rates for drugs other than cannabis are generally very low and classes are often used as sampling units, raising questions about the possibility of intra-class correlations.

School-aged children are not the only special target population selected for assessing drug use levels: surveys of military conscripts have been conducted in some countries, while at-risk groups such as out-of-school youth, the homeless and sex workers have also been targeted for surveys.

21.5.2 Household surveys

Less commonly available for the developing world, but a mainstay for reporting on drug use in North America, Australia and Europe, are national household surveys on the health habits of the general population, like the U.S. National Survey on Drug Use and Health (NSDUH). Such surveys are costly and methodologically complex, but they include numerous approaches developed to reduce reporting biases, such as the use of computer-aided interviewing. Despite these state-of-the-art methods, general population surveys are generally regarded as inadequate for measuring stigmatised and infrequent drug use behaviours (e.g. injecting drug use), which are disproportionately found in marginalised communities. For this reason a number of statistical techniques (e.g. capture-recapture and benchmark-multiplier methods) have been developed that try to extrapolate from known data sources to estimate the unknown, or 'hidden', proportion of drug users (Hickman & Taylor, 2005). Nevertheless, well-conducted household surveys are useful for examining the relative prevalence of illicit drugs, and they can provide time series data on more commonly used drugs, which is important for evaluating trends and compensating for other data limitations.

21.5.3 Treatment and health data

Drug information systems also report on people who are identified as having a drug problem through their contact with health care services or the criminal justice system. In the United States, approaches in this area include drug testing among arrestees (Arrestee Drug Abuse Monitoring – ADAM) and reported drug use among medical emergency patients (Drug Abuse Warning Network – DAWN).

More common is the practice of monitoring the characteristics of people seeking drug treatment, which provides a convenient tool for analysing global drug trends. The Treatment Demand Indicator is one of the key epidemiological measures adopted by the EMCDDA, while similar treatment demand monitoring systems have been established in a number of non-European countries. Clearly, information on the characteristics of those seeking help for drug problems is influenced by the availability of drug treatment services and factors such as court-mandated treatment. Nonetheless, this type of data is useful in monitoring problematic drug use (see EMCDDA, 1997) and shifts in treatment demand. Other key indicators include monitoring drug-related deaths (by acute poisoning) and levels of infectious disease (principally HIV and hepatitis C) among injecting drug users. Finally, data from ad hoc research studies and more qualitative information from interviews with researchers, health care providers and social workers, and drug users themselves – all contribute to the global information base on drug use trends.

In Europe, a distinction is made between first treatment demand and all treatment demands in a given year (Hartnoll et al., 1989). This is because the characteristics of those who have never been in treatment before (first treatment) is considered likely to be more representative of new cases and thus more helpful for identifying new trends than the numbers of those who have already been in contact with treatment services. The numbers actually taken on for treatment might just reflect the capacity of services, whereas the numbers requesting help are more likely to reflect demand. Treatment demand can also be considered a 'lagged' indicator, as there tends to be a considerable delay between initial substance use and application for treatment (Griffiths et al., 2000).

21.5.4 Drug seizures and law enforcement data

For supply-related drug interdiction efforts, intelligence and law enforcement authorities monitor trends on drug seizures and arrests for drug-related offences, as well as market price and purity information. Seizures of illicit drugs, in particular the total amounts seized, tend to be used to monitor the illicit drug market, which, in turn, is assumed to reflect to a certain extent levels of consumption (Hartnoll et al., 1989). Methodological approaches vary, as does the quality of the information available, with data on price and purity being generally poor or unavailable. Because reporting on the number and quantity of illicit drugs seized is obligatory for countries that are signatories to the United Nations drug control conventions, this data set is generally relativity robust at the international level. Nonetheless, seizure data are problematic to interpret because they are heavily influenced by large volume seizures, most of which relate to drugs in transit rather than being reflective of local drug consumption trends. At the 'user' level, the number of seizures is more significant than the quantities seized. The significance of quantities seized is questionable, unless considered in conjunction with other market indicators. In reality, both the number and size of drug seizures depend to a large extent on the priorities and resources of the enforcement agencies, and a single large seizure can distort figures.

Police **arrests** are also used as an indicator of trends in illicit drug use. Yet, once again, their utility is questionable unless police practices and priorities are taken into account (Hartnoll et al., 1989).

21.5.5 Key informant panels and surveys and other approaches sensitive to new trends

It is not possible to cover all the possible sources of information on drug use here, but it is worth noting a growing interest in the role of drug information systems as early warning networks and a corresponding focus on what can be regarded as sensitive sources of information. Among the approaches most commonly used for this purpose is simply to ask people who are close to or part of the behaviour of interest. As a component in monitoring systems, key informants tend to be used either via panel studies with in-depth interviews or via surveys with semi-structured questionnaires. In some models, these are professionals working closely with drug users (Hando et al., 1998; Kemmesies & Hess, 2001), and in others they represent a mix of professionals, cultural companions and drug users themselves (Korf & Nabben, 2000; Mounteney & Leirvåg, 2004). Panel studies are particularly useful in answering questions about the drug using context and dynamics of change. Care and attention needs to be given to how the panel is recruited as the characteristics of the informants will influence their perspective and experience of drug use. For example, a key informant recruited to comment on injecting drug use may not be appropriate for collecting information on recreational cocaine or ecstasy use.

Other approaches have also been used to identify new trends, and unusual findings from forensic science data play an important role in the European early warning system, for example (see Box 21.2). Another source of interest has been the youth media and the internet. An analysis of historical changes in drug use patterns (Griffiths et al., 2000) suggests that information is often available in the specialist media, a considerable time before it is picked up in more formal monitoring sources. Monitoring of youth and local media is included in some information systems (see Box 21.1) although in practice it is both methodological and practical challenging (EMCDDA, 2005). Some projects have begun to monitor drug use discourse and drug advertisements on the internet, as this area is likely to become more developed in the future. It is also worth noting that if the results of random drug testing become more commonly available, perhaps due to an increase in surveillance of drug-impaired driving, this might also prove a useful if somewhat controversial source of information. Innovations may also open up new opportunities. Recent work, for example, has pointed to the possibility of detecting trends in real time in overall levels of drug use through the analysis of biological residues in waste water systems (EMCDDA, 2008).

Box 21.2   An international case study: the European early warning system on new drugs

The European early warning system (EWS) on new psychoactive substances is a multi-agency, interdisciplinary action, which aims to detect and report new drugs as soon as they appear on the European drug market. When a new substance is first identified, detailed information on the manufacture, traffic and use is generated by the European countries and rapidly shared between the EMCDDA, European Police Office and the European Medicines Agency. The information includes a chemical and physical description of the new psychoactive substance; the circumstances in which it is encountered; the chemical precursors, methods of manufacture and trafficking and the involvement of organised crime; indications of the health and social risks associated with the new psychoactive substance; as well as the user groups and the patterns use of the new substance. The main information sources at national level are the heath and care system (emergency rooms, treatment centres, low threshold, outreach and street work agencies, drug prevention centres, drug help lines, etc.) and the main law enforcement agencies are police, customs, border guards, etc. One of the main strengths of the EWS is that it bridges the gap between the health and law enforcement practitioners in the drug field and the forensic science and toxicological findings in the laboratory establishments.

In the last decade, the EWS was able to detect and is monitoring more than 90 new psychoactive substances, among them a number of piperazine derivatives such as BZP (benzylpiperazine). BZP is a stimulant drug with some similarities to amphetamine. From around 2005, BZP had begun to be marketed by internet-based retailers as a legal alternative to ecstasy (3,4-methylenedioxymethamphetamine) and was often misrepresented as a 'natural' product. The early warning system has three components: information exchange, which may trigger a formal risk assessment exercise, with then the possibility of a political-level decision to control. For BZP risk assessment conclusions led to a decision in March 2009 that the drug should be controlled throughout the European Union (EMCDDA, 2008).

21.6   Issues for the interpretation and analysis of data

Some data sources, such as national household surveys and school surveys, may be used to monitor drug patterns and trends in their own right. However, it has become increasingly common to collect together multiple drug-related information sources into networks or drug information systems in order to provide a comprehensive picture for policy-making purposes. An interesting example here is the French TREND project, which utilises a broad set of sources, with a focus on identifying new trends and significant changes in patterns of drug use (Cadet-Taïrou et al., 2008). Most drug trend monitoring systems combine sources to some extent – the key questions are which sources and how? Mounteney et al. (2009) propose five key dimensions that need to be reviewed if a source's validity as a component in a drug monitoring system is to be ascertained. These are reliability, timeliness, directness, drug specificity and coverage.

Data *reliability* puts the focus on consistency and the extent to which the data can be taken as an accurate record of the events they were supposed to record. On the whole, administrative data collection systems such as treatment databases and criminal justice data come with already built checks for reliability. More ad hoc information sources such as youth media and informant reports have clear reliability challenges. *Timeliness* refers to how rapidly individual sources are able to identify and report on a drug phenomenon. There are two dimensions to timeliness, first, an operational level – how quickly or slowly data are collected, analysed and reported publicly. Secondly, how sensitive a source is to new developments, how rapidly it can identify an emerging trend or changing

---

Box 21.3   A national case study: the Australian Illicit Drug Reporting System (IDRS)

The IDRS is intended to provide an early warning system for identifying important emerging trends in drug use at either the local or national level in Australia (Stafford et al., 2005). The reporting system is based on three distinct sources of information: (i) interviews with injecting drug users, (ii) interviews with key experts who have contact with drug users as part of their work and (iii) analysis of various indicator data related to drug use, including survey data, market indicators and information on morbidity and mortality related to drug use (Black et al., 2007).

   The system is intended to provide a sensitive and timely reporting system that can trigger further investigation of important new developments rather than provide a representative picture of drug use in Australia. An example of this is provided by the reporting of a sustained heroin shortage that was initially identified in three Australian states (Degenhardt et al., 2005) and subsequently attracted considerable academic interest. The IDRS data showed that in early 2001 there was a sudden decrease in heroin availability, reflected in increased prices and a decrease in purity. This provided an interesting natural experiment of what happens when a drug like heroin suddenly becomes scarce. In this case, a reduction in fatal and non-fatal opioid overdoses, a possible decrease in overall levels of drug injection and possibly reduced levels of drug-related crime.

---

drug consumption pattern. The use of terms, such as 'lagged' and 'leading edge' indicators, risks conflating these two aspects of a data source's reporting speed and sensitivity (Box 21.3).

For monitoring purposes, it can be useful to differentiate between *direct and indirect measures* of drug consumption – with direct measures relating specifically to drug consumption patterns and indirect measures relating to some broader aspect such as drug markets or drug-related harms. Direct measures generally refer to those in which a group of participants are asked about their own drug consumption (often survey data), indirect measures can be subdivided into those which report primarily on availability and drug markets (price, purity, seizures), those say something about consequences of drug use (arrests, overdoses, hospital admissions) and those which reflect levels of public interest and concern (helpline calls, internet chatrooms, newspaper reports).

Drug specificity – whilst many sources (such as surveys, seizures data) provide drug-specific information, others utilise collective data categories such as 'stimulants', 'opiates' and 'benzodiazepines', which are less useful for monitoring trends in individual substances. For monitoring purposes, sources which provide drug-specific data are generally more useful than those which provide generic information on drug consumption or its consequences.

Coverage refers both to the population covered by a measure (e.g. general population, illicit drug users) and to the range of drugs reported on. Some data sources reflect, to some extent, drug trends in the general population, for example household surveys, hospital admissions data, drink/drug driving data and seizure data. Others focus on specific populations such as drug user surveys, school surveys and key informant panels linked to nightlife environments. It can be important for monitoring systems to ensure a broad coverage of both population and the range of substances used.

In reality, no single data source comes close to meeting all these criteria, and thus at a system level, selection of a mix of sources with strengths across these five dimensions can be desirable. For monitoring purposes, data reliability is paramount; however, for rapid reporting purposes – a source's speed and sensitivity to new and emerging trends is crucial. A challenge for those building systems remains, that reliable measures are often slow and less valid in terms of timeliness, whilst sensitive measures are rapid on the identification of emerging trends, but low on reliability (Mounteney et al., 2009).

A number of other important factors determine the choice of indicators incorporated into systems and the mix of methods adopted. The policy context and underlying premise for the system will influence selection of sources – is the primary goal one of harm reduction or early intervention? Particular populations or subgroups may be prioritised. Source selection is also likely to be different for the identification of emerging trends compared to more routine monitoring.

21.7 Mixed methods

Whilst drug trend monitoring has largely developed within an epidemiological research tradition, most drug information systems that have some focus on monitoring emerging drug trends utilise a mixed method approach whether acknowledged or not. They combine both quantitative methods and qualitative approaches to achieve their aims. Mixed method research is closely linked with a pragmatic paradigm, which amongst other things allows for a pragmatic selection of sources and methods required to best achieve a study's aims. The research problem is most important, and researchers use a variety of approaches to understand the problem (Rossman & Wilson, 1985). It does not require commitment to any one philosophical system (Creswell, 2003), and researchers are free to choose methods that best meet their needs and purposes. This approach developed as *rapid assessment and response* has been widely used for assessing health, and social infrastructure, intervention needs in developing countries and more recently for dug uses and HIV issues (Rhodes et al., 1999).

   Mixed method research is underpinned by the principle of 'triangulation' (Denzin, 1989) – the employment of several approaches aiming to enhance confidence in findings. Creswell (2003) provides a decision choice framework, which can be useful for monitoring systems. At the study implementation stage, clarity is important as to whether a concurrent or sequential strategy is followed. If sequential – which method will be prioritised? Will quantitative data be collected first and prioritised, setting the framework for the study or qualitative? For mixed method approaches, it is important to decide whether the overall framework for merging variables will be conceptual or statistical. Mitchell (1986) suggests that each type of data should be analysed separately in accordance with required principles for that research paradigm.

21.8 Triangulation

The use of multiple indicators and mixed methods brings with it challenges at the data analysis stage. Should all sources be given equal weight in the analysis? To what extent do sources measure the same phenomenon – drug consumption, health consequences, availability, public concern? How do we triangulate? Are sources analysed as part of a dynamic process or simultaneously?

   In the context of monitoring systems, triangulation usually refers to the combination of two or more data sources, approaches or methods, with the aim of increasing validity of findings (Denzin, 1989; Kelle, 2001). It is common to use both triangulation of a range of routine datasets (generally for mutual validation purposes) as well as, or alongside, triangulation of qualitative and quantitative approaches (typically, for completeness purposes). A major challenge for systems is to be more explicit on the reason for triangulation of data and the way this is undertaken. Mutual validation is most common and involves cross-checking findings from multiple sources against each other, on the grounds that any result identified by divergent approaches is likely to be more valid than one found by a single method. The usefulness of triangulation for mutual validation purposes depends on the extent to which results relate to the same drug-related phenomenon. If, as is common with drug-related indicators, they relate to different populations or aspects of drug use, then different results can be expected. For example, a school survey might show a decrease in cannabis use amongst younger pupils, whilst key informants report increased levels of cannabis use by drug injectors. The complementarity approach involves the use of two or more methods to provide a more comprehensive picture. A combination of methods can provide more complete insight into the varied dimensions of a phenomenon, with each source contributing an additional piece to the puzzle and in that way complement each other (van de Mheen et al., 2006). Triangulation can also be simultaneous/concurrent – with different sources and methods being used at the same time, or it can be sequential – with the findings from one approach being used for the planning of the next. Concurrent triangulation will require a common unit of analysis and data transformation, either quantifying qualitative data to allow comparison (e.g. coding) or qualifying of quantitative data (e.g. factor analysis) (Creswell, 2003).

Mounteney et al. (2009) propose a number of steps useful for analysis and data triangulation in trend monitoring systems:

1. Undertake a 'pragmatic' selection of sources on the basis of system's primary objective, as well as availability, reliability and validity.
2. State explicitly the theoretical framework(s) used for data collection and analysis.
3. Clarify the method used for analysis, in particular how qualitative and quantitative methods are triangulated, stating whether:
    (a) Data are collected and analysed concurrently or sequentially.
    (b) Triangulation is used for mutual validation, for complementarity or both. For example, if statistical datasets are triangulated for convergent validity, and then qualitative data are included for completeness, this needs to be made explicit.
    (c) Data are transformed and if so how. In addition, what common unit of analysis is utilised?
4. Make explicit how sources are weighted in comparison with each other and state how divergent results are handled.
5. Ensure findings are presented and disseminated in such a way as to be 'real world' and practice relevant.

21.9   Reliability and validity

Indicators are approximate and often imperfect measures of the nature and extent of particular drug-related events or outcomes. There is a need to systematically check the quality of data sources as a prerequisite for their selection within a system. Quantity of data sources used does not in itself provide a more valid system. Data sources reflect different aspects of the phenomenon. It is important to include sources that are as close as possible to the drug-using population (e.g. data that have passed through less filtering) and to differentiate measures' validity as indicators for rapid reporting of emerging trends as distinct from their validity for longer-term drug monitoring sources.

Drug trend monitoring has multiple challenges in terms of reliability and validity of data used. By data reliability we are referring to the extent to which a measurement procedure yields the same answer, however and whenever it is carried out (see Chapter 2; Kirk & Miller, 1986). It refers to a measure of 'repeatability' or 'consistency'. Trend monitoring using a single source or indicator needs to take into account whether the source says something real about drug consumption patterns (**validity**) and how good the instrument is at reporting (**reliability**). Models combining multiple sources or methods will need to give some consideration as to the reliability of individual sources as well as the validity of the composite picture provided by the chosen mix.

Reliability of measures will be important to consider when selecting them for use in a system. Their ability to detect differences or changes over time is influenced by the size of the sample as small numbers (e.g. the number of new hepatitis C cases in a month), and can cause problems in ascertaining statistically significant differences over time. It is possible to explore the reliability of such measures, particularly prevalence surveys and key informant reports, using test–re-test for reliability studies (Day et al., 2004). Data can also be reviewed and adjusted for seasonal patterns, for example increased alcohol sales during Christmas festivities, in order to iron out short-term data behaviours that do not constitute new trends.

The **construct validity** of measures – the extent to which they are able to reflect the emerging drug trend construct – will have implications for whether they are selected in the first place and for the weighting they are given in an overall analysis. Issues pertaining to *internal validity* are relevant to development of survey instruments. In addition, factors such as key informant panel dropout or mortality can influence the internal validity. The *convergent validity* of findings from individual measures will be important for triangulation and mutual validation purposes. Convergent validity enhances our confidence, but the possibility of error remains. Non-convergence of findings from sources challenges us to explore results more deeply. What underlying factors cause this divergence? *External validity* or a finding's generalisability will be strengthened with repeated measures over time or with confirmation by the same model in another geographical context. Many data sources show short-term fluctuations and variations from 1 year to the next, and this cannot be taken as a reliable sign of change (Hartnoll et al., 1989). Transferability refers to the generalisability of qualitative results from one specific context to another.

Reliability and validity challenges for drug trend monitoring systems, or potential for error, lie in two broad areas: at the level of individual sources and at the whole system level. A type 1 error – finding something that is not there would involve identifying a trend that does not exist. A type 2 error – missing something that is there would involve a system failing to identify a new drug trend. Short-term and rapid reporting systems are more vulnerable to type 1 errors – seeing something that is not there, and less robust than the slower monitoring systems who are more at risk of type 2 errors – missing something that is there, the start of a new trend – due to lack of sensitivity. For further details on reliability and validity, see Chapter 2.

21.10   Reflections in a broken mirror: Pragmatic and imperfect solutions to an intractable problem

In many respects, drug information systems can be seen as a practical rather than scientific accomplishment. No perfect methods exist for studying trends in illicit drug use, and even the definition of the object of subject itself can prove somewhat illusive. What has emerged is a pragmatic set of approaches to a methodologically demanding topic. As we have seen, researchers have had to use a diverse set of information sources and approaches and consider carefully how these can be analysed and their reliability and validity can be assessed. Multi-methods dominate and conclusion must always be drawn with caution. Nonetheless, this way of working can be seen to deliver useful results. Policy making, programme design and the need to respond rapidly to emerging problems are all better informed by information, even if it is imperfect or incomplete. Looking to the future, as more complex and new patterns of substance use emerge, and drug problems continue to profligate in the developing and transitional world, having even a distorted image of the underlying phenomenon is likely to become increasingly important.

Exercises

1. National and international policy agendas often drive the development of drug monitoring systems. Which data sources would you prioritise in a system focused on monitoring drug control and supply factors, as compared with a system monitoring public health and harm reduction factors?
2. If you were developing a drug monitoring system in your own city/locality, what information sources would you include and why? Which of these sources do you consider most reliable? Which sources are most sensitive to new trends?
3. The most commonly used data sources for monitoring drug use include surveys (school and household), drug treatment data and drug seizures data. Name some of the shortcomings of these sources as measures of drug consumption.
4. How might you successfully monitor drug use trends amongst clubbers and trendsetter populations? What particular challenges exist here?
5. Take a look at the data sources you identified in Question 2 for your local monitoring system. Choose four different sources and discuss their reliability, timeliness, directness, drug specificity and coverage. Make a judgement as to which sources you would consider to be the strongest or most useful in the light of these discussions.
6. Taking the example of a city-level monitoring system which incorporates a school survey, a key informant panel and a mix of routine data sources, what analysis challenges does such a model present, and how might these be addressed?
7. How might triangulation be used in the context of a national alcohol monitoring system? What might be the strengths and weaknesses of an approach based on triangulation in this context?

References

Anderson, D., Beckerleg, S., Hailu, D. & Klein, A. (2007) *The Kat Controversy*. Berg: Oxford International Publishers.

Bergeron, H. & Griffiths, P. (2006) Drifting towards a more common approach to a more common problem: epidemiology and the evolution of a European drug policy. In: R. Hughes, R. Lart & P. Higate (eds) *Drugs: Policy and Politics*. England: Open University Press.

Black, E., Roxburgh, A., Degenhart, L., Raimondo, R., Campell, G., De Graaff, B., Fetherston, J., Kinner, S., Moon, C., Quinn, B., Richardson, M., Sindicich, N. & White, N. (2007) *Findings from the Illcit Drug Reporting System (IDRS)*. Australia: Australian Drug Trends series No 1., NDARC.

Cadet-Taïrou, A., Gandhilon, M., Toufik, A. & Evrard, I. (2008) *Phénomènes émergents liés aux drogues en 2006*. France: OEDT.

Courtwrite, D. (1992) A century of American narcotic policy. In: D. R. Gerstein & H. J. Harwood (eds) *Treating Drug Problems*, Vol II. Washington: Institute of Medicine.

Creswell, J. W. (2003) *Research Design: Qualitative, Quantitative and Mixed Method Approaches*. Thousand Oaks, CA: Sage.

Day, C., Collins, L., Degenhardt, L., Thetford, C. & Maher, L. (2004) Reliability of heroin users' reports of drug use behaviour using a 24-month timeline follow-back technique to assess the impact of the Australian heroin shortage. *Addiction Research and Theory*, 12(5), 433–443.

Degenhardt, L., Day, C., Dietze, P., Pointer, S., Conroy, E., Collins, L. & Hall, W. (2005) Effects of a sustained heroin shortage in three Australian States. *Addiction*, 100, 908–920.

Degenhardt, L. & Dietze, P. (2005) *Monograph No. 10: Data Sources on Illicit Drug Use and Harm in Australia*. DPMP Monograph Series. Fitzroy: Turning Point Alcohol and Drug Centre.

Denzin, N. K. (1978) *The Research Act: A Theoretical Introduction to Sociological Methods*, 2nd edn. New York: McGraw-Hill.

Denzin, N. K. (1989) *The Research Act: A Theoretical Introduction to Sociological Methods*, 3rd edn. Chicago: Aldine.

EMCDDA (1997) *Estimating the Prevalence of Problem Drug Use in Europe. EMCDDA, Scientific Monograph 1*. Luxembourg: Office for Official Publications of the European Communities.

EMCDDA (2001) *Monograph – Number 6: Modelling Drug Use: Methods to Quantify and Understand Hidden Processes*. Luxembourg: Office for Official Publications of the European Communities.

EMCDDA (2005) *EMCDDA Thematic Papers – Youth Media*. Lisbon: European Monitoring Centre for Drugs and Drug Addiction.

EMCDDA (2008) Insights 9. *Assessing Illicit Drugs in Wastewater, Potential and Limitations of a New Monitoring Approach*. Luxembourg: Office for Official Publications of the European Communities.

Griffiths, P., Lopez, D. & Gotz, W. (2008) *Monitoring Trends in Illicit Drug Use in Europe: An Overview of the Work of the European Monitoring Centre for Drugs and Drug Addiction (EMCDDA). Psychiatrie und Psychotherapie*, 4, 58–65.

Griffiths, P., Vingoe, L., Hunt, N., Mounteney, J. & Hartnoll, R. (2000) Drug information systems, early warning and new drug trends: can drug monitoring systems become more sensitive to emerging trends in drug consumption? *Substance Use Misuse*, 35(6–8), 811–844.

Hando, J., Darke, S. & O'Brien, S. (1998) The development of an early warning system to detect trends in illicit drug use in Australia: the illicit drug reporting system. *Addiction Research*, 6(2), 97–113.

Hartnoll, R. (2003) Drug epidemiology in the European institutions: historical background and key indicators. *Bulletin on Narcotics*, LV 1&2, 53–71.

Hartnoll, R. (2004) *Drugs and Drug Dependence: Linking Research Policy and Practice. Lessons Learned and Challenges Ahead*. Strasbourg: Pompidou Group, Council of Europe.

Hartnoll, R., Avico, U., Ingold, F., Lange, K., Lenke, L., O'Hare, A. & de Roij-Motshagen, A. (1989) A multi-city study of drug misuse in Europe. *UNODC Bulletin*, 41, 3–27.

Hartnoll, R., Hendriks, V. & Morrival, M. (1998) *The Assessment of Drug Problems*. Copenhagen: WHO Regional Office for Europe.

Hibell, B., Andersson, B., Bjarnason, T., Ahlstrom, S., Balakireva, O., Kokkevi, A. & Morgan, M. (2004) *The ESPAD Report 2003, Alcohol and Other Drug Use Among Students in 35 Countries*. Stockholm, Sweden: Swedish Council for Information on Alcohol and Drugs.

Hibell, B., Guttormsson, U., Ahlström, S., Balakireva, O., Bjarnason, T., Kokkevi, A. & Kraus, L. (2007) *The 2007 ESPAD Report, Substance Use Among Students in 35 European Countries*. The Swedish Council for Information on Alcohol and Other Drugs (CAN), The European Monitoring Centre for Drugs and Drug Addiction (EMCDDA, Council of Europe, Co-operation Group to Combat Drug Abuse and Illicit Trafficking in Drugs (Pompidou Group). Available online: http://www.espad.org/espad-reports (accessed 13 October 2009).

Hickman, M. & Taylor, C. (2005) Indirect methods to estimate prevalence. In: Z. Sloboda (ed.) *Epidemiology of Drug Abuse*. Akron, OH: Institute for Health and Social Policy.

Kelle, U. (2001) Sociological explanations between micro and macro and the integration of qualitative and quantitative methods. *Forum: Qualitative Social Research*, 2(1).

Kemmesies, U. & Hess, H. (2001) *MoSyd. Monitoring-System Drogentrends*. Frankfurt: Centre for Drug Research.

Kirk, J. & Miller, M. (1986) *Reliability and Validity in Qualitative Research*. Newbury Park, CA: Sage Publications.

Korf, D. & Nabben, T. (2000) *Antenna: A Multi-method Approach to Assessing New Drug Trends in EMCDDA Understanding and Responding to Drug Use: The Role of Qualitative Research*. Lisbon: European Monitoring Centre for Drugs and Drug Addiction.

Mitchell, E. (1986) Multiple triangulation: a methodology for nursing science. *Advances in Nursing Science*, 8, 18–26.

Mott, J. (1994) Notification and the home office in heroin addiction and drug policy. In: J. Strang & M. Gossop (eds) *The British System*. Oxford, UK: Oxford University Press, pp. 270–289.

Mounteney, J., Fry, C. L., McKeganey, N. & Haugland, S. (2010) Issues of reliability, validity & triangulation in the rapid identification and monitoring of emerging drug trends. *Substance Use & Misuse*, 45(1&2), 266–287.

Mounteney, J. & Haugland, S. (2009) Earlier warning: a multi-indicator approach to monitoring of trends in the illicit use of medicines. *International Journal of Drug Policy*, 20, 161–169.

Mounteney, J. & Leirvåg, S.-E. (2004) Providing an earlier warning of emerging drug trends: the føre var system. *Drugs: Education, Prevention and Policy*, 11(6), 449–471.

Musto, D. (1973) *The American Disease: Origins of Narcotic Control*. New Haven: Yale University Press.

Musto, D. & Sloboda, Z. (2003) The influence of epidemiology on drug control policy. *Bulletin on Narcotics*, 1&2, 9–22.

Parry, C., Myers, B. & Plüddemann, A. (2004) Drug policy for methamphetamine use urgently needed. *South African Medical Journal*, 94, 964–965.

Rhodes, T., Stimson, G., Fitch, C., Ball, A. & Renton, A. (1999) The Rapid assessment, injecting drug use, and public health. *LANCET*, 354, 65–68.

Rossi, C. (2002) A critical reading of the World Drug Report 2000. *International Journal of Drug Policy*, 13, 221–231.

Rossman, G. & Wilson, B. (1985) Numbers and words: combining quantitative and qualitative methods in a single large-scale evaluation study. *Evaluation Review*, 9(5), 627–643.

Sloboda, Z. & Kozel, N. (2003) Understanding drug trends in the Unites States of America: the role of the Community Epidemiology Work Group as part of a comprehensive drug information system. *Bulletin on Narcotics*, 1&2, 41–51.

Sloboda, Z. (ed.) (2005) *Epidemiology of Drug Abuse*. New York: Springer.

Sloboda, Z. & Kozel, N. (1999) Frontline surveillance in the community epidemiology work group on drug abuse. In: M. Glantz & C. Hartel (eds) *Drug Abuse Origins and Interventions*. Washington, DC: American Psychological Association Press, pp. 47–62.

Stafford, J., Degenhardt, L., Black, E., Bruno, R., Buckingham, K., Fetherston, J., Jenkinson, R., Kinner, S., Newman, J. & Weekley, J. (2005). *Australian Drug Trends 2005: Findings from the Illicit Drug Reporting System (IDRS)*. National Drug and Alcohol Research Centre. NDARC Monograph No. 59, Australia.

Taylor, C. & Griffiths, P. (2005) Sampling issues in drug epidemiology. In: Z. Sloboda (ed.) *Epidemiology of Drug Abuse*. New York: Springer.

UNGASS (1998) *United Nations General Assembly Special Session: Declaration on Guiding Principles of Drug Demand Reduction*. Available online: http://www.un.org/ga/20special/demand.htm (accessed 12 November 2009).

United Nations (1961) *Single Convention on Narcotic Drugs, 1961, As Amended by the 1972 Protocol Amending the Single Convention on Narcotic Drugs, 1961*. Available online: http://www.unodc.org/pdf/convention_1961_en.pdf (accessed 12 November 2009).

United Nations (1971) *Convention on Psychotropic Substances, 1971*. Available online: http://www.unodc.org/pdf/convention_1971_en.pdf (accessed 12 November 2009).

United Nations (1988) *Convention against the Illicit Traffic in Narcotic Drugs and Psychotropic Substances, 1988*. Available online: http://www.unodc.org/pdf/convention_1988_en.pdf (accessed 12 November 2009).

United Nations Office of Drugs and Crime (2002) *Bulletin on Narcotics: The Science of Drug Abuse Epidemiology*, Volume LIV, Nos. 1 and 2. Vienna: United Nations Office of Drugs and Crime.

United Nations Office of Drugs and Crime (2003) *Bulletin on Narcotics: The Practice of Drug Abuse Epidemiology*, Volume LV, Nos. 1 and 2. Vienna: United Nations Office of Drugs and Crime.

United Nations Office on Drugs and Crime (2006) *East Asia and the Pacific 2005 Regional Profile*. Bangkok: United Nations Office on Drugs and Crime Regional Centre for East Asia and the Pacific.

Van de Mheen, H., Coumans, M., Barendregt, A. & van der Poel, A. (2006) A drug monitoring system: keeping a finger on the pulse by triangulation of qualitative and quantitative methods. *Addiction Research and Theory*, 14(5), 461–473.

Recommended websites

International

HBSC – Health Behavior in School-Age Children Survey
www.hbsc.org
INCB – International Narcotics Control Board
www.incb.org
UNODC – United Nations Office on Drugs and Crime
www.unodc.org
UNAIDS – United Nations Program on HIV/AIDS
www.unaids.org
WHO – World Health Organization
www.who.int
World Health Organization page for Rapid Assessment and Action Planning Process (RAAPP)
http://www.who.int/school_youth_health/assessment/raapp/en/

Drug conventions and related materials

United Nations (1961) *Single Convention on Narcotic Drugs, 1961, As Amended by the 1972 Protocol Amending the Single Convention on Narcotic Drugs, 1961.*
http://www.unodc.org/pdf/convention_1961_en.pdf (accessed 12 November 2009)
United Nations (1971) *Convention on Psychotropic Substances, 1971.*
http://www.unodc.org/pdf/convention_1971_en.pdf
United Nations (1988). *Convention against the Illicit Traffic in Narcotic Drugs and Psychotropic Substances, 1988.*
http://www.unodc.org/pdf/convention_1988_en.pdf
UNGASS (1998) *United Nations General Assembly Special Session: Declaration on Guiding Principles of Drug Demand Reduction*
http://www.un.org/ga/20special/demand.htm
United Nations – Annual Report Questionnaire
http://www.unodc.org/unodc/en/cnd_questionnaire_arq.html
Lisbon Consensus
http://www.unodc.org/unodc/en/drug_demand_gap_datacollection.html#core

Americas

CICAD – Inter-American Drug Abuse Control Commission
www.cicad.oas.org

North America

ADAM – Arrestee Drug Abuse Monitoring
www.ojp.usdoj.gov/nij/adam/
CCSA – Canadian Centre on Substance Abuse
www.ccsa.ca
CEWG – Community Epidemiological Working Group
http://www.drugabuse.gov/about/organization/CEWG/CEWGHome.html
DAWN – Drug Abuse Warning Network
www.dawninfo.samhsa.gov
Monitoring the Future
www.monitoringthefuture.org

NIDA – *National Institute of Drug Abuse*
www.drugabuse.gov
NSDUH – *National Survey on Drug Abuse and Health*
http://www.oas.samhsa.gov/nhsda.htm
SAMHSA – *Substance Abuse and Mental Health Services Administration*
www.samhsa.gov

Europe

EMCDDA – *European Monitoring Centre for Drugs and Drug Addiction*
www.emcdda.europa.eu
ESPAD – *European School Survey Project on Alcohol and Other Drugs*
www.espad.org

Asia

ACCORD – *ASEAN and China Cooperative Operations in Response to Dangerous Drugs*
http://www.aseansec.org/645.htm

Africa

SACENDU – *South African Community Epidemiology Network on Drug Use*
http://www.sahealthinfo.org/admodule/sacendu.htm

Australia

AODTS-NMDS – *Alcohol and Other Drug Treatment Services National Minimum Data Set*
http://www.aihw.gov.au/drugs/datacubes/index.cfm
ADIN – *Australian Drug Information Network*
http://www.adin.com.au
DUMA – *Drug Use Monitoring in Australia*
http://www.aic.gov.au/research/duma/
IDMS – *Illicit Drug Monitoring System*
http://www.ndp.govt.nz/moh.nsf/indexcm/ndp-publications-idms
IDRS and EDRS – *Illicit Drug Reporting System and the Ecstasy and Related Drugs Reporting System*
http://ndarc.med.unsw.edu.au/
NDSHS – *National Drug Strategy Household Survey*
http://www.aihw.gov.au/

Chapter 22
DRUG POLICY RESEARCH

Jonathan P. Caulkins and Rosalie Liccardo Pacula

22.1 Introduction

Drug policy research is the application of policy analysis in the substance use and 'addiction' domain with a level of rigor that merits publication in academic journals on the grounds that the methods and/or results can provide foundational insights upon which subsequent analyses might draw.

Policy analysis in turn is an interdisciplinary field that strives to objectively and empirically understand the consequences of different public policy interventions, including both retrospective evaluation of past interventions and prospective projections of contemplated interventions.

It is useful to distinguish three types of policy analysis:

1. Analysis of net effects on society as a whole (a 'social planner's perspective')
2. Distributive analysis of effects on each significant group of stakeholders
3. Political analysis of what convergence of forces can push through a piece of legislation or other policy change

The following example illustrates the differences. Many analysts believe increases in 'sin taxes' on tobacco, alcohol and gasoline would be welfare enhancing. Consumption of these goods generates 'externalities', meaning costs suffered by people other than the producers and consumers. Society would be better off if consumers substituted some consumption into other goods that did not generate such large external costs. A so-called Pigouvian tax that 'internalises those externalities' can create the right incentives for people to reduce consumption down to socially optimal levels. That sort of thinking is an example of societal-level policy analysis.

However, even if raising excise taxes improved aggregate social welfare, not everyone would benefit; there would be winners and losers and that is where distributive analysis fits in. In the case of alcohol, winners include those who are not killed by drunk drivers or assaulted by inebriated drinkers. Losers include responsible and casual drinkers who must pay more for their alcohol, the brewery/distillery that sells less alcohol due to higher prices and distillery workers whose jobs come under threat. Distributive analysis projects outcomes not only in aggregate but also for each significant stakeholder.

From a social planner's perspective, the cases for increasing tobacco and alcohol taxes are similar. Indeed, the alcohol case may be stronger because tobacco is so effective at killing smokers that they often die before collecting retirement or social security benefits. Furthermore, with the significant exceptions of second-hand smoke and fires, most of the social costs of smoking fall on the smoker, not on other people. Nevertheless, at least in the United States it has been easy to raise tobacco excise taxes, while alcohol taxes are rarely increased, so inflation gradually erodes their real value. Why? A political analysis might begin with the observation that in the United States, smokers are a relatively poor, uneducated, ostracised and politically marginalised minority, whereas alcohol consumption is mainstream. Both alcohol and tobacco industry groups try to rally opposition to proposed taxes, but the alcohol lobby has been more successful because most drinkers like their drink, whereas most smokers are intensely ambivalent about the companies whose products have addicted them (Kleiman, 1992). Such discussion of why certain policies do and do not get enacted is the third type of policy analysis.

One contribution of policy analysis can be helping to overcome limitations inherent in less systematic approaches to debating policy. Policy analysis does this in part by providing analytical frameworks that encourage systematic thinking about the issues and the alternative perspectives that might be taken on the issues. Classic examples include MacCoun and Reuter (2001) for illegal drugs and Kleiman (1992) for psychoactive substances more generally. Another key contribution is providing methods for quantitatively comparing the benefits and costs of various policy alternatives, a topic to which we turn next.

22.2 Methods for quantitatively comparing an intervention's benefits and costs

Over the last 40 years, there have been increasing demands to view policy interventions as 'investments' in the public good and to hold them accountable for yielding favourable returns in the way that private investors expect their financial investments to yield a favourable financial return. The analogy is not perfect. For example, in Australia it is common to recognise a triple bottom line of economic, social and environmental outcomes. Nevertheless, programmes are more likely to garner support if legislators can reassure voters that, with respect to some objective, quantifiable metrics, the expenditure of taxpayer dollars is yielding a good 'return on investment'.

Many drug policy analyses seek to assess the quality of these investments using economic evaluation methods, employing metrics such as a 'benefit–cost ratio' (BC), 'cost-effectiveness ratio' (CE), or cost per 'quality-adjusted life year' (QALY) saved. There are several such metrics, some with similar sounding names (see Table 22.1). Thus, it is important to clarify what are their common elements and principal differences.

22.2.1 Cost-identification analysis

All these metrics begin with a 'cost-identification' (also referred to simply as cost analysis), which estimates the value of all resources consumed by the programme, intervention or policy (Gold et al., 1996).[1] Although cost identification might seem like a simple exercise in accounting, important conceptual issues arise that can influence the results. We defer discussion of them until the next section, both because similar issues arise with respect to estimation of benefits and to keep the present focus on contrasting the methods listed in Table 22.1.

22.2.2 Cost-offset analysis

Cost-offset analysis counts not only costs generated by the programme but also cost savings. A classic example would be providing preventive care that obviates the need for more expensive treatment (e.g. screening for hepatitis, allowing treatment to begin before the disease has progressed). Sometimes the cost offsets (reductions) are bigger than the original programme costs, so implementing the programme actually saves money. That might be the case, for example, when non-violent offenders are diverted into treatment in lieu of expensive incarceration. In that case, it may not be necessary

Table 22.1 Common forms of economic evaluations used in addiction studies

Name	Acronym	Outcome measure
Cost offset	—	Currency
Cost-effectiveness analysis	CEA	Any single outcome (e.g. initiation, past-month prevalence, drug-free days, clean urine samples, length of time in treatment)
Cost–utility analysis/quality of life	CUA/QoL	Psychometric indicators of quality of life or extension of life with a disability or illness vs shorter life without the illness/disability
• Cost per quality of life saved • Cost per disability-adjusted life year • Health-year equivalent • Quality-of-life index	• QALY • DALY • HYE • QOLI	
Cost–benefit analysis	CBA or BC	Currency

to take on the more challenging task of quantifying the non-monetary benefits; as long as they are positive, no matter whether they are large or small, a programme that saves money is a good investment.

While identifying costs and offsets is necessary, programme costs are usually not fully offset through future cost savings, so one must also evaluate what these resources contribute in terms of the desired outcome or outcomes. Furthermore, policy makers are frequently forced to choose between alternative programmes that accomplish similar goals. That is where the other forms of evaluation come in.

22.2.3 Cost-effectiveness analysis

Cost-effectiveness analysis (CEA) is the most common form of economic evaluation (Gold et al., 1996; Drummond et al., 1997). CEA evaluates costs and outcomes simultaneously by comparing ratios of the cost of a programme relative to its effectiveness at producing a specific desirable outcome. For example, if the key outcome were overdoses (ODs) averted, then

$$\text{Cost} - \text{effectiveness ratio} = \frac{\text{Cost with intervention} - \text{Cost without intervention}}{\text{ODs averted with intervention} - \text{ODs averted without intervention}}$$

Thus, the CEA ratio indicates how much one has to 'pay' in order to 'purchase' one unit of the benefit (e.g. cost per OD). Expressed in this format, smaller ratios are better, indicating less expensive ways of purchasing a given benefit. Some literatures prefer the inverse of this ratio so that larger numbers are better (more benefits purchased per million dollars spent). CEA provides a measure of a programme's cost per unit of outcome, which can be compared directly to competing projects that produce the same outcome. The biggest limitation of CEA is that many interventions produce multiple benefits in disparate proportions. Hence, one programme may have the best CEA ratio when focusing on one outcome, while a different programme appears superior when focusing on a different outcome.

22.2.4 Cost–utility analysis

When an intervention generates multiple benefits that are health related, cost–utility analysis (CUA) can be used to assess effectiveness using a singular outcome (Yin & Forman, 1995; Drummond et al., 1997). Like CEA, CUA considers the costs and outcomes simultaneously by forming and comparing ratios. The outcome of interest, however, is expressed in terms of expected utility or general well-being with respect to health, not in terms of a single outcome such as overdose. Changes in utility are expressed in terms of healthy-year equivalents (HYEs), disability-adjusted life years (DALY), or, most commonly, in QALYs (Gold et al., 1996). The HRQoL (health related quality of life) approach requires that each health state of interest be assigned a numerical weight that reflects preferences for that health state, ranging from 0 (death) to 1 (optimal health). The effects of an intervention can then be represented as changes in health states where the quality-adjusted score for each health state is multiplied by the expected time in the state and then summed over the expected time of life.

A number of methods have been used to obtain preference weightings for health states. Specialists in this area grapple with issues like the fact that prospectively people think an adverse health outcome (e.g. loss of a limb) will be much worse than do people who have suffered that outcome and had time to adjust to it. Two particular methods that have been widely adopted include The Healthy Days Measures (CDC, 2000) and the EuroQol-5D (Kind et al., 1998; Rabin & de Charro, 2001). However, neither fully captures the cognitive, behavioural or physical limitations of addiction; nor do they capture all the non-health dimensions of improved well-being (e.g. better family relations, improved employment situation and less criminal involvement). Hence, scientists continue working on new measures of well-being (e.g. the 'quality-of-life index' or QOLI or the Personal Well-Being Index or PWI) that more accurately capture these dimensions for substance use disorders (French et al., 2002; Cummins, 2003; Jofre-Bonet & Sindelar, 2004; Daley et al., 2005).

22.2.5 Cost–benefit analysis

There remains another fundamental limitation of CUA when applied to substance abuse, namely, that substance abuse creates and drug control interventions avert a wide range of important non-health-related costs and benefits. Policy analysts generally incorporate non-health outcomes into their analyses of other societal issues. For example, when analysing the possibility of damming a river, policy analysts would factor in outcomes such as electricity production, enhanced recreational outcomes and flood control (including protection of property as well as lives). These are at best awkward to include within a CUA because they are not naturally thought of in terms of health states. Hence, policy analysts working beyond the domain of health interventions generally view cost–benefit analysis (CBA) as the preferred tool. CBA is similar to CUA inasmuch as it too attempts to convert diverse outcomes into a common metric so that they can be added up to get a full accounting of benefits. The principal difference is that in CBA that common metric is currency (dollars in the United States, euros in the Eurozone, etc.).

Just as with CUA, there is an entire subliterature devoted to the question of how one assigns reasonable values to various outcomes. This is easy if the outcomes are priced directly in a market, and in modern industrial societies a remarkable range of things are. Nevertheless, a number of key drug-related outcomes are not traded in markets or are traded in highly imperfect markets (e.g. safety and family bonds). Social policy researchers in the addiction field spend a lot of time debating how to deal with these complications. Box 22.1. briefly summarises the debate surrounding how best to value some of these outcomes.

Box 22.1   Outcomes whose valuation poses special challenges

Property crime: What is the societal cost of a burglar stealing something? The old answer is zero on the grounds that theft merely transfers wealth from one person to another, with no net loss to society. Sometimes allowance is made for the possibility that someone who actually bought an object might value it more, on average, than someone who got it for free (stole it). That still skirts the real issue, namely, that the public, and policy makers accountable to the public, vehemently object to the idea that there is no social cost to property crime. The more modern approach is to focus on the 'willingness to pay' to avoid such criminal victimisation. That is, if an average person were willing to pay $1000 to avoid being burglarised (as evidenced, e.g. by analysis of investments in household alarm systems), then preventing a burglary should be valued at $1000.[2]

Violent crime: A similar conundrum surrounds violent crime. The old approach counted primarily victims' hospital bills for treating injuries and days of work lost while recuperating, but as with property crime, this led to valuations that struck the public as absurdly low. Estimates based on jury awards and willingness-to-pay principles can incorporate the 'intangible' costs of pain and suffering as well as the much smaller 'tangible' costs associated with receiving medical care.[3]

Premature death: How does one value a human life, such as one saved by a drug policy intervention? An often contentious measure employed in many studies is the human capital approach, where the value of a human life is calculated as the present discounted value of expected future earnings (Rice, 1967). A central criticism of this approach is that individuals who choose not to work (e.g. stay at home parents) or those who earn lower wages (e.g. workers in developing countries) are presumed to have less worth than those who earn more, and this seems morally wrong. The willingness to pay approach has been adopted by economists to get around this issue. It calculates the statistical value of life based on market purchases people make to reduce their risk of death, or premiums they must be paid to accept additional risk of mortality.[4] Examples of such market transactions include the purchase of safety devices (cars with airbags, home security systems) and wage premiums for working in risky jobs (e.g. mining or construction). These measures, however, remain contentious as they too can be influenced by the wealth and income of the population in which they are assessed.

Cost of addiction itself: Conventional economic reasoning holds that when people buy something, there is a 'consumer surplus', meaning, the monetary valuation of the satisfaction derived from consuming the product must exceed its purchase price, otherwise the consumer would not have freely chosen to pay for it. Non-addicted users are presumably choosing to consume drugs of their own volition, but most of the expensive drugs (heroin, cocaine and amphetamines) are used by people who are dependent. Are those dependent users more like a typical consumer or more like a prisoner, compelled by the addiction to consume something from which they do not derive much satisfaction? To date, many economic analyses still assume that even dependent users are like conventional consumers and so recognise no cost of addiction per se. Likewise, very few consider the psychological pain and suffering addiction causes the family and friends of those who are addicted because the unit of analysis in many economic studies is the household, not the individual, so the entire household's consumption decisions are assumed to be welfare enhancing for the household as a unit. Some suggest that when the purpose of the economic analysis is to compare drug interventions to interventions in other policy domains, all analyses must be done using the traditional, common methods. However, when the analysis is only meant to inform choices within the domain of drug policy, then the standard methods should be adopted to domain-specific idiosyncrasies, such as a need to discard standard assumptions that consumption always enhancing the consumer's welfare.

Table 22.2 Some issues to consider when identifying costs and benefits

Perspective	Payer
	Provider
	Government (taxpayer)
	Society
Costs and benefits included	Programme costs
	• Accounting cost
	• Economic (opportunity) cost
	Client costs and cost savings
	Intangible costs and benefits
Time	Evaluation period
	Discount rate

22.3   Issues that arise in quantifying an intervention's benefits and costs

Box 22.1 discusses challenges in valuing outcomes that are related to addiction. Distinct from those difficulties are conceptual issues that complicate analyses regardless of one's position on the value of a life or the cost of crime. These include issues related to the perspective from which costs are evaluated, the costs and benefits considered, and the time horizon over which they are evaluated (see Table 22.2).

22.3.1   Perspective

Perspective refers to whose shoes the analyst steps into when deciding which outcomes to include. Common perspectives for economic analysis include the payer, the provider and society as a whole. When private insurance pays for treatment provided by a hospital or non-profit treatment agency, these three perspectives are all distinct. When the government provides services in its own facilities (e.g. treatment provided through the US Veterans Administration or the British National Health Service), the three perspectives are one and the same. However, even when the public sector is both payer and provider, perspective can still matter if costs borne by one department or ministry produce benefits or cost savings for another department or ministry. For example, when treatment reduces criminality and, hence, associated law enforcement costs, the Ministry of Justice rarely expresses its appreciation by writing a check to the Ministry of Health, so the payer/provider's perspective (the Ministry of Health) differs from the social welfare perspective (which would encompass both ministries).

In addiction services, costs have traditionally been evaluated from the payer's perspective. Because so many services and programmes are paid for by the public sector and because they often have impacts beyond the payer and the provider, a U.S. Public Health Service panel now advocates that economic evaluations be conducted from the societal perspective, rather than just from a payer's or provider's perspective. While the societal perspective has been widely adopted for cost-of-illness studies (Collins & Lapsley, 2002; Single et al., 2003; ONDCP, 2004), some doubt this is truly desirable when considering programmes that will only be adopted if they are financially viable for the agency delivering them (Humphreys et al., 2008). Unfortunately, agencies are not frequently evaluated in terms of the savings they generate for other agencies; they are usually evaluated only in terms of costs and performance within their own silo. So, the choice in perspective may depend somewhat on the goal of the evaluation. For an academic audience, the societal perspective may be preferred, but if the goal is to inform real policy makers, a more local perspective (e.g. that of a single agency or provider) may be more influential.

22.3.2 Economic versus accounting costs

Another issue to consider is whether resources should be evaluated in terms of their cost in that use or in terms of their full economic value. Payers and providers have traditionally focused on the accounting or monetary cost of the goods and services they purchase. However, sometimes the price paid for a resource may be more or less than its true market value. A good example would be supplies or volunteer hours donated to a non-profit provider. Although the provider's cash flow accounting statements will contain no entry for donated items, economists prefer to value these resources in terms of their full value (referred to as 'opportunity cost'), as these resources could have been used for other things. The argument is that resources are inherently limited in society, and when they are used for one purpose, they can no longer be used for another purpose. For example, a volunteer who donates time, assisting patients in a neighbourhood treatment clinic, might have a paid job to do similar activities in a hospital. The wage she could have earned if she did a similar job represents the opportunity cost of her time or true economic value of the labour. Similarly, when a teacher uses class time to teach students drug prevention, this represents a real opportunity cost since that time could have been used to teach traditional academic subjects. So the cost of the drug prevention programme, to economists, includes the cost of time taken away from other subjects in addition to the monetary cost of the programme materials and teacher training.

An economic evaluation may also consider costs incurred by the individual receiving the programme (i.e. the client's costs). Individuals who have to miss work or need to employ daycare to watch children in order to attend treatment incur real costs to participate in the programme above and beyond any monetary co-payments. If the goal is to consider costs from a societal perspective, then these additional costs should be considered. One challenge when moving beyond accounting costs is that it can be like opening a Pandora's box of indirect effects that are hard to quantify. Suppose someone attending a 30-day inpatient programme lost their job because they did not have enough accrued vacation and did not want to or could not claim short-term disability. Or suppose that inpatient treatment created strain on a family due to 30 days of separation. In theory, one should include such costs, particularly if the corresponding long-term effects of improved employment and family functioning are included on the benefit side. Analysts with an agenda can (perhaps unconsciously) distort results by judging that the evidence base concerning some costs is insufficient to support quantification while patching together estimates for other, favourable, effects for which the evidence base is no better. Likewise, bias can enter one step earlier if the programme evaluation works harder to document anticipated programme benefits than unintended adverse consequences.

22.3.3 Time horizon

A third issue is the time horizon over which a programme's cost and benefits are to be evaluated. Although formal drug treatment (and programme costs) might end after a 30-day period, the benefits of that drug treatment can continue to accrue for months and years after the treatment episode has been completed (Zarkin et al., 2005). If a drug treatment programme is assessed only in terms of its costs and benefits for the period in which treatment took place, the costs could easily exceed the benefits. However, simply extending the evaluation period by 6 or 9 months can dramatically change the net result. Likewise, targeted law enforcement initiatives like reductions in the availability of precursor chemical laws might have large effects if evaluated within a relatively short time horizon (e.g. months within their adoption), but have no lasting effect when evaluated over a longer time horizon (e.g. 2 years post). Thus, consideration of the time horizon is important when measuring effectiveness and will likely be partially dependent on the policy being evaluated.

When evaluations are done over periods longer than 1 year, it is important to make sure that both outcomes (benefits) and costs are discounted to reflect their net present value. Choice of discount factor can have important implications if the horizon over which things are to be evaluated is long, as high discount rates will reduce the benefit (loss) associated with outcomes far off in the future, while low discount rates will increase their values.

22.4   Methods for estimating an intervention's effects

The previous sections explained how policy analysts aggregate quantitative projections of an intervention's beneficial and costly outcomes into a summary performance measure. The next question is, how does one project programme outcomes in the first place? The general answer is, 'by any means necessary' or, perhaps more precisely, by any accepted, replicable, objective method that is suitable to the context and evidence. In other words, policy analysis is happy to borrow tools from statistics, econometrics, epidemiology, operations research or any other science. Some of the most common methods are highlighted in Table 22.3.

This ecumenicalism with respect to methods is admirable; it lets policy analysts grapple with a wide range of issues. However, it is also a source of misunderstanding and sometimes even mistrust from scientists who work within a discipline where one method dominates. For example, some disciplines view randomised controlled trials (RCTs) as not just the gold standard but almost as the *only* reputable form of inquiry. However, it would not make much sense to use RCTs as the basis for estimating the benefits of space exploration, for example.

22.4.1   Randomised controlled trials

Nevertheless, there are good reasons why RCT is the gold standard, and other methods should be employed only when an RCT is not feasible. For treatment and other interventions aimed at dependent users, policy analysis usually builds directly on a clinical RCT. For example, a group of imprisoned drug users are randomly assigned to standard treatment in prison, treatment plus half-way

Table 22.3   Statistical tools for evaluating outcomes in policy analyses

1. Random assignment study design
2. Quasi-experimental methods

   - Propensity score methods
   - Instrumental variables techniques
   - Difference-in-difference techniques
   - Regression discontinuity approach

3. Modelling approaches

   - Microsimulation
   - Agent-based modelling

house support after prison, or a no-treatment control condition. Study subjects are followed up at various times, perhaps 6, 12 and 18 months post-release. Health and criminal justice outcomes might be tracked through administrative data and/or by self-report. The effect of the intervention is judged to be the difference in the average number of events of a particular type experienced or reported by the treatment group relative to the control group (sometimes only recording such differences when the difference is statistically significant). There are limitations to how broadly RCTs can be applied in social research, however. Some interventions, including media-based prevention campaigns and community coalition building, operate at the community level, not at the individual level. It is hard to randomly assign communities to one treatment condition or another, and sample sizes when this is done are generally smaller. The problem becomes even more acute when the intervention's impact would be felt nationally, as with changes in national sentencing policy, border control or interventions undertaken in source countries (e.g. Colombia or Afghanistan) with the goal of constraining supply in final market countries.

RCT designs also do not always measure long-term and spillover effects. School-based drug prevention programmes typically address 10–14 years old youths, yet most of the social costs of drug use stem from use later in life. Twenty-year follow-up data collection is both expensive and rare. Even when possible, it inevitably produces dated information and usually suffers sample selection bias (because people who stay in a study for 20 years are different than those who drop out). The challenge with spillover effects is that they can be diffuse and manifest in the behaviour of people not in the programme. For example, cracking down on drug dealing in a particular neighbourhood might yield tangible, readily apparent benefits for that neighbourhood not so much by reducing drug use as by displacing it. If the displaced activity were spread over ten other neighbourhoods (or into social network-based rather than place-based selling), the displaced activity might be hard to detect, leading to an overestimate of the net benefits of intervening. Similarly, if harm reduction programmes directed at dependent adult users had an adverse effect on initiation by teens, it would be very hard to detect that with typical RCT designs that focus on outcomes experienced by programme participants.

22.4.2   Quasi-experimental methods

Although randomised experiments remain the gold standard, observational studies using non-random population data are often necessary due to practical considerations. In observational studies, systematic differences can exist between the 'treated' and 'untreated' groups with respect to both observable and unobservable characteristics. Hence, direct comparisons of the observed outcomes from the two groups may not be appropriate and can lead to biased or misleading conclusions. Fortunately, quasi-experimental methods have emerged from a variety of disciplines to assist with the identification of programme or policy effects when randomisation is not possible. The methods most useful for addiction research include: propensity score methods, instrumental variable techniques, difference-in-difference estimation and regression discontinuity approaches.

Propensity score methods

Propensity score methods (e.g. propensity score weighting, nearest neighbour matching) are an increasingly common approach for handling biases associated with non-random assignment to programmes, policies or treatment conditions. The methods involve adjusting the comparison group members in terms of their observational characteristics so that they become observationally equivalent to the treated population before the policy (programme, treatment) takes place. Assuming no unobserved factor differs systematically between these two groups once this adjustment takes place, analysis of these adjusted data provides a good estimate of the effect of the treatment on the treated population. A variety of methods for adjusting the data have emerged, from 'matching' algorithms making use of a small subset of the comparison group to 'reweighting' methods that make full use of the comparison group by adjusting the distribution of multiple observed characteristics across the two groups so that they are nearly identical.

Instrumental variables approaches

Instrumental variables (IV) methods are frequently used for inferring causal associations from observational data, particularly when the explanatory variable is known to be correlated with the error term (i.e. 'endogenous'). Standard regression techniques (ordinary least squares, logistic regression, and so on) require that the error term be uncorrelated (or more technically 'orthogonal') to all the independent variables for unbiased and consistent estimation of the parameters to occur. If this condition is not met, then the estimated coefficients and their standard errors from these techniques will be biased (the direction of which depends on the nature of the correlation with the error term). Endogeneity results from common unaccounted for third factors that influence both participation in the programme/policy (the key independent variable) and the error term. The advantage of IV methods is that they generate statistically consistent estimates of beta coefficients, enabling the researcher to answer the same question as regression methods (i.e. 'what is the average effect of the programme?'). IV techniques depend critically on the ability to identify an instrument that (1) is highly correlated with the endogeneous explanatory variable, conditional on the other variables in the model, and (2) is not correlated with the error term itself or directly influences the outcome (dependent) variable being modelled (except through the explanatory variable being instrumented). IV estimates are usually obtained through two-step modelling. In the first step, the endogenous variable (e.g. programme participation) is estimated as a function of all the other variables and the instrument(s) used for identification. In the second stage, the original regression of interest is estimated, but instead of putting actual programme participation in the regression, the analyst replaces that variable with the predicted value obtained from the first-stage regression and adjusts the variance-covariance matrix appropriately. Occasionally, reduced form methods are used where the instrument replaces the policy or programme variable in the second regression. This allows the researcher to determine if a causal association exists, although they cannot then determine the true magnitude of the association.

Difference-in-differences methods

Difference-in-differences (DD) techniques attempt to ascertain the average treatment effect of a programme or policy by looking at how changes in the outcome of interest differ between the treatment and control groups over time. Because treatment and control groups could differ in both observable and unobservable ways, it is critical to have data on the outcome variable of interest for at least three different periods: (1) some time before the policy/programme took place, (2) right before the policy/programme took place and (3) some time after the policy/programme. With information from these three points, one can look at the average change in the outcome of interest for both groups before the policy or programme (to see if they had similar rates of change even before the policy took place) and after (to see if the programme or policy influenced the rate of change in the outcome variable after it took place). By examining changes in the control group as well as the treatment group, analysts can isolate the true programme effect by taking out the average change that would have taken place (based on the controls) even if the programme or policy did not take place. Simple examination of mean differences and sophisticated regression methods have been used to construct DD estimates, but the principal idea is the same: to understand if the programme or policy influenced the rate of change in the outcome variable for the treatment group beyond what it would have otherwise had the programme never taken place (known from the pre-programme data and the overall changes observed for the control group).

Regression discontinuity approaches

Like DD methods, regression discontinuity methods involve a pretest–posttest group comparison. Groups, however, are assigned not by the programme or policy but rather by the analyst based on an observed covariate that is expected to be impacted by the programme or policy, and that has values on either side of a critical fixed threshold (e.g. the poverty line, 0.08 blood alcohol content level, or possession of 1 ounce of marijuana). Observations in the data are assigned to groups based on the cut-off score of the measured covariate. Observations below the cut-off are assigned to one group, and observations above the cut-off are assigned to the other group. The effect of the programme or policy is estimated by the disconnect in the regression lines (slopes) or functions (for higher order polynomials) obtained from separate models estimated on each of these groups below and above the threshold value. Unlike DD, regression discontinuity does not provide an estimate of the average effect but rather identifies whether a difference in average behaviour exists at the critical threshold value. Thus, it can identify if a programme or policy had an effect, but it cannot provide a good estimate of the average effect of the programme or policy on the populations as a whole.

22.5 Modelling methods

Quasi-experimental methods can be useful for evaluating past interventions when suitable data are available. However, sometimes policy makers want to project the results of trying something new or replicating something for which suitable data have not been collected in the past. In such cases, modelling may still be possible if researchers have a good understanding of the structure of the system and the cause and effect rules that it follows. Modelling is rather common in engineering. Space scientists do not estimate how much fuel a rocket will need by collecting data on how much fuel rockets used in the past and running a regression; they build a model of the rocket's dynamics from first principles, such as Newton's laws of motion.

Individual people are rarely as predictable as rockets, but sometimes they behave predictably in aggregate. For example, queueing theory provides a set of models that might do a very good job of predicting how expanding the number of treatment slots would reduce waiting times for people seeking treatment (Kaplan & Johri, 2000). Likewise, product diffusion models from marketing may help predict the spread of a drug that has recently become available within a particular population (Caulkins, 2008), and models of infectious diseases may help predict how certain drug control interventions will affect the spread of hepatitis or HIV (Kaplan, 1995; Pollack, 2001, 2002). So-called risks and prices models of drug markets try to estimate how changes in law enforcement might affect retail drug prices in equilibrium (Reuter & Kleiman, 1986) and, when coupled with estimates of the 'elasticity' (responsiveness) of demand to price changes, how prices changes could affect drug initiation and use (e.g. Caulkins et al., 1997). Short descriptions of two of the many modelling methods are as follows:

Microsimulation models. A microsimulation is a computer programme that projects the behaviour of an individual entity (typically, a person, but could be a household or business) within a 'synthetic' environment, conditional on that entity's characteristics (e.g. gender, age, income and criminal proclivity). The simulation is then run for a large number of heterogeneous agents whose character-istics match some population of interest (e.g. a birth cohort or the population of a city). The goal is to weight and aggregate the individual agents' outcomes to understand results for the population as a whole (in terms of average behaviour or distribution of outcomes). Running the entire process twice, with different environmental conditions perhaps representing different policy regimes, produces an estimate of how that change would affect population-level outcomes. Static simulations explore a fixed population that does not change. Dynamic models can 'age' the population for many years (decades) into the future, applying appropriate rules for demographic and economic processes, such as death rates, high school completion rates and retirement rates. Thus, dynamic models allow one to assess both the immediate and longer-term effects of a policy or programme on the population as it changes over time.

Agent-based models. Agent-based models (ABMs) are similar to microsimulation models, except that all the individuals (called 'agents') move through the simulation at the same time, and interact with each other, as they follow their behavioural rules (Agar & Wilson, 2002; Perez et al., 2006). For example, in ABM models of traffic flow, the agents are drivers and a general rule common to all drivers might be 'drive along the quickest route to work'. Individual characteristics might include where the individual agent lives and works. Because the agents interact, and in many models can even learn from these interactions over time, the population-level outcomes are not just the summation of the projections for individuals. The agents' behavioural rules can be quite complex, combining elements of game theory, social contagion and complex systems. Likewise, in data-rich environments (e.g. traffic modelling), ABM models can give quite detailed projections. More often though the goal is to discover 'emergent' system behaviours that manifest even when the agents are modelled in a very stylised fashion and follow only very basic rules. Thus, agent-based models allow us to examine dynamic systems with complex interactions in a way that other models cannot allow (due to the inability to track all the possible interactions).

22.6 Summary

Policy analysis strives to understand (often quantitatively) the effects of implementing policies and programmes by projecting their outcomes, both intended and unintended, in aggregate and from the perspective of each relevant stakeholder. There are a variety of particular techniques associated with policy analysis, including CEA, CUA, and CBA. All strive to provide summary metrics that concisely capture and balance the good and the bad consequences of a past or planned action. Hence, policy analysis builds a bridge between scientific understanding of a policy domain and evidence-based decision-making concerning how best to intervene in that domain.

Policy analysis in the addictions field presents a number of special challenges that make this type of research exciting, and its findings sometimes controversial. Addiction-related issues span many levels of aggregation, from the molecular, to the individual, agency, community, national, and even international level. Some involve relatively simple logic models; others involve complicated endogeneity (e.g. market behaviour), lags and/or nonlinear feedback. Hence, the best policy analyses are often conducted by interdisciplinary teams that can usefully borrow and adapt methods from many different disciplines.

Acknowledgements

This work was funded in part by the Robert Wood Johnson Foundation, the Qatar Foundation and the National Institute on Drug Abuse (1R01 DA019993).

Excercises

1. *(Stakeholder identification)*
   Give one example each of a policy that would be good for society that has not been implemented because it lacks political support, and a policy that is bad for society overall but which has nonetheless been implemented because a coalition of stakeholders pushed for it. In each case, list the stakeholders who are or who would be helped or hurt by that policy.

2. *(Discounting future outcomes)*
   (a) Imagine two hypothetical polices (A and B) that are mutually exclusive. Policy A will save 100 lives over the next 24 months, and Policy B will save 200 lives in 10 years. Which would you prefer?
   (b) Now consider two policies that would have no effect on health outcomes, but the first (Policy C) will save taxpayers $100 million (or pounds, or euros) over the next 24 months, and the other (Policy D) will save $200 million in 10 years. Which would you prefer?
   (c) For the money-saving policies (C and D), find your indifference point. That is, if you preferred C (saving $100 million soon), how large would the savings in 10 years under Policy D be in order for you to be indifferent between choosing Policies C or D? Similarly, if you initially preferred D, how much could the $200 million figure be reduced before you would become indifferent between choosing Policies C or D?
   (d) Repeat Exercise (c) but for Policies A and B, for which the outcomes are lives saved.
   (e) Do you get the same numerical value of the indifference point in parts (c) and (d)? Many people do not, but Keeler and Cretin (1983) prove that policy analysis must make intertemporal trade-offs consistently for monetary and non-monetary outcomes to avoid logical traps.

3. *(Event trees)*
   There is enormous heterogeneity in drug consumption 'careers', with most people using drugs only occasionally and a small subset progressing to prolonged, frequent use. A full model of this would capture dynamics over time and the use of different types of substances, but many of the policy implications of heterogeneity can be elucidated even by a simple event tree such as the one in Figure 22.1. Circles in event trees represent random events. For instance, the first circle in Figure 22.1 represents a situation in which half of all people in the population of interest (e.g. a birth cohort) try drugs (lifetime prevalence is 50%). Probabilities on subsequent branches are conditional, so the probability of reaching any given 'leaf' (the tip of a set of branches on the far right) can be obtained by multiplying the probabilities along the path leading to that leaf. For example, in Figure 22.1, $1/2 \times 1/2 \times 1/3 = 1/12$ of the population will escalate and use an average of 300 days per year for 10 years. Leaves are customarily annotated with one or more outcomes. In this case, the outcome is the total number of times drugs are used over the lifetime.

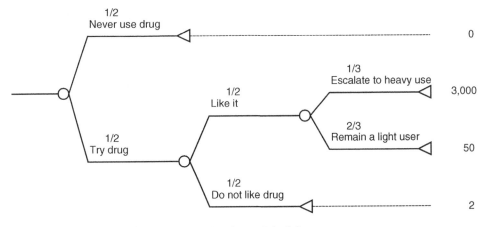

Figure 22.1 Event tree for Exercise 3: simple model of drug use careers.

(a) How many times does the average person in this population use drugs?

(b) Among those who ever use drugs, what is the average number of times drugs are used?

(c) Show that 96.6% of drug use is attributable to the 1/6 of all users who escalate to heavy use. That is, heterogeneity in this model is even more extreme than the classic 'Pareto law' that says that often 80% of an activity is attributable to the 20% of people who participate most actively.

(d) How many times more use would be prevented by convincing a light user not to escalate (secondary prevention) versus preventing a typical person from trying drugs the first time (primary prevention)?

4. *(Breakeven analysis)*

Models of drug use careers become even more useful for policy analysis if they can be augmented by estimates of the social cost or harm associated with each state, transition or event over the course of that career. To illustrate this, suppose that in the previous problem's model, every day of heavy drug use generated $100 in social costs, and costs associated with other drug use are negligible. This implies that the social cost per year of heavy use is $30 000, which is not an unreasonable figure for dependent use of stimulants, particularly by people who are criminally involved.

(a) Suppose a universal prevention programme cost $100 per student. What proportion of participants would the programme have to persuade not to use drugs in order for the programme's benefits to equal its costs? (For now, ignore discounting and assume that those whose initiation is prevented are typical of all users in the population.)

(b) How would your answer in Part (a) change if prevention only worked on people who would not have escalated to heavy use anyhow?

(c) How would your answer in Part (a) change if the programme is administered to 13-year-olds, the average year of heavy use occurs at age 28, and future events are discounted at a compound annual rate of 5% per year?

(d) Now consider a treatment intervention that costs $2000 per person admitted. If, on average, people enrol in the programme half-way through their career of heavy drug use and the only programme outcome were permanent abstinence for a subset of those treated, how high would that treatment effectiveness rate have to be in order for the programme to have a favourable benefit–cost ratio?

(e) Today, treatment programmes rarely think in terms of achieving permanent abstinence. Instead, consider a treatment programme that costs $1000 per month and whose only effect is to reduce use during treatment (no long-term effects). By what proportion would such a programme have to reduce use in order to have a favourable benefit–cost ratio?

(f) Some interventions seek to reduce harm, not use. If such a programme cost $1000 per month, by what proportion would it have to reduce harm in order to have a favourable benefit–cost ratio?

Notes

1. We will henceforth use the term 'programme' to refer to a programme, policy or intervention that might be considered by the government or treatment (prevention) service provider.
2. Miller et al. (1996) is a classic reference to this more modern approach.
3. Again, Miller et al. (1996) is a classic reference.
4. See Viscusi and Aldy (2003) for a review.

References

Agar, M. H. & Wilson, D. (2002) Drugmart: heroin epidemics as complex adaptive systems. *Complexity*, 7(5), 44–52.

Bardach, E. (2000) *A Practical Guide for Policy Analysis: The Eightfold Path to More Effective Problem Solving*. New York: Chatham House Publishers.

Caulkins, J. P. (2008) Implications of inertia for assessing drug control policy: why upstream interventions may not receive due credit. *Contemporary Drug Problems*, 35(2–3), 347–369.

Caulkins, J. P., Rydell, C. P., Schwabe, W. L. & Chiesa, J. (1997) *Mandatory Minimum Drug Sentences: Throwing Away the Key or the Taxpayers' Money?* MR-827-DPRC. Santa Monica, CA: RAND.

Centers for Disease Control and Prevention (CDC) (November 2000) *Measuring Healthy Days*. Atlanta, GA: CDC.

Collins, D. J. & Lapsley, H. M. (2002) *Counting the Cost: Estimates of the Social Costs of Drug Abuse in Australia in 1998–1999*. National Drug Strategy Monograph Series No. 49, Canberra, Australia: Commonwealth Department of Health and Ageing.

Cummins, R. A., Eckersley, R., Pallant, J., van Vugt, J. & Misajon, R. (2003) Developing a national index of subjective wellbeing: the Australian unity wellbeing index. *Social Indicators Research*, 64, 159–190.

Daley, M., Shepard, D. S. & Bury-Maynard, D. (2005) Changes in quality of life for pregnant women in substance user treatment: developing a quality of life index for the addictions. *Substance Use and Misuse*, 40(3), 375–394.

Drummond, M. F., O'Brien, B., Stoddart, G. L. & Torrance, G. W. (1997) *Methods for the Economic Evaluation of Health Care Programmes*. Oxford: Oxford University Press.

French, M. T., Salome, H. J., Sindelar, J. L. & McClellan, A. T. (2002) Benefit-cost analysis of addiction treatment: methodological guidelines and empirical application using the DATCAP and ASI. *Health Services Research*, 37(2), 433–455.

Gold, M. R., Siegel, J. E., Russell, L. B. & Weinstein, M. C. (1996) *Cost-effectiveness in Health and Medicine*. Oxford: Oxford University Press.

Humphreys, K., Todd, H. W. & Mistry, G. (2008) *Is it in medical centers' self-interest to provide substance use disorder treatment? A cost-consequence analysis in a national health care system*. Paper presented at the ISSDP Conference in Lisbon, 4 April 4 2008.

Jofre-Bonet, M. & Sindelar, J. L. (2004) Creating an aggregate outcome index: cost-effectiveness analysis of substance abuse treatment. *The Journal of Behavioral Health Services and Research*, 31(3), 229–241.

Kaplan, E. H. (1995) Probability models of needle exchange. *Operations Research*, 43(4), 558–569.

Kaplan, E. H. & Johri, M. (2000) Treatment on demand: an operational model. *Health Care Management Science*, 3, 171–183.

Keeler, E. & Cretin, S. (1983) Discounting of life-saving and other nonmonetary effects. *Management Science*, 29, 300–306.

Kind, P., Dolan, P., Gudex, C. & Williams, A. (1998) Variations in population health status: results from a United Kingdom national questionnaire survey. *British Medical Journal*, 316, 736–741.

Kleiman, M. A. R. (1992) *Against Excess: Drug Policy for Results*. New York: Basic Books.

Kleiman, M. A. R. & Teles, S. N. (2006) Market and non-market failures. In: M. Michael, R. Martin & E. G. Robert (eds) *The Oxford Handbook of Public Policy*. Oxford: Oxford University Press.

MacCoun, R. & Reuter, P. (2001) *Drug War Heresies*. New York: Cambridge University Press.

Miller, T. R., Mark, A. C. & Brian, W. (1996) *Victim Costs and Consequences: A New Look*. National Institute of Justice Report NCJ 155282. Washington, DC.

Office of National Drug Control Policy (2004) *The Economic Costs of Drug Abuse in the United States, 1992–2002*. Washington, DC: Executive Office of the President (Publication No. 207303).

Perez, P., Dray, A., Ritter, A., Dietze, P., Moore, T. & Mazerolle, L. (2006) SimDrug: a multi-agent system tackling the complexity of illicit drug markets in Australia. In: P. Perez & D. Batten (eds) *Complex Science for a Complex World – Exploring Human Ecosystems with Agents*. Canberra: ANU E Press, pp. 193–224.

Pollack, H. (2002) Methadone maintenance as HIV prevention: cost-effectiveness analysis. In: E. H. Kaplan & R. Brookmeyer (eds) *Quantitative Evaluation of HIV Prevention Programs*. New Haven, CT: Yale University Press.

Pollack, H. A. (2001) Can we protect drug users from hepatitis C? *Journal of Policy Analysis and Management*, 20(2), 358–364.

Rabin, R. & de Charro, F. (2001) EQ-5D: a measure of health status from the EuroQol Group. Annals of Medicine, 33, 337–343.

Reuter, P. & Kleiman, M. (1986) Risks and prices: an economic analysis of drug enforcement. In: N. Morris & M. Tonry (eds) *Crime and Justice: An Annual Review of Research*, Vol. 7, pp. 289–340.

Rice, D. P. (1967) Estimating the costs of illness. *American Journal of Public Health*, 57, 424–440.

Single, E., Collins, D., Easton, B., Harwood, H., Lapsley, H., Kopp, P. & Wilson, E. (2003) *International Guidelines for Estimating the Costs of Substance Abuse*, 2nd edn. Geneva, Switzerland: World Health Organization.

Stokey, E. & Zeckhauser, R. (1978) *A Primer for Policy Analysis*. New York: Norton.

Viscusi, K. W. & Aldy, J. E. (2003) The Value of a Statistical Life: A Critical Review of Market Estimates Throughout the World. National Bureau of Economic Research Working Paper #9487. Cambridge: National Bureau of Economic Research.

Yin, D. & Forman, H. P. (1995) Health care cost-benefit and cost-effectiveness analysis: an overview. *Journal of Vascular and Interventional*, 6(3), 311–320.

Weimer, D. L. & Vining, A. R. (2005) *Policy Analysis: Concepts and Practice*. Upper Saddle River: Prentice Hall.

Zarkin, G. A., Dunlap, L. J., Hicks, K. A. & Daniel, M. (2005) Benefits and costs of methadone treatment: results from a lifetime simulation model. *Health Economics*, 14, 1133–1150.

Recommended readings

Bardach (2000) offers the classic, readable introductory text on policy analysis. Stokey and Zeckhauser (1978), Weimer and Vining (2005), and Kleiman and Teles (2006) are also highly recommended. Policy analysis is sometimes best learnt by example. The exercises give the reader a chance to try doing some policy analysis for well-structured questions, and we close with references to some organisations and websites that are good sources of policy research that can serve as models for further work.

Academic conferences

International Society for the Study of Drug Policy
www.issdp.org

Independent research organisations

Including the Drug Policy Modelling Program
www.dpmp.unsw.edu.au/
National Drug and Alcohol Research Centre
www.ndarc.med.unsw.edu.au/
RAND's Drug Policy Research Center
www.rand.org/multi/dprc

International policy agencies

European Monitoring Centre on Drugs and Drug Addiction
www.emcdda.europa.eu/
United Nations Office on Drugs and Crime
www.unodc.org/unodc/

National policy agencies

U.K. Home Office
www.drugs.homeoffice.gov.uk/
U.S. Office of National Drug Control Policy
www.whitehousedrugpolicy.gov/

Online libraries, bibliographies and other sources

Schaffer Library of Drug Policy
www.druglibrary.org/toc.htm
Substance Abuse and Mental Health Data Archive (SAMHDA)
www.icpsr.umich.edu/SAMHDA/
*Substance Abuse and Mental Health Services Administration's (SAMHSA's) National Clearinghouse
   for Alcohol and Drug Information (NCADI)*
http://ncadi.samhsa.gov/

Section VI
Beyond Research

Chapter 23
CONCLUDING REMARKS

Peter G. Miller, John Strang and Peter M. Miller

The preceding chapters have demonstrated the wide-ranging nature of the study of addiction and its related topics. Because of this very broad field of study, the research methods available to answer research questions are highly varied and there is no one correct method for each issue under study. In fact, while the researcher must be careful and deliberate in his or her approach to research questions, flexibility is also the key to successfully conducted scientific investigations. The coverage of *Addiction Research Methods* has been purposely comprehensive and all-encompassing, ranging from basic tools and methodologies to applications from tightly controlled investigations in laboratory settings to qualitative research in real-world clinical venues.

Even with the most deliberate planning, research projects do not typically follow a smooth path. For example, subject recruitment can be unpredictably slower than anticipated, requiring novel or more aggressive recruitment strategies or even different statistical analytic methods due to a smaller sample size. In addition, unexpected logistical problems can be encountered early in the project, requiring changes in research methodology. Hopefully, these issues will arise early and not after significant time and energy have been expended. This is the main reason why sufficient pre-study planning time, including extensive discussion of what might go wrong, is an absolute necessity.

We hope you have also been encouraged to try newer methods, particularly using multidisciplinary approaches. Determining which methodology is most appropriate to answer a specific scientific inquiry requires an open-minded approach that is often as much an art as it is a science. The successful scientist knows well that an in-depth knowledge of basic methodology combined with research experience, trial and error and a little luck is all involved in conducting addiction research. The goal of *Addiction Research Methods* is to provide the necessary framework upon which these elements can be merged to enable researchers to find the most appropriate solutions to their questions. The future of addiction science lies in translational, collaborative, interdisciplinary research since it is more and more evident that addictions constitute complex phenomena that cut across disciplinary lines.

23.1 Publishing addiction science

Science is meaningless unless the lessons learnt from it are communicated. Publication communicates scientific findings, and is also the hallmark of a productive scientific career (Babor et al., 2008). At the core of this infrastructure lie the peer-reviewed scientific article and the expanding network of journals that publish such articles. Science is also meaningless unless it maintains a high level of integrity. This must ultimately be embodied in the behaviour of individuals, groups and institutions. Throughout *Addiction Research Methods* we have focused on methods which are of a standard to publish as scientific papers in peer-reviewed journals because this is a key part of the meaning of scholarship. Ideally, publishing allows the scientist to take a position and operate in a forum that encourages the free exchange of ideas and findings.

There are now close to 90 journals in 17 languages that specialise in addiction science as part of their broader mission. Despite these expanding opportunities, getting research published can be complex, if not impossible, and involves a raft of issues including choosing a journal and a host of potential language, authorship, citation and ethical issues. It might be assumed that, in these concluding remarks, we will discuss how to write research proposals and articles and delve into the best ways in which to present scientific findings. However, we have decided not to do this in *Addiction Research Methods* for two reasons.

First, having covered so many different disciplines, it would be difficult to present such information comprehensively for all readers without substantially adding to the size of the book. Instead, we recommend looking to discipline-specific texts such as Bryman (2004) for social research methods or Stevens (1951) for experimental psychology. We would also refer the reader to recommended readings at the end of each chapter for information on seminal studies and examples on the way each discipline reports results.

Second, there already exists an excellent text, which covers the major issues related to reporting addiction science and more. *Publishing Addiction Science* (Babor et al., 2008) has been written by the editors of the major journals in the addiction field under the auspices of the International Society of Addiction Journal Editors and can be downloaded free of charge from http://www.parint.org/isajewebsite/isajebook2.htm. *Publishing Addiction Science* is a comprehensive guide for addiction scientists – especially novice researchers – facing the complex process of publishing in scholarly journals. It tackles such issues as choosing a journal, publishing qualitative research, responding to reviewers' reports, becoming a reviewer yourself and appropriatly responding to ethical issues common to addiction science publishing.

23.2 Final thoughts

In conclusion, our hope is that this text will provide the young researcher with a basic primer in addiction research methodology and the more experienced addiction scientist with food for thought about newer methodologies that are cutting-edge. The overarching aim of our efforts and the efforts of our contributors is to advance the science of addiction and eventually improve our understanding of the nature, treatment and prevention of these disorders. Ultimately, of course, the goal is to improve the lives of those who are addicted and to prevent addiction in at-risk individuals throughout the world.

References

Babor, T. F., Stenius, K., Savva, S. & O'Reilly, J. (eds). (2008) *Publishing Addiction Science: A Guide for the Perplexed*, 2nd edn. Rockville, MD: International Society of Addiction Journal Editors. Available online: http://www.parint.org/isajewebsite/isajebook2.htm (accessed 7 October 2009).
Bryman, A. (2004) *Social Research Methods*. New York: Oxford University Press.
Stevens, S. (1951) *Handbook of Experimental Psychology*. New York: John Wiley & Sons.

INDEX

Note: Italicized b, f and t refer to boxes, figures and tables

Printed and bound by CPI Group (UK) Ltd, Croydon, CR0 4YY

09/06/2025

14685998-0004